ENCYCLOPEDIA OF
FAMILY HEALTH

THIRD EDITION

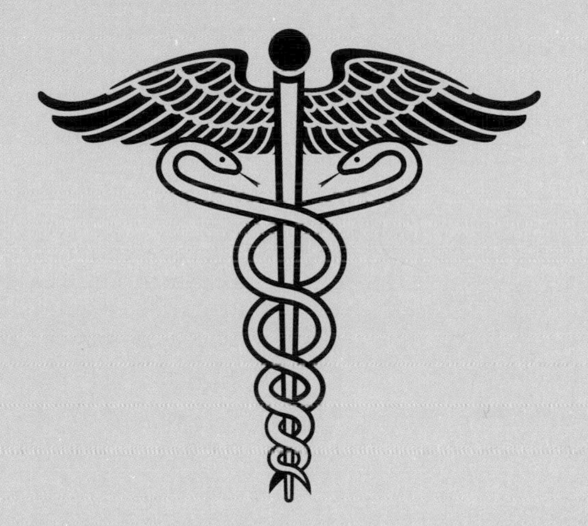

CONSULTANTS

David B. Jacoby, M.D.
Johns Hopkins School of Medicine

Robert M. Youngson, M.D.
Royal Society of Medicine

VOLUME 10

MUSCULAR DYSTROPHY — OSTEOARTHRITIS

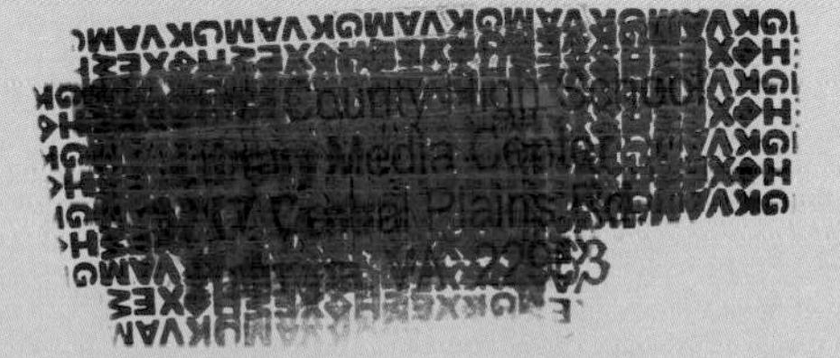

MARSHALL CAVENDISH
New York • London • Singapore

MEDICAL CONSULTANTS

Second Edition
David B. Jacoby, M.D.
Johns Hopkins School of Medicine
Associate Professor of Pulmonary and Critical Care Medicine

Third Edition
Robert M. Youngson, M.D.
Fellow of the Royal Society of Medicine
Officer of the Order of St John of Jerusalem
Diploma in Tropical Medicine and Hygiene
Fellow of the Royal College of Ophthalmologists

CONTRIBUTORS TO THIRD EDITION

David Arnot
Deborah Evans
Leon Gray
Joanna Griffin
Tim Harris
John Jackson
Tom Jackson
Nathan Lepora
Fiona Plowman
Alison Tarrant
Aruna Vasudevan

Picture Credits
(b – bottom; t – top; r – right; l – left; c – center)

Cover: Corbis: Leland Bobbé c; Dynamic Graphics: John Foxx & Images 4 Communication b/l, b/r; PhotoDisc: Don Farrall b/c, Keith Brofsky t/r.

Alan Hutchison Library: 1305t/l; ARS: Doug Wilson 1418, Keith Weller 1379, Scott Bauer 1419; A-Z Collection Ltd: 1359; Biophoto Associates: 1305t/r, 1349t/l, 1377c/r, 1410; Brown Reference Group: Clare Newman 1369; Bruce Coleman Ltd: Jonathan T Wright 1373t/r; Bubbles: 1318; Charles Day: 1426 all, 1427b, 1429t/l; Charles Thackeray: 1406b; C James Webb: 1431; Colorific: Carl Perutz 1389; Corbis: Annie Griffiths Belt 1386, Ariel Skelley 1413, Bettmann 1337, Cat Gwynn 1429b, Children's Hospital & Medical Center 1350, Chuck Savage 1322b, Dick Clintsman 1387, Helen King 1405b, James A Sugar 1351, Jeff Zaruba 1353, Jim Craigmyle 1343, John Henley 1320, Jose Luis Pelaez Inc 1404, Lester V Bergman 1313, Michael Keller 1414, 1416, Philip Harvey 1368, Roger Ressmeyer 1344, Rolf Bruderer 1334b, 1335b, Ronnie Kaufman 1340, Roy Morsch 1425, Ted Horowitz 1336, Warren Morgan 1401; Corbis Royalty Free: 1391, 1392t, 1392b, 1393, 1394; Corbis Sygma: Dung Vo Trung 1421, Pierre Perrin 1357; Dynamic Graphics: John Foxx & Images 4 Communication 1329, 1356, 1406t; Getty Images: 1308t, 1310, 1326, 1328, 1349t/r, 1360, 1363, 1365t/l, 1366t, 1390, Donna Day 1385, Michael Krasowitz 1366b, Romilly Lockyer 1377t/r; Hammersmith Hospital: Dr C A Sewry 1301; Homecraft Supplies: 1437; Image State: James Davis 1376, Stock Images 1423; Imagingbody.com: 1349c, 1402, 1433; Ingram Publishing: 1319, 1377t/l, 1405t; Kim Sayer 1380; Kobal Collection: 1358; London Scientific Fotos: 1373b; Muscular Dystrophy Group of Great Britain: 1303 all; Paul Windsor: 1315, 1316t, 1316c/r, 1317 all; PHIL: Dr Mae Melvin 1409; PhotoDisc: Keith Brofsky 1312, 1429t/r, Steve Mason 1339; Photo Library International: 1362; Rex Features: Bob Crandall 1403, Burger/Phanie Agency 1334t, John Lodge 1428t, Mykel Micolaou 1388, Nils Jorgensen 1316c/l, Peter Brooker 1306, PGE 1308b, Phanie Agency 1375, 1424, Simon Roberts 1307, Sipa Press 1367, Stewart Cook 1365b; Robert Harding: 1338, 1407; Roger Payling: 1365t/r; Ron Sutherland: 1412; Science Photo Library: 1311, 1322t, 1342, Alex Dex/Publiophoto Diffusion 1435, Biophoto Associates 1384, Brad Nelson 1432, CC Studio 1408t, Hank Morgan 1398t/l, James King-Holmes 1309, John Greim 1397, 1398t/r; Sue Ford: 1408b; Syndication International: 1323; Topham Picturepoint: The Image Works 1381; Transworld Features: 1321, 1324; Vision International: Anthea Sieveking 1373t/l, CNRI 1354, 1436 all; Wellcome Photo Library: 1302; Zefa: 1304, 1330, 1331, 1335t, 1341, 1352, 1382, 1396 all, 1434, 1430.

Marshall Cavendish
99 White Plains Road
Tarrytown, NY 10591-9001

www.marshallcavendish.com

Library of Congress Cataloging-in-Publication Data

Encyclopedia of family health / David B. Jacoby, Robert M. Youngson.--
3rd ed.
p. cm.
Includes bibliographical references and index.
ISBN 0-7614-7486-2 (set)
ISBN 0-7614-7496-X (vol 10)
1. Medicine, Popular--Encyclopedias. 2. Health--Encyclopedias. 1. Jacoby, David B. II. Youngson, R. M. III. Marshall Cavendish Corporation. IV. Title
RC81.A2E5 2004
610'.3--dc22 2003065554

Printed in China
08 07 06 05 04 5 4 3 2 1

Marshall Cavendish

Editor: Joyce Tavolacci
Editorial Director: Paul Bernabeo
Production Manager: Alan Tsai

The Brown Reference Group

Project Editor: Anne Hildyard
Editors: Jane Lanigan, Sally McFall
Designers: Jeni Child, Reg Cox, Karen Frazer
Picture Researcher: Clare Newman
Indexer: Kay Ollerenshaw
Illustrations: Samantha J. Elmhurst
Managing Editor: Tim Cooke
Art Director: Dave Goodman

CONTENTS

KEY TO COLOR CODING OF ARTICLES

- HUMAN BODY
- DISEASES AND OTHER DISORDERS
- TREATMENTS AND CURES
- PREVENTION AND DIAGNOSIS OF DISEASE
- HUMAN BEHAVIOR

Muscular dystrophy

Questions and Answers

The little boy next door has muscular dystrophy, but there is no history of it in his family. How did this happen?

Inherited diseases occur when there are abnormal genes in a person's makeup; these are passed on to his or her child. Sometimes, an abnormal gene is formed when an egg or sperm is produced, a process known as mutation. Some people with inherited diseases suffer from them as a result of a new mutation passed on by a parent when there is no family history of the disease.

My brother has Duchenne muscular dystrophy. Could I possibly be a carrier?

As a sibling of an affected person, you have a 50 percent chance of being a carrier. You will have to have a blood test for an enzyme called CPK (creatine phosphokinase), which is released from muscle into the blood and is present at a raised level in people who carry the disease.

My nephew has muscle weakness and was diagnosed as having muscular dystrophy. Could the diagnosis be incorrect?

It is unusual to find muscle weakness in children. When it occurs, muscular dystrophy is a common cause. This together with positive blood tests suggest that it is unlikely the diagnosis is wrong. His weakness will not just go away.

My brother-in-law had Duchenne dystrophy. Will my children inherit it?

This disease is carried on the X chromosome, and your husband has only one of these. If it had been a carrier chromosome, he would have the disease.

Like most inherited diseases, muscular dystrophy tends to strike early in life. The age at which the symptoms first appear is one way of distinguishing the many different types of this uncommon disease.

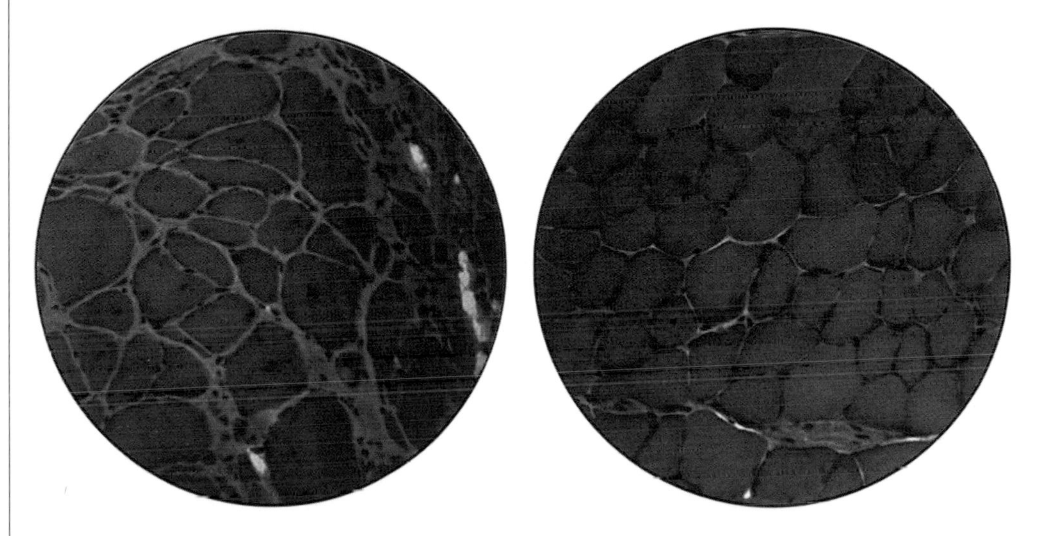

▲ *Muscle cells (left) of a normal person and (right) those of a patient with dystrophy.*

The term "muscular dystrophy" describes a group of disorders that produce muscle weakness, rather than a weakness resulting from disorders of the nerves that make the muscles work (see Muscles). The dystrophies make up only a small number of all disorders that affect the muscles alone and are characterized by two factors: they do not seem to be a consequence of disease elsewhere in the body, and they are always inherited.

Causes and symptoms

Although the cause of the disorder is unknown, it is fairly certain that the problem arises in the muscle cell. When the muscles of people affected with the disease are examined under a microscope, the cells are seen to be in varying stages of destruction.

Just like any other cell in the body, a muscle cell must convert oxygen and food into energy. In addition, it has to convert energy into physical power by contracting. An abnormality in any one of the many processes involved in this activity could result in muscular dystrophy. Also, it seems very likely that the various types of the disease each result from a different abnormality.

The symptoms depend on the type of dystrophy that is present. In general, symptoms appear earlier in the more severe types than in the less severe forms. There are approximately 20 different types of the disease but only four of them commonly occur: they are Duchenne, Becker's, Landouzy-Dejerine (fascioscapulohumeral dystrophy), and myotonic dystrophy.

Duchenne dystrophy is the most severe form of the disease and may occur in very young children. About one in every 5,000 male babies is affected. It is a sex-linked disease inherited on the X chromosome, so that when only one X chromosome is present, as it is in boys, the disease becomes evident. When two X chromosomes are present (in girls), it is prevented by the other normal chromosome, although 12 cases have been reported in girls. However, girls can carry the disease and pass it on to their sons. The disease starts with weakness of the thighs and pelvic muscles, which causes difficulty in standing, walking, and climbing. Weakness may be obvious at a very early stage, even before the child can walk. However, it is more usually noticed between the ages of two and seven. Continuing progression affects the neck, shoulders, and back so that loss of power may eventually lead to deformities of the spine and difficulties in breathing. The heart may become involved, and difficulties in breathing and heart function can lead to an early death, often before the age of 20. An unusual characteristic of Duchenne dystrophy in its early stages is

Common types of muscular dystrophy

DISEASE	TYPE OF INHERITANCE*	CHARACTERISTICS
Duchenne	X-linked	Starts early in childhood, often before the age of two. The calves may show hypertrophy (overdevelopment). Survival beyond 20 is unusual.
Becker's	X-linked	Like Duchenne, except that it starts later and sufferers may live into middle age.
Landouzy-Dejerine (fascioscapulo-humeral)	Autosomal dominant	Most variable in its effects, ranging from minor weakness of the face and cheeks to severe disability. Face, arms, and shoulders are affected.
Myotonic	Autosomal dominant	Weakness of the face muscles and inability to relax muscles. Affected people often go bald. Children of affected mothers may be worse than those of affected fathers.

*With X-linked inherited dystrophies, only boys tend to be affected; girls are usually carriers (although a girl could be affected if her father had the disease and her mother was a carrier and passed on the abnormal X chromosome); with autosomal dominant, children of an affected person have a 50 percent chance of inheriting the disease.

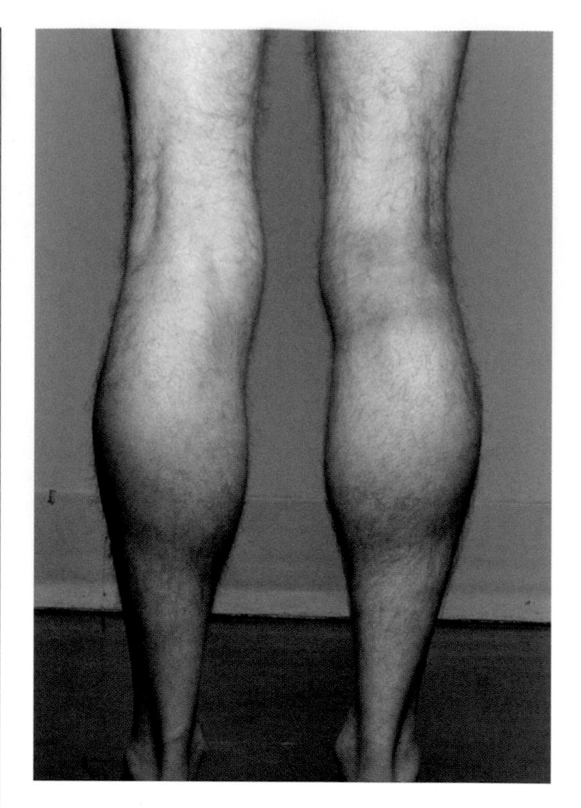

▲ *The muscles in the legs of a patient with muscular dystrophy look deceptively strong.*

X-LINKED INHERITANCE

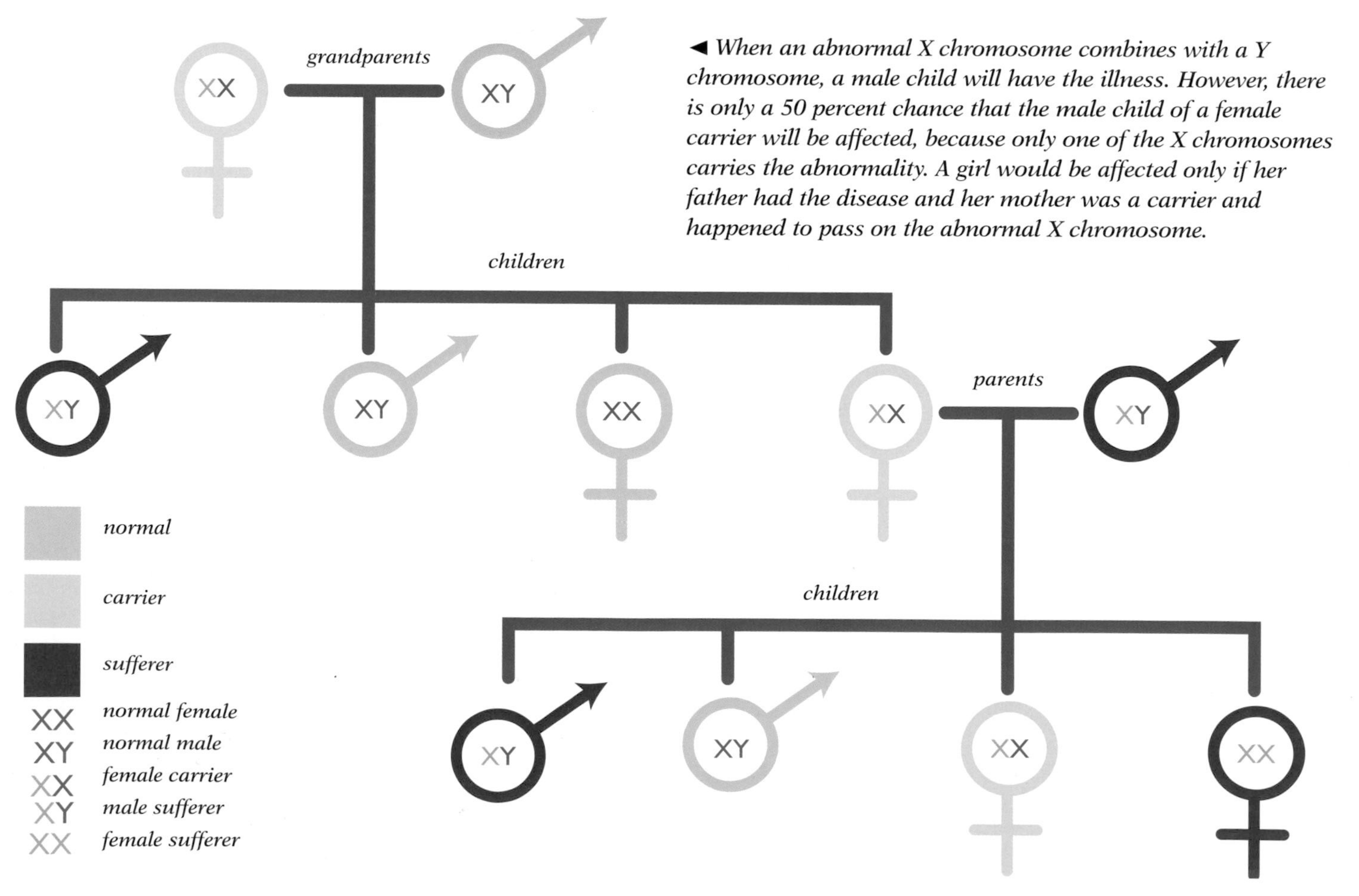

◄ *When an abnormal X chromosome combines with a Y chromosome, a male child will have the illness. However, there is only a 50 percent chance that the male child of a female carrier will be affected, because only one of the X chromosomes carries the abnormality. A girl would be affected only if her father had the disease and her mother was a carrier and happened to pass on the abnormal X chromosome.*

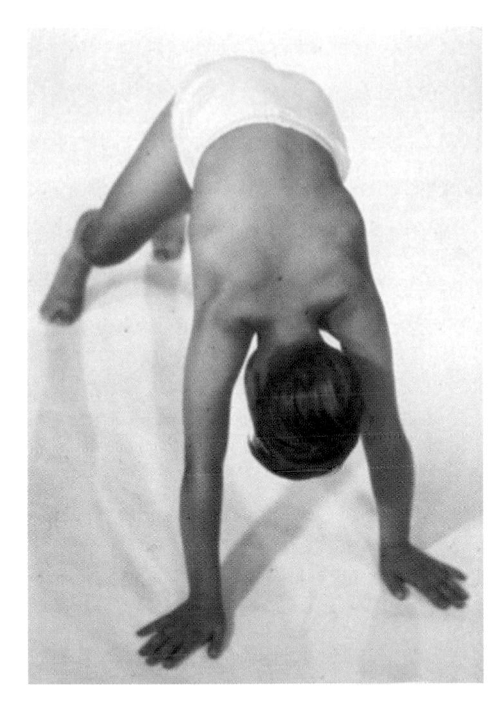

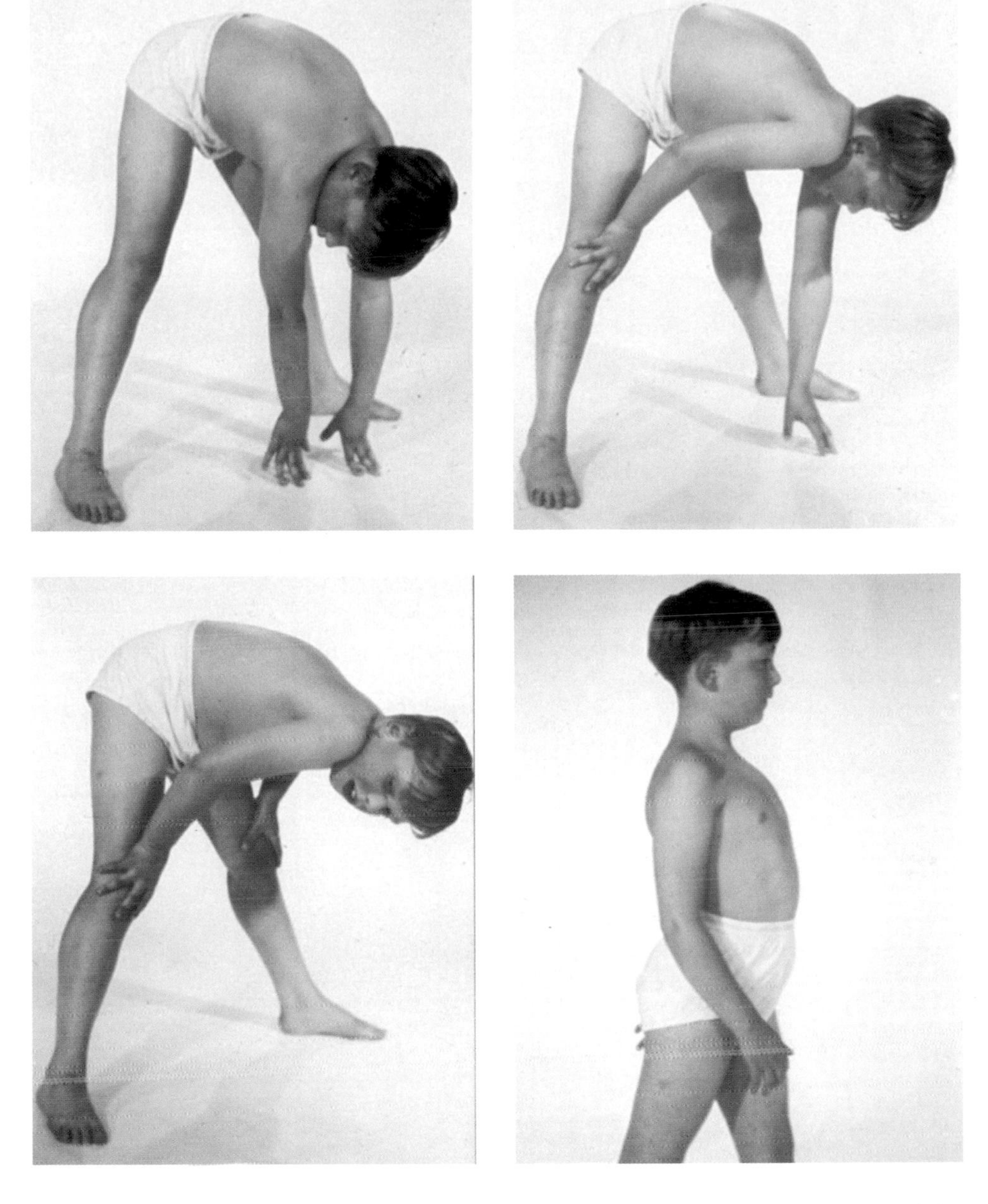

▲ *Although girls can be carriers of Duchenne dystrophy (and only rarely get the disease), it usually afflicts boys. Weak leg muscles, particularly those in the thighs, result in difficulties in walking and climbing in the early stages of the disease. An inability to stand up after a fall is another sign. The patient shown illustrates how children are taught to get off the ground into a standing position. After raising himself up on all four limbs, he balances on his legs and places his hands on his knees. From there he helps himself into an erect position by walking up his legs with his hands.*

that the muscles involved are not necessarily wasted and shrunken but large and powerful-looking, even though weak.

A similar type of dystrophy, Becker's pseudohypertrophic dystrophia, develops usually after the age of 10. People are much less severely affected and can live until their thirties and forties.

The face, shoulders, and upper arms are the areas worst affected in Landouzy-Dejarine dystrophy. It can occur in men and women, and affected individuals will have at least one parent with the disease. Anyone with this type of dystrophy has a 50 percent chance of passing it on to each of his or her children. The face is affected first, and difficulty in puffing out the cheeks is an early sign. The symptoms appear during the teens, but signs of the disease can appear in people in their fifties who were unaware they were ill. The heart is usually unaffected, although people with this condition can have all the problems associated with Duchenne-type dystrophy.

Myotonic dystrophy, or dystrophica myotonica, differs from the dystrophies already described. It is the type people are most familiar with. Myotonia means an inability to relax a muscle after it has contracted. This is an early symptom, which may occur in the teens. The disease often affects the hands. Later in life, the muscles of the face, neck, and hands may become wasted and weak, and this effect may spread to the legs. Unlike other types of the disease, myotonic dystrophy may cause baldness in men and women, and cataracts. It is also the most variable of the dystrophies, with symptoms ranging from a minor degree of failure in muscle relaxation, in a person who lives out a normal life span, to severe weakness that begins in early life.

Treatment and outlook

No treatment can stop the progression of weakness in the dystrophies, although drugs such as quinine are used to aid relaxation in myotonia. Patients should be encouraged to exercise as much as possible to keep the muscles that are in good condition functioning normally. The gene that causes Duchenne muscular dystrophy has been isolated, although it may be years before this knowledge leads to effective treatment. Until this happens, prevention through genetic counseling is the best option.

See also: **Genetics; Relaxation**

Mutation

Mutations, or the changes in the DNA that determine human physical and mental makeup, may sometimes be advantageous; however, they are also responsible for a number of inherited disorders.

A mutation is a change in the DNA that is contained within a living cell. Mutations occur in body-cell DNA all the time, but most of them never have any serious effect. Occasionally, however, a mutation may be passed on, in an egg or sperm cell, to a baby; the baby will then have the mutation in each of his or her body cells. The mutation may in turn have a detectable effect on the child that can vary from a slight change in hair color or nose shape to a serious disease or defect. The child may also pass the mutation on to some of his or her own children in the years to come, and they too may show its effects.

All of the physical differences between individual human beings, and also between humans and other animal species, are the result of mutations that have occurred continually over millions of years. This is because some mutations have advantageous effects and tend to be

▼ *These white kangaroos exhibit albinism, an absence of pigment in skin, hair, and eyes.*

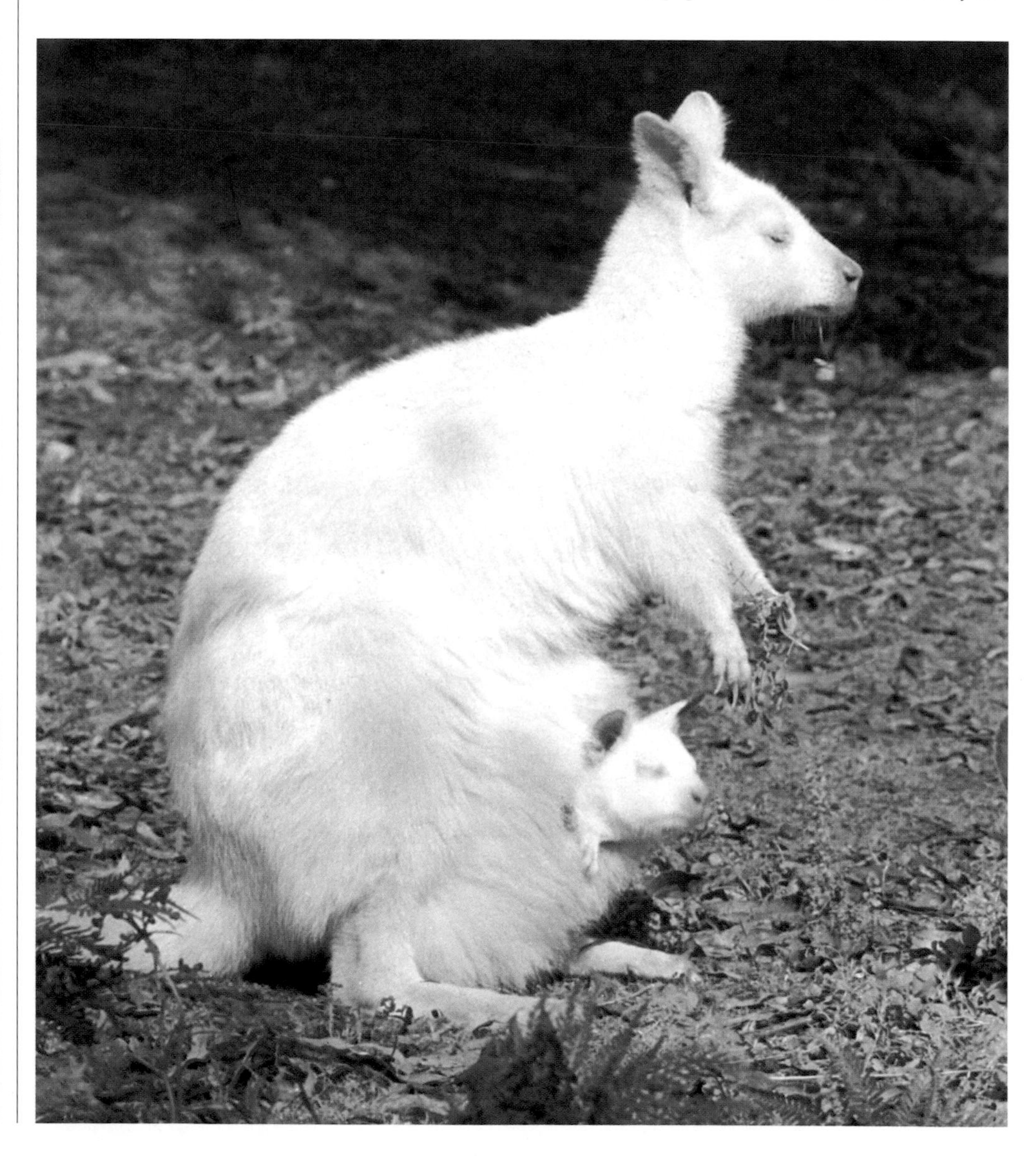

Questions and Answers

Both my husband and my daughter have webbed fingers. Will my daughter's future children have webbed fingers, too?

Many defects that affect the fingers are caused by dominant mutant genes. Those who have such a gene will exhibit the defect, although they usually carry it on only one of the gene pair. Your daughter will have the mutant gene in about half of her egg cells; thus her children will have a 50-50 chance of inheriting the gene and exhibiting the defect.

Similarly, about half of your husband's sperm cells carry the mutation, so any more children you have together will have an even chance of inheriting the defect.

Can mutations cause cancer, and if so, can they be inherited?

The causes of cancer are not fully understood, but at least some types may be due to mutations that cause body cells to grow and divide in a disorganized manner. However, the mutant genes responsible cannot be inherited by the victim's children.

In other cases a person may inherit a mutation that predisposes him or her to a type of cancer, but the growth of a tumor is actually triggered by some other factor, such as a virus infection. This type of mutation may explain why some cancers tend to run in families.

Are mutations ever deliberately engineered?

Yes, but not in humans. One example involves the mold that produces penicillin. If the mold is irradiated with X rays, several mutant strains are produced, some of which give a slightly higher yield of penicillin. Selecting and growing these, followed by further irradiation and further selection, can produce a strain that gives a useful yield of penicillin.

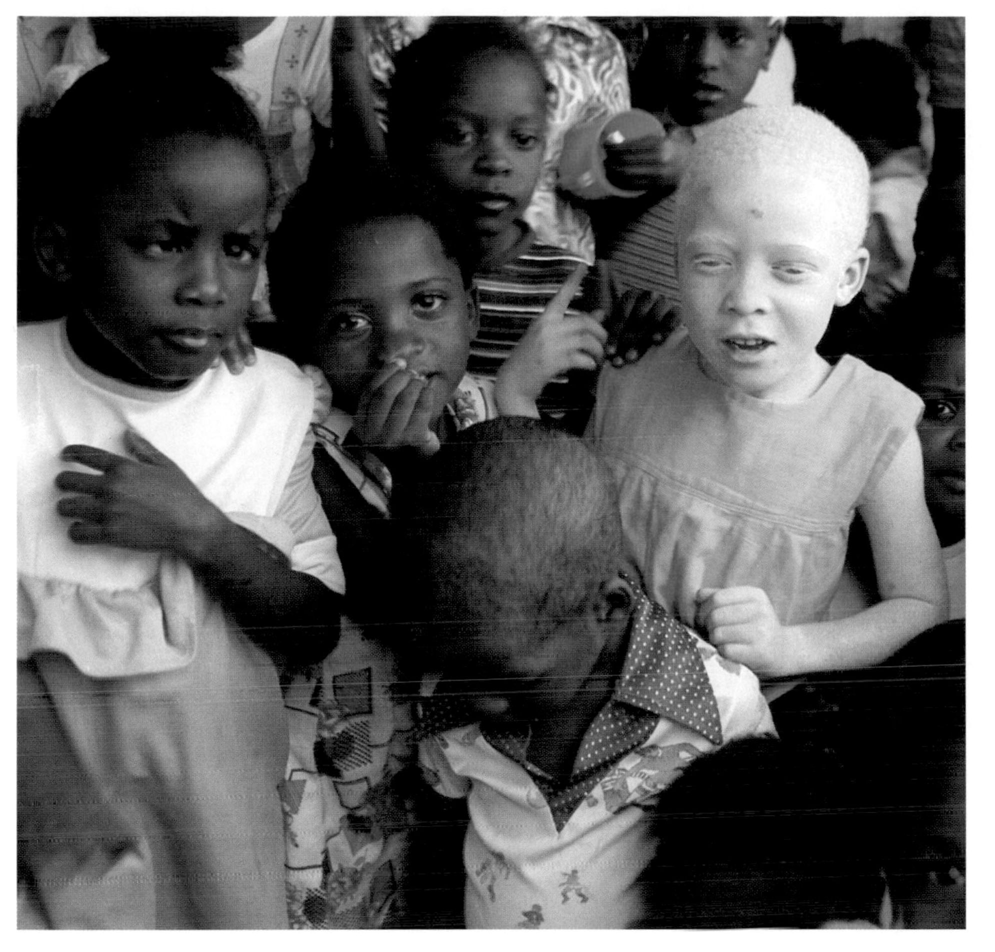

▲ *Albinism is due to a recessive mutant gene. For the mutation to be expressed outwardly, as it is in this pale Ugandan child, the mutant gene must be inherited in a double dose—that is, one mutant gene must be inherited from each parent. Because the gene is recessive, the parents may not exhibit the mutation themselves.*

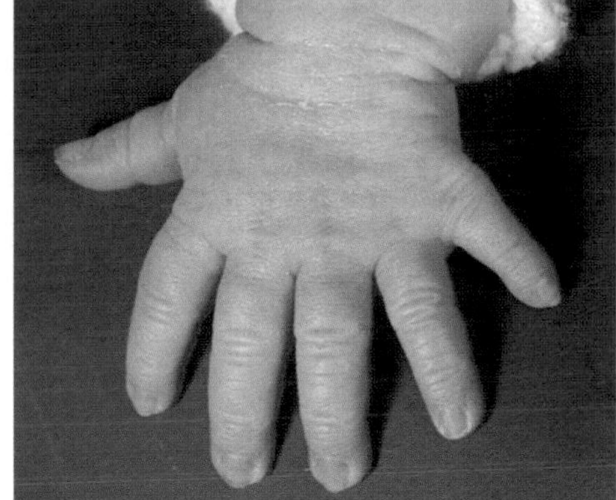

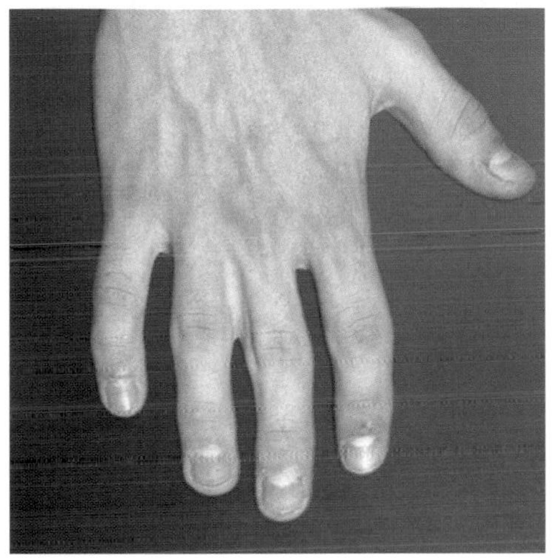

▲ *People who inherit a dominant mutant gene may exhibit its effects in the form of extra fingers (top) or webbed fingers (bottom).*

transmitted from generation to generation, gradually increasing in their frequency; however, advantageous mutations are far less frequent than mutations with harmful effects.

How mutations affect cells

Cells are affected in one of two ways. Gene mutations involve the rearrangement of the sequence of nucleotide bases in a gene, the substitution of one base for another, or the addition or deletion of one or more bases. Such mutations usually affect the activity of only one gene. Similar effects are produced by chromosomal abnormalities. However, such abnormalities involve the addition or deletion of whole, or sections of, chromosomes, and may result in a cell with extra—or missing—copies of several genes. As a result, chromosomal abnormalities tend to have more serious and widespread effects than gene mutations.

Gene mutations

A great majority of genes are the codes for enzymes, so gene mutations usually produce defective or missing enzymes. The effect of the mutation will depend on the normal role of the enzyme. If the enzyme is involved in growth, the mutation may cause a growth disorder; if it is involved in retinal cell function, it may cause blindness; and so on.

However, all human genes come in pairs, and the production of a defective enzyme by a mutant gene may be masked by the production of a normal enzyme by its normal twin gene. Such mutant genes are known as recessive and have to be present in a double dose—one mutant gene must be inherited from each parent—to have a significant effect. Mutant genes that cannot be masked are said to be dominant and need only to be present to have an effect.

Chromosome abnormalities

Whole chromosomal abnormalities are likely to be serious and are often lethal, causing miscarriage. An additional chromosome 21 in each cell causes Down syndrome (see Down Syndrome). A missing X chromosome in girls causes Turner's syndrome.

Another defect, caused by an extra X chromosome, has little effect in girls but in boys causes a condition called Klinefelter's syndrome. The condition mainly affects sexual development.

How new mutations arise

During the formation of cells, new mutations may arise that are caused by the miscopying of genetic material (DNA) from their parent cells. Genes seem to differ in the extent to which they are liable to mutations of this type, and thus they each have characteristic mutation rates.

Questions and Answers

Are mutations always a handicap?

Not at all. Many mutations are disadvantageous, but sometimes one may occur that is beneficial. For example, if the Earth's atmosphere became polluted by poisonous carbon monoxide, a mutant gene that gave immunity to carbon monoxide poisoning would obviously be an advantage. Individuals who carried the mutation would tend to survive longer and have more children than other people, and many of their children would also possess the mutation. Over a number of generations the mutant gene would gradually become more common until immunity to carbon monoxide poisoning would be a feature of human physiology.

My brother has hemophilia. I don't have the disease, but if I have children will they be affected?

Because hemophilia is a sex-linked condition, that depends on whether you are male or female. If you are male, you can't have the mutant gene, so your children are safe. However, if you are female, there is a 50-50 chance that you are a carrier of the mutation, in which case some of your sons may be affected by the condition, and some of your daughters may be carriers.

Before having any children you should discuss the situation with a doctor or a genetic counselor. You may also be able to have tests that can help to establish whether or not you are a carrier.

I suffer from gout. Is this because of a mutation?

Gout runs in some families and is probably due to a mutant gene, or perhaps as a result of a number of mutant genes acting together to produce the high level of uric acid in the blood that directly causes gout. In many people who have the mutation, uric acid levels are not actually high enough to cause deposits of uric acid crystals in the joints. For this reason, the disease often skips one or more generations.

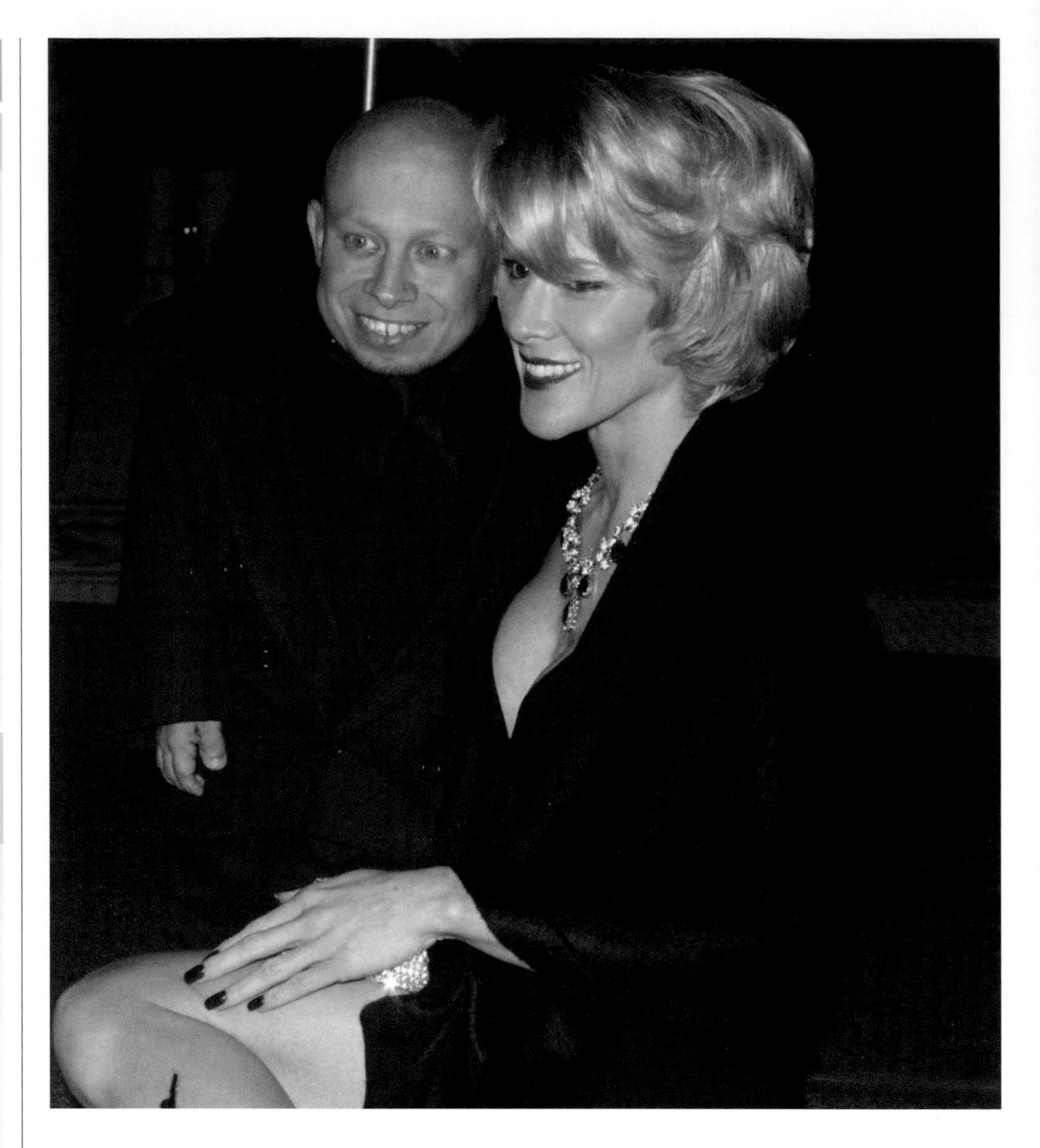

▲ *Achondroplasia—a form of dwarfism characterized by short limbs, small face, and normal trunk—is due to a dominant mutant gene.*

Other mutations are thought to be caused by external factors, such as certain chemicals, and—more importantly—by ionizing radiation, such as X rays or the radiation from nuclear explosions and fallout (see Radiation Sickness; X Rays). During a lifetime, most people are not exposed to sufficient X rays for the mutation rates of their genes to be increased significantly; doctors and medical staffs are careful never to expose the germ cells in the ovaries of female patients, or the testes of male patients, to any unnecessary X rays.

Some mutations are inherited more frequently the older people (particularly women) are when they decide to have a child; the reason why this should happen is not fully understood.

Prevention

At the present time there is no practical means of eradicating genetic mutations from the human population. This is because it is believed that each person carries several recessive mutant genes, and in a double dose these are capable of producing serious effects (see Hemophilia).

However, genetic defects can be kept to a minimum by genetic counseling, by prenatal screening in cases of high risk, and by having children earlier in life rather than later.

Anyone who fears that he or she might pass on a hereditary disease to a future child should see a genetic counselor.

See also: **Genetic diseases and disorders; Genetic engineering; Genetics**

Mutism

Questions and Answers

My first child is deaf and mute. If I have another child is it likely that he or she will be affected?

Unless deafness runs in the family, it is very unlikely that you will have another child who is affected in the same way.

Since her stroke four years ago my mother can say only "yes" and "no," though she understands well. Will her speech ever return?

It is now unlikely that her speech will return. Most speech recovery following a stroke happens in the first six months and then more slowly during the next 18 months.

Can mute babies cry?

Yes. Speech is far more complex than crying. Crying uses the voice but not the speech muscles.

My young son has a learning disorder. He is very friendly but is mute. Will he ever learn to speak?

Over the years he may learn some basic speech and language. However, it is unlikely that he will ever speak as well as children with normal learning ability.

My daughter was born soon after my husband left me, when my son was four. He is now six and will speak only to me. I am worried that he will fall behind in school by refusing to speak.

Your son is an elective mute as a result of the shock of rejection by his father and by the baby's disrupting his relationship with you. When he has built up trust with other people again, normal speech should return. You may need to give him extra help with his schoolwork until then. If the problem persists, ask your doctor to refer you for further help.

Speech is something people often take for granted. However, for a variety of reasons some children and adults do not have this natural ability; they have to be taught how to talk or must learn other methods of communication.

Mutism, which used to be called dumbness, is an inability to pronounce words and speak normally. The condition can affect both children and adults, and it may be caused by physical problems or psychological difficulties.

Causes in children

Deafness: Children learn to talk by listening to their parents speak and from the noises they make themselves. A deaf baby will make all the usual baby noises for the first few months of life. At approximately six months old, when babies normally start repeating the sounds they hear, a deaf baby will become silent (see Deafness). Deafness, however, is usually detected early, and

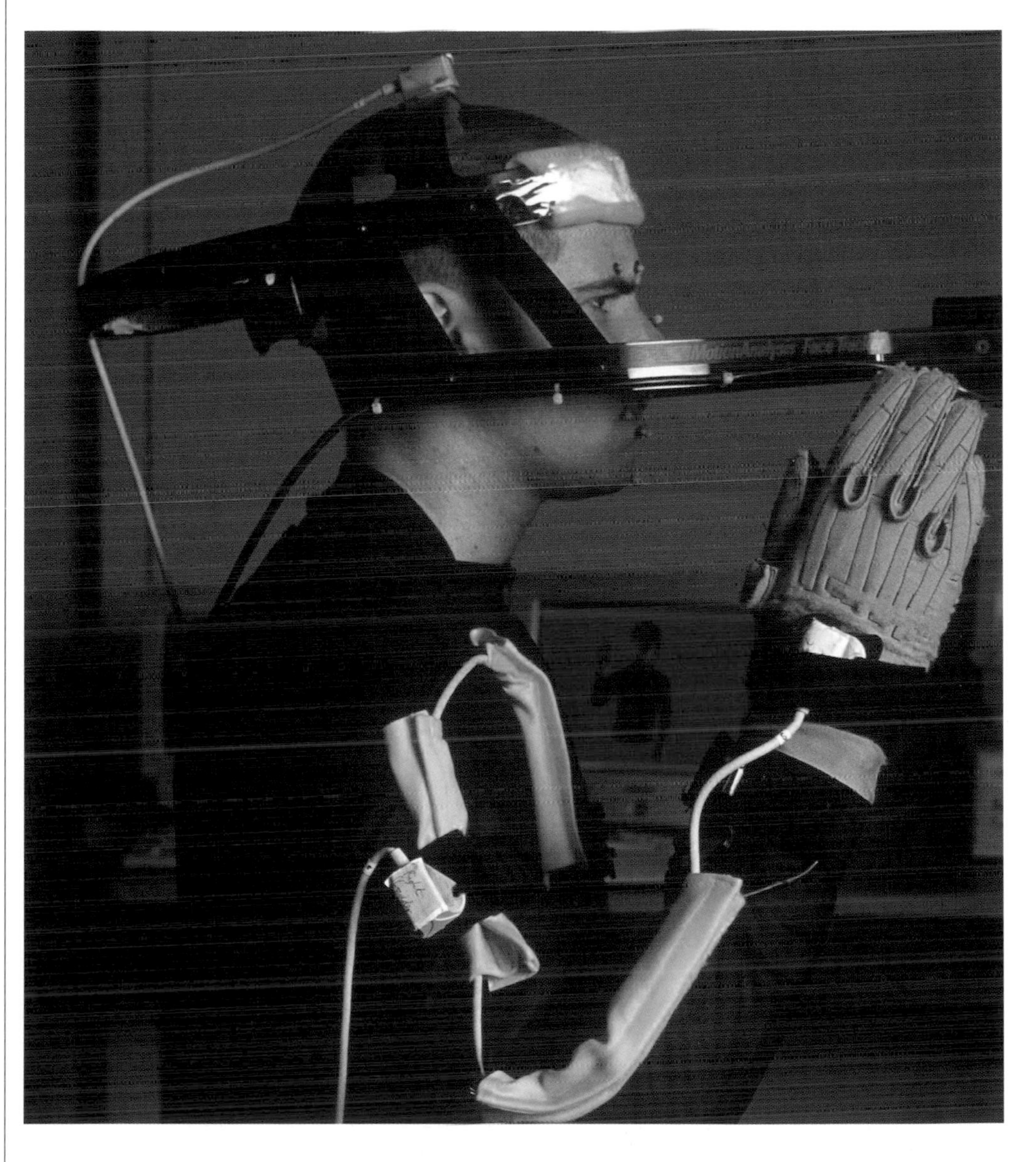

▲ *A young man with mutism learns sign language at Tessa Virtual Sign Language Computer Facility for the Deaf in the United Kingdom.*

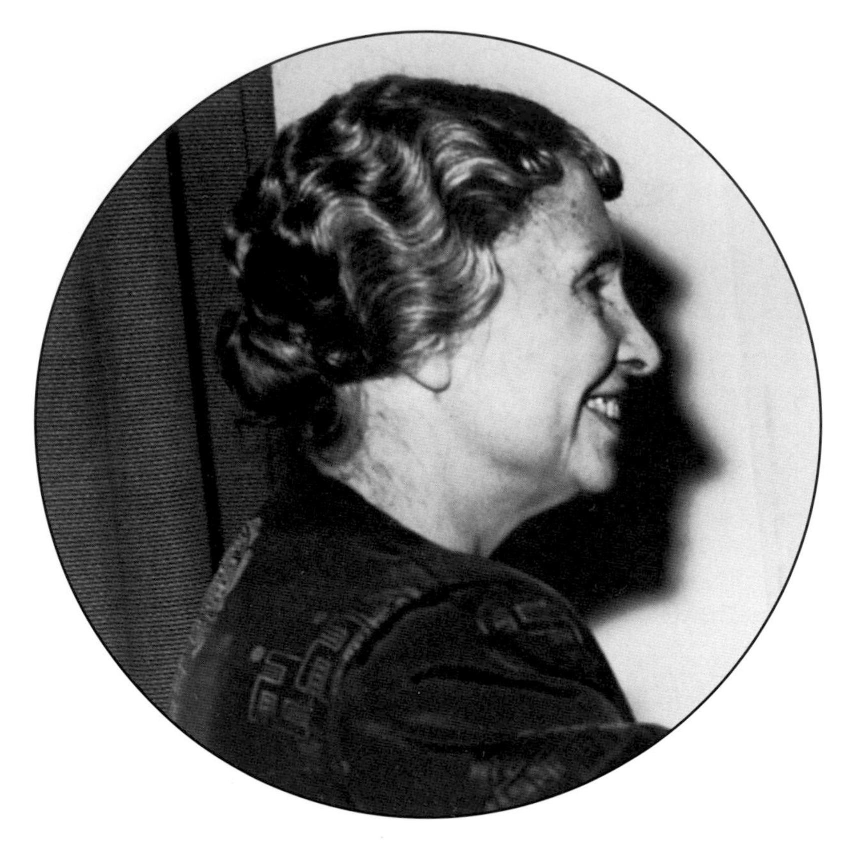

◄ *The American Helen Keller (1880–1968) was born blind, deaf, and mute; in spite of her difficulties, she became a celebrated author.*

infants can learn to speak with the help of hearing aids or by learning to read lips. Some deaf children, especially if they have other problems such as low intelligence or emotional difficulties, never learn to speak.

Autism: Because of their mental disturbance, autistic children do not learn to speak normally. They either are mute or fail to use language to communicate with other people. Instead they merely repeat meaningless phrases. Autistic babies do not babble as much as normal babies, nor do they use a large range of sounds. Research suggests that lack of language is the major difficulty for an autistic child; other problems then occur because of the child's difficulty in understanding other people or being understood him- or herself.

Learning difficulties: Children with learning disabilities often also have difficulty in fully understanding speech. As a result, they can be limited to learning simple speech only. Even with a degree of understanding, these children do not learn to speak normally, and many children with severe learning difficulties can be mute or almost mute (see Learning Disabilities).

Spastic disorders: Cerebral palsy might be the cause of muscular spasms, and these might prevent the lips, tongue, and palate from moving sufficiently accurately and fast enough for normal speech. If the condition is severe, the child is completely unable to control or coordinate the muscles of speech and cannot make speech sounds.

Brain damage: Mental aphasia—a failure to develop the speech process and understanding and forming of words—can develop as a result of brain damage. The infant may babble a little or may be completely silent. One or two words may be used during the first three years of life, but building up a vocabulary develops slowly, if at all. If brain-damaged children do develop language, they often have characteristic difficulties, such as putting words in the wrong order, leaving words out, and adding words that should not be there. Older children can also mispronounce words.

Emotional difficulties: In a rare condition, children who have perhaps experienced a traumatic event, such as the death of a parent, can develop "elective mutism." In such cases, the refusal to speak cannot be related to any physical cause. When children with elective muteness do start to speak again, they usually speak normally.

Causes in adults

Aphasia: This disorder usually follows a stroke, when the part of the brain controlling speech is damaged. In "motor" aphasia the speech of other people continues to be understood by the patient. However, in "global" aphasia both language and speech are affected.

Voice disorders: Actual damage to a person's vocal cords rarely causes a complete loss of voice. However, damage to the nerves in his or her neck or chest can paralyze the vocal cords and lead to loss of voice. Speech is also lost if part of the larynx is removed—for example, because of cancer.

Psychological problems: Losing the power of speech can occur after an emotional upset, and more women than men tend to be affected. Muteness that is intermittent can occur and is often caused by mental disturbances.

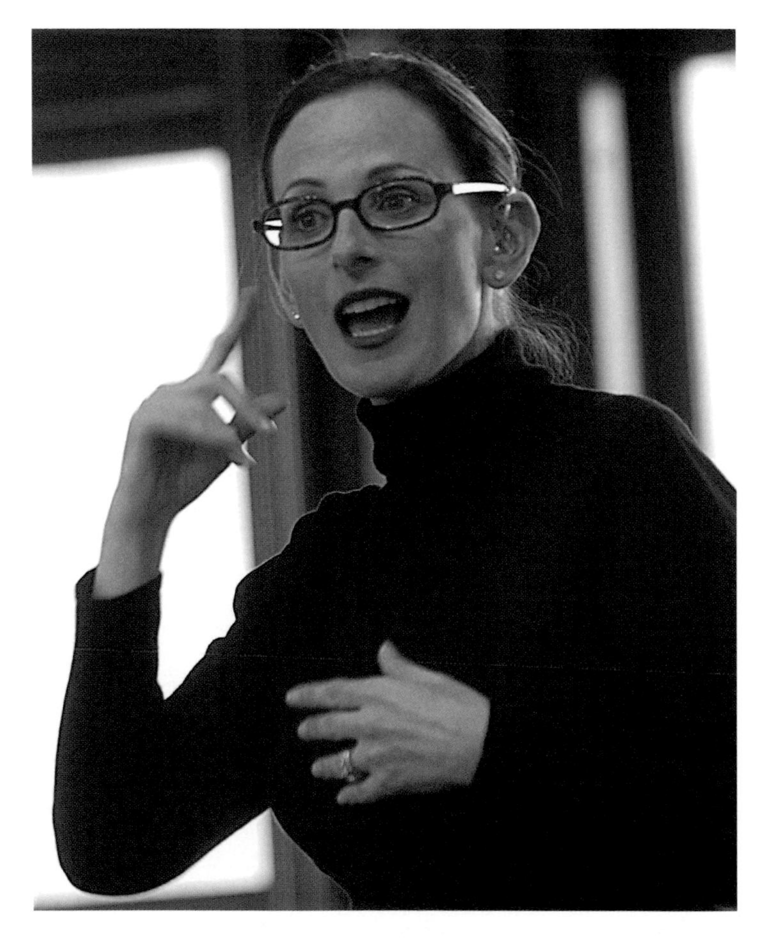

▲ *For many deaf people sign language is a vital, and sometimes their only, means of communicating with others.*

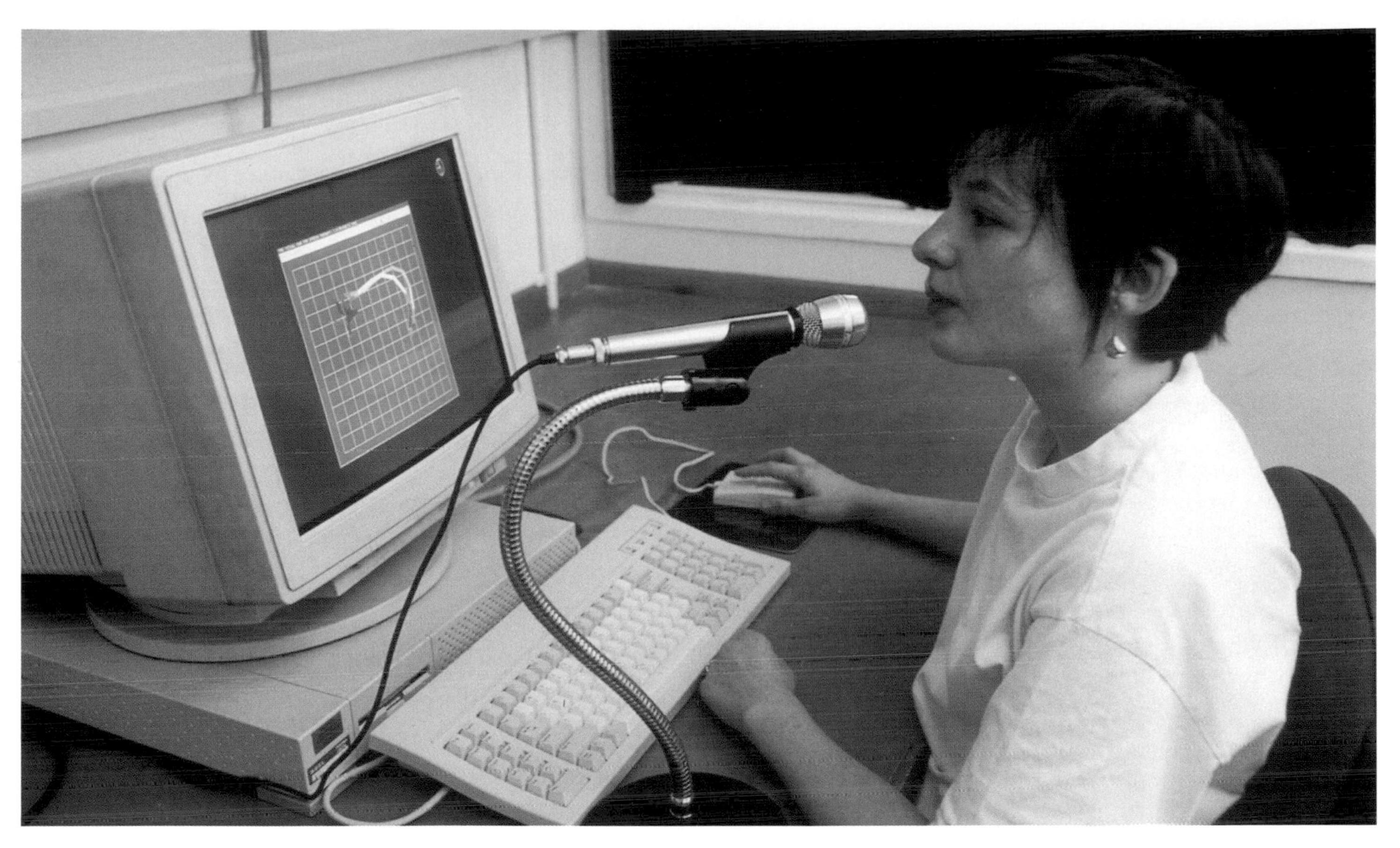

▲ *Computers are often used as an aid to speech therapy for people with hearing impairment.*

Treatment for children

With such diverse causes there is no general outline of treatment for mutism. When the causes are physical and attempts at teaching speech have failed or are progressing very slowly, sign language can be a successful supplement or alternative. For example, severely deaf, autistic, and spastic children may be able to use sign language to replace or augment their attempts at speech.

The most important consideration with mute children who are unable to communicate in conventional ways is to give them a means of successfully relating to other people. Without this, they are unable to express themselves, they become frustrated, and they may stop trying to communicate or interact with others altogether.

The initial treatment and speech therapy for autistic children, children with learning difficulties, and children with brain damage encourage understanding of simple language through, for example, play. Later on, words associated with familiar objects may be taught through imitation. Any attempts at speech made by a child are always praised.

Individual differences between mute children are great, and there is no general rule for the length of treatment. Treatment may be given by teachers of the deaf, speech therapists, and sometimes, in the case of elective muteness, by a psychiatrist.

In elective muteness, the refusal to speak is actually a symptom of emotional disturbance. The treatment involves either changing the child's environment, if that is causing the disturbance, or helping him or her to come to terms with and to cope with the emotional problems that have caused the silence.

Treatment for adults

Treatment for aphasia usually starts about four weeks after a stroke. When the patient is mute, the problem may be caused by a language difficulty, a speech difficulty, or both. In the first case he or she may not be able to remember what words mean; in the second, the patient does not know how to make the sounds of speech.

A patient is taken back to the basic understanding of language through pointing to pictures by name, matching pictures to pictures and objects to pictures at a basic level, and progressing to basic reading comprehension. The ability to make the sounds of speech can be relearned through diagrams that show how to make the sounds, and by having a therapist demonstrate them to the patient.

Voice problems can be treated through relaxation, breathing exercises, and exercises such as humming and sighing. When the voice box has been removed, it is possible to teach a person to speak again by using his or her esophagus.

When muteness occurs because of an emotional disturbance, the voice often returns when a patient begins to relax and accept what has happened. If muteness is caused by a serious psychological problem, psychiatric treatment may be necessary.

Outlook

Mutism is not a common condition, yet it can often be treated successfully. When speech does not develop or return, the patient may learn sign language as an alternative. A mute child or adult is unlikely to stop communicating altogether unless his or her intelligence is severely impaired.

See also: Aphasia; Autism; Cerebral palsy; Speech; Speech therapy; Stroke

Myalgia

Questions and Answers

My sister complains of muscle pain and fatigue. What is wrong?

She may have fibromyalgia, a muscle disorder that causes tender, painful muscles. Your doctor can arrange blood tests to eliminate other disorders, and the pain can be helped by ultrasound treatment and deep tissue massage.

I have fibromyalgia syndrome. How can I prevent flare-ups?

First, learning stress management techniques can be helpful. It is also important to get as much restful sleep as possible. A daily exercise and stretching routine will help reduce the pain and stiffness, and relaxation techniques should also help.

Since my hip surgery a few months ago, I have experienced a bad case of fibromyalgia. Could the surgery be the problem?

Most likely the anesthesia, the emotional and physical stress associated with undergoing surgery, or your body mechanics following the surgery caused fibromyalgia to flare up. Auto accidents and whiplash injuries can cause post-traumatic fibromyalgia. In such cases, the condition appears after about six months and slowly spreads.

I always feel tired when I wake up. My feet are sore, and I hurt all over with throbbing and burning pains. Do I have fibromyalgia?

Your symptoms of pain and fatigue may indicate fibromyalgia. Many victims of this syndrome claim to hurt all over every day. Feeling tired may be due to inadequate amounts of deep, restful sleep. It is best to discuss your concerns with a doctor, who may refer you to a rheumatologist for further testing and treatment.

Myalgia is muscle pain that can occur anywhere in the body. Fibromyalgia syndrome is a chronic disorder with symptoms of widespread pain and stiffness in the muscles and connective tissues. It may be associated with headaches, numbness and tingling, and depression.

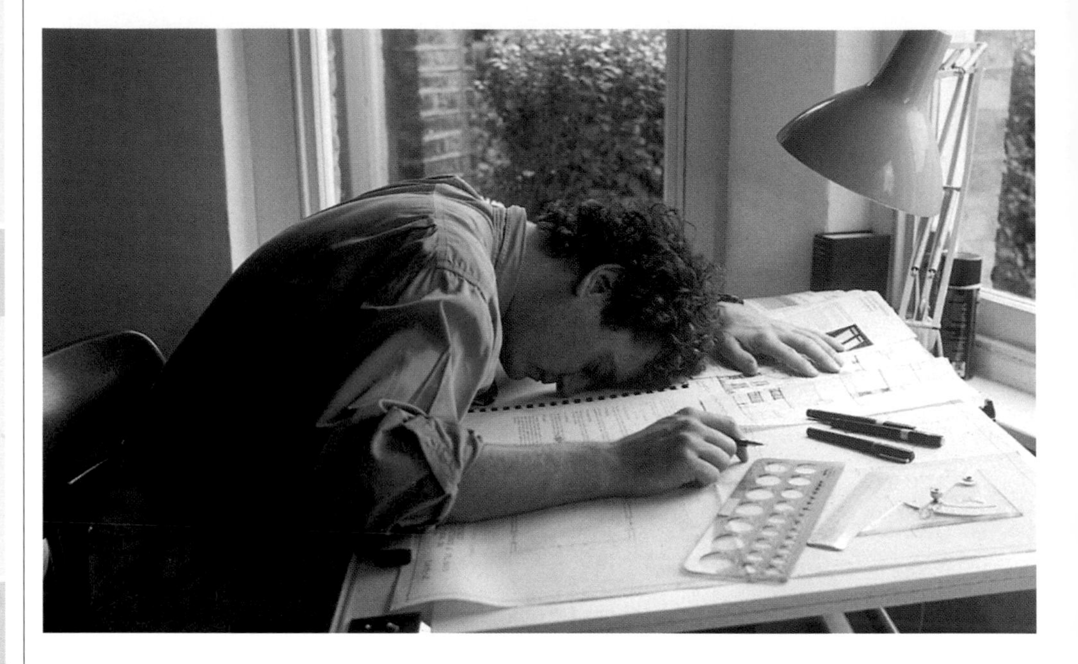

▲ *People with fibromyalgia experience pain and stiffness in the muscles and connective tissues. This complex and incapacitating disorder causes extreme fatigue in most cases.*

Fibromyalgia syndrome (FMS) is a common and often poorly understood clinical condition that afflicts as many as three million to eight million people in the United States alone. Most FMS patients are women, although men also experience this chronic, painful, and frequently incapacitating disorder. There is no certain cause nor any definite cure for FMS.

Symptoms and causes

Fibromyalgia syndrome is characterized by diffuse aches that are poorly localized and are perceived by the patient to be in the muscles, joints, nerves, and bones. This constant, widespread pain is felt as deep muscular aching, and as burning, shooting, and stabbing pains. The flare-ups can fluctuate in intensity, may last for days or months, and are never completely relieved.

Most patients experience their most severe symptoms—such as stiffness in the neck, spine, shoulders, or hips—upon waking in the morning, or after spending several hours in a fixed position. Symptoms of stiffness tend to disappear as the muscles warm up. The sufferer may require up to an hour to become limber; taking a warm bath and doing exercises such as stretches will often speed up the process.

Other symptoms associated with FMS include dryness in the eyes or mouth, premenstrual syndrome (PMS), painful periods, skin sensitivities, chronic headaches, morning stiffness, a feeling of swollen extremities (without swelling), dizziness, and impaired coordination.

Fibromyalgia syndrome should never be diagnosed until all possible organic causes have first been eliminated. Symptoms often begin rather insidiously between the ages of 20 and 40 years. They can develop following some traumatic event, such as an acute sprain, a nerve root irritation, or traumatic shock; after prolonged exposure to environmental stressors, such as cold drafts and dampness; following physical stresses, such as repetitive activities; or as a result of long-term emotional stressors related to home or work (see Stress).

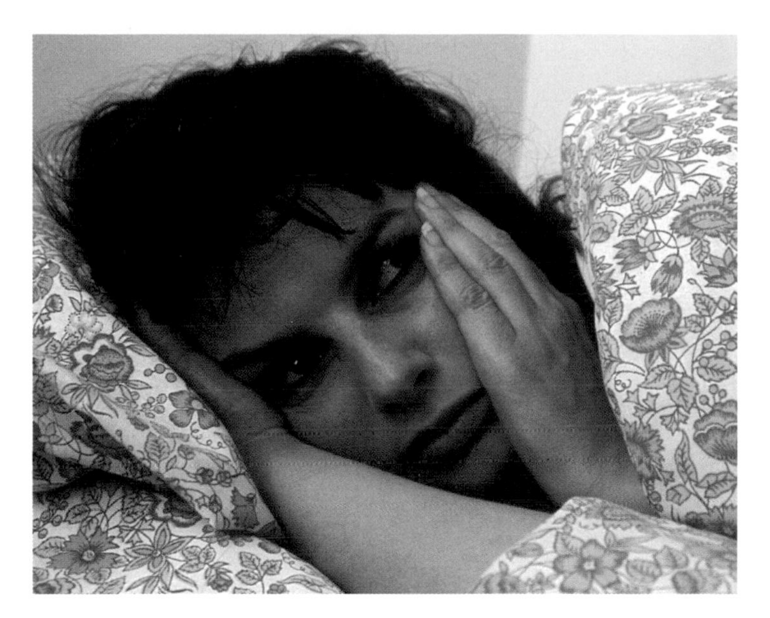

▲ *Women are particularly prone to develop fibromyalgia, which can be associated with chronic headaches, premenstrual syndrome, and painful periods.*

Dangers

Fibromyalgia syndrome often complicates diagnosis and treatment of other arthritic conditions such as rheumatoid arthritis, tennis elbow, biceps tendinitis, and regional myofascial pain. When FMS is severe, even those patients who are receiving good treatment can become incapacitated and unable to work.

Medications such as corticosteroids, immunosuppressive drugs, narcotics, and sedative-hypnotics—which are used to manage other conditions—should never be used to treat FMS. Withdrawal from these drugs often induces a similar condition to FMS; it can also worsen existing pain for FMS patients. Routine use of sleeping pills should also be avoided, as they may be habit-forming. However, doctors may be able to prescribe less addictive sleeping medications.

Attempts made by sufferers at self-diagnosis and self-medication, although common, can be problematic.

Diagnosis

FMS is often confused with chronic fatigue syndrome (CFS), arthritis, and rheumatism. FMS has symptoms that overlap many of these conditions. Nearly 75 percent of CFS patients also have FMS. However, the criteria for FMS are more clearly established than those for CFS.

To be diagnosed with FMS, a patient must experience widespread pain in all four quadrants of his or her body for at least three months, and must suffer in at least 11 of the 18 different sensitive pressure areas of the body, defined as "tender points." These 18 tender points are specific to the diagnosis of FMS; they cluster around the neck, shoulders, hips, knees, and elbows. When a doctor palpates the tender points with his or her thumb, applying steady, uniform pressure, patients who are suffering from FMS will say they feel pain; they will grimace, flinch, withdraw, or jump aside.

Treatment

Treatment for FMS is many-faceted, and the most important aspect is education. Before patients diagnose themselves, it is always wise for them to discuss their concerns with a doctor. They should also ask for printed literature and any information on support groups and other organizations, such as the Fibromyalgia Alliance of America in Ohio.

There is no definite cure for FMS, but with proper treatment, pain and fatigue can be decreased and patients can learn to manage their symptoms. Traditional treatments are often designed to improve the patient's quality of sleep, as well as reduce the level of pain and fatigue he or she suffers. Sleep management, pain management, and lifestyle management are all vital steps.

Patients should keep an FMS diary similar to a migraine diary to help identify the factors that increase their pain and fatigue. These factors can include physical, psychological, or environmental stress; disrupted sleep; or a poor state of physical fitness. After assessing possible causes, the individual may have to make the appropriate lifestyle changes (see Stress Management).

The use of medications has proved useful for some, but not all, FMS sufferers. Tricyclic antidepressants, such as amitryptyline and cyclobenzaprine, provide some relief and thus improve the quality of sleep. Continued use of these medicines, as well as antidepressants such as Prozac, Zoloft, Paxil, and Serzone, increases the level of serotonin—an important neurotransmitter—in the body, to modify the patient's attitude toward pain.

However, the use of tricyclic medications only eases the symptoms of fibromyalgia; it does not relieve them altogether. As always, caution must also be used with any chemical treatment, since many patients develop an increased sensitivity to both the therapeutic and the unwanted side effects of medications, as well as the precipitating environmental stressors.

A program of stretching and exercise is essential and helpful for the majority of patients. Anyone can learn beneficial routines to build muscle tone and improve his or her overall level of aerobic fitness. Gentle exercises, such as walking, use of stationary exercise equipment, swimming, and stretching, all help FMS patients to maintain flexibility and increase vigor (see Exercise).

Other treatments that can be beneficial for FMS sufferers include therapeutic massage, heat or hot baths, ice massage, biofeedback and other relaxation techniques, behavior modification, stress reduction, body mechanics and posture training, meditation, acupuncture, and chiropractic and osteopathic treatments.

Outlook

If a patient follows the advice and instruction of a knowledgeable, experienced physical therapist and accepts the help of support groups, it is possible for him or her to learn how to adapt to the pain and fatigue of FMS, and to live a better, healthier life.

It is important to take charge of FMS, and education is essential for this process. Self-management techniques allow FMS patients to handle their symptoms more effectively, so patients should be willing and able to take responsibility for their own health and well-being as much as possible. Support from family and friends is also paramount.

Until fibromyalgia is better understood, patients should, with the agreement of their doctor, attempt to exercise regularly so that they can maintain more flexibility and muscle tone. Most sufferers do make a full recovery, but the condition can recur.

See also: **Alternative medicine; Arthritis; Chronic fatigue syndrome; Depression; Fatigue; Muscles; Pain; Pain management; Rheumatism; Sleep and sleep problems**

Myasthenia gravis

Questions and Answers

My wife is 32 and has recently developed a condition called myasthenia. What does this word mean, exactly?

Any medical term containing the root "myo-" has something to do with muscles. *Myo* is a Greek word meaning "of muscles." *Asthenia* is also a Greek word; it means "weakness" or "loss of strength." So myasthenia means loss of power in the muscles. Myasthenia gravis does not cause permanent paralysis of muscles, however, and when episodes of weakness do occur, they can be effectively treated.

My middle-aged daughter has complained to her doctor several times of weakness and fatigue but has just been told to pull herself together and get more exercise. Recently I have noticed that her eyelids are drooping. Could she have myasthenia gravis?

Doctors are so used to hearing complaints of weakness and tiredness, and myasthenia is so rare, that this possibility may not have occurred to your daughter's doctor. If she tells her doctor that she has episodes of blepharoptosis (drooping eyelids) and thinks she may have myasthenia gravis, the doctor may then take her seriously and arrange for appropriate tests.

My sister was thought to have myasthenia and had a tensilon test, which involved injections. The first injection had no effect, but the second abolished her weakness within seconds. Does this suggest that there may be doubt about the diagnosis?

No. The psychological effect of an intravenous injection can be very strong, so it is usual to do a control test with a harmless saline solution before giving the tensilon shot. If the saline has no effect but the tensilon works, the diagnosis of myasthenia is virtually proved.

Myasthenia gravis is a disease that causes severe weakness and abnormally rapid tiring of muscles when they are used. Although the basic cause remains unknown, doctors now understand exactly what happens in the disease and are able to control it effectively.

Myasthenia gravis can begin to affect people at any age but most commonly starts between the ages of 15 and 50. It affects about one person in 25,000 and is twice as common in women as in men. Initially, the disease may be very mild and difficult to distinguish from other causes of tiredness and weakness. However, it is typical of the condition that the muscle weakness becomes progressively worse toward the end of the day and after exercise.

Symptoms

When myasthenia first appears, it is usually intermittent, and all the patient appreciates is that he or she gets tired more rapidly than normal. The muscles that move the eyes and that close the eyelids are often affected early, typically causing drooping of the eyelids in the absence of sleepiness. Patients often complain of double vision and may be referred to ophthalmologists (see Double Vision). In the early stages, patients may notice that, during meals, their chewing

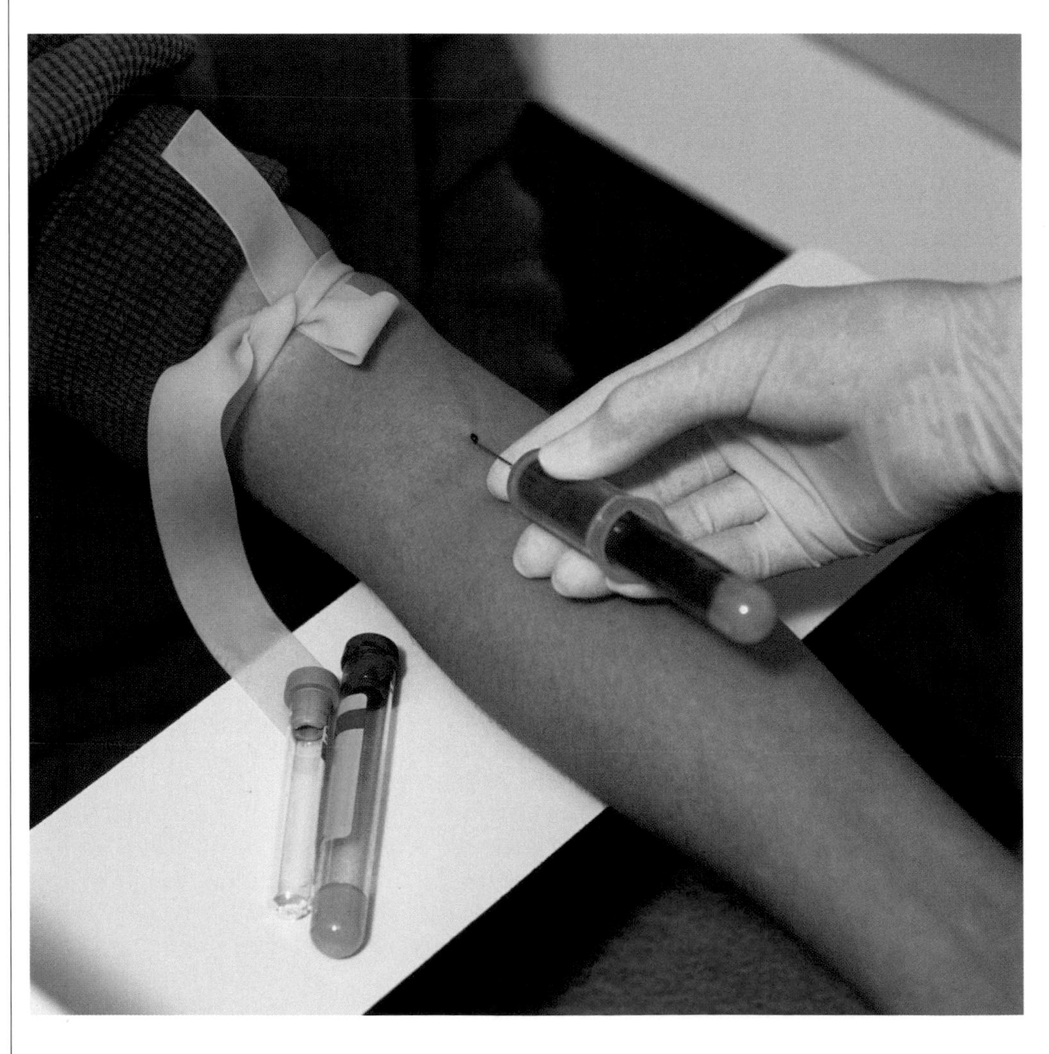

▲ *A diagnostic blood test is taken to check for the specific acetylcholine receptor antibodies that attack the muscle receptors in myasthenia gravis.*

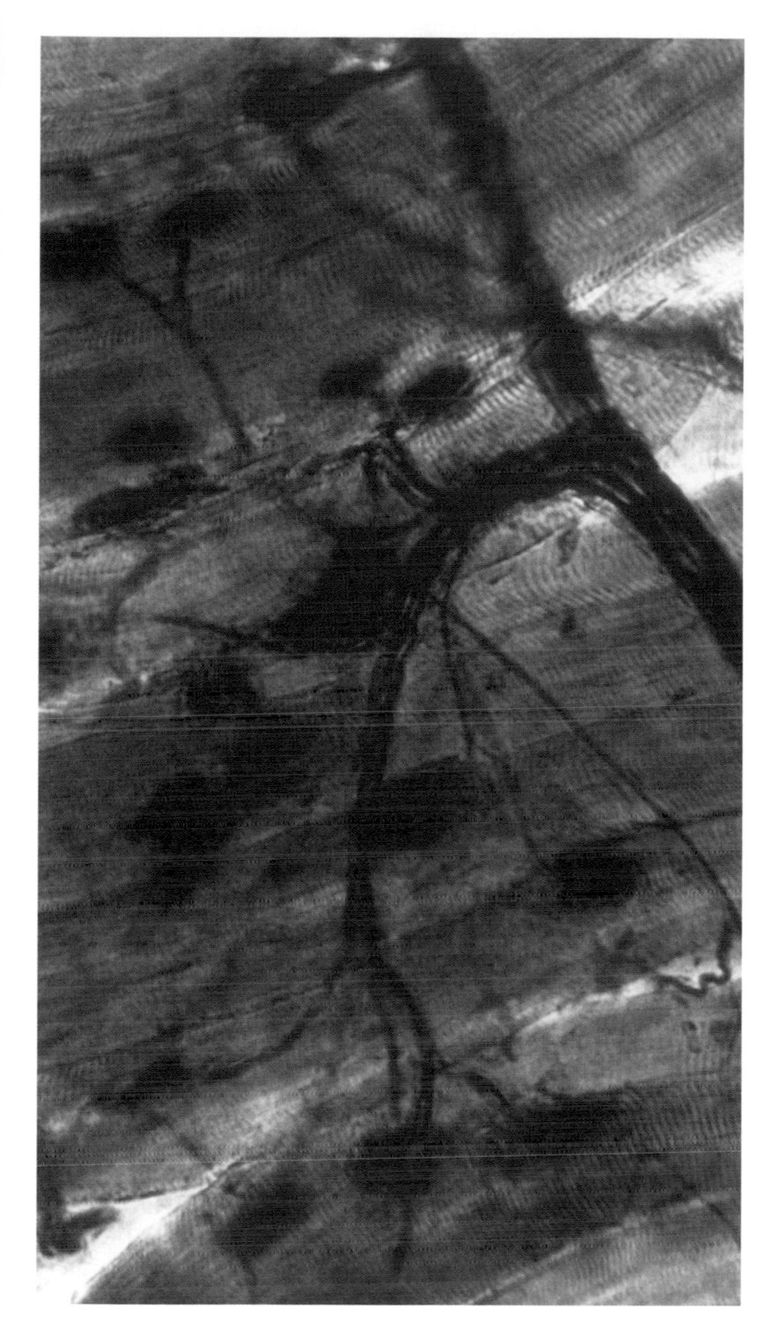

▲ *This magnified image of a neuromuscular junction shows the synaptic knobs in the muscle tissue that serve as receptor sites for messages from the nerves. In patients with myasthenia gravis, abnormal antibodies attach themselves to these muscle receptor sites and block the neurotransmitters that convey nerve messages, thereby preventing the muscles from contracting.*

muscles get tired rapidly. Some may even find that it is difficult to swallow. The muscles involved in speech may also be affected, so that it becomes difficult to go on speaking. General weakness of the limb muscles may also be an early sign.

More dangerous is weakness affecting the muscles used for breathing—those between the ribs and the muscle sheet, the diaphragm, that forms the floor of the chest cavity (see Breathing). Weakness of these muscles may endanger life. Before that stage is reached, however, affected people are likely to be aware that their ability to cough is severely reduced. This is a dangerous development calling for urgent medical attention. The inability to cough can lead to asphyxia from the blockage of the air passages by the accumulation of lung secretions (see Coughing).

Causes

To understand myasthenia gravis it is necessary to know that voluntary muscles cannot contract unless an electrical signal passes to them along the nerve that activates them. The point at which a nerve fiber contacts a muscle fiber is called the neuromuscular junction. When the nerve impulse reaches the end of the nerve, it causes the release of a substance called acetylcholine. This is known as a neurotransmitter, and it passes to specific sites on muscle fibers called receptor sites. The arrival of acetylcholine at these receptor sites triggers the contraction of the muscle fibers.

In myasthenia gravis, abnormal antibodies are formed by the immune system. These antibodies attach themselves to the muscle receptor sites, thereby blocking them so that the acetylcholine cannot operate to cause the muscle fibers to contract. The reason for the formation of the antibodies is still unknown, but myasthenia gravis is a clear example of an autoimmune disease.

Some cases of myasthenia are known to be due to an abnormality in the thymus gland in the neck, which processes the immune system cells called T lymphocytes. Although these cells do not themselves produce antibodies, they have an important part to play in the production of antibodies by the B lymphocytes. In about 10 percent of cases of myasthenia a benign tumor can be found in the thymus gland.

Diagnosis and treatment

The neurotransmitter acetylcholine is important in the body, and much is known about it. So that acetylcholine does not cause muscles to go on contracting, the body breaks it down with a powerful enzyme called cholinesterase. Several drugs that antagonize cholinesterase exist. Such drugs can be used both to diagnose and to treat myasthenia. Once the suspicion of myasthenia has been aroused, the condition can be diagnosed by giving an injection of the anticholinesterase drug tensilon (edrophonium). The effect of this shot is briefly to abolish the muscle weakness and restore strength to normal. An additional diagnostic test is to demonstrate the presence of specific acetylcholine receptor antibodies. These are not found in any other disease.

The action of tensilon is too short to make it useful in the treatment of myasthenia, but other anticholinesterase drugs have a longer action. The drug pyridostigmine can be taken by mouth and has a duration of action of about four hours. The dosage has to be determined by observing the patient's response to a trial dose and adjusting it accordingly. Surgical removal of the thymus is also helpful, especially when myasthenia is present in women under 40 with a positive antibody result. In addition, drugs that damp down the action of the immune system (immunosuppressants) are often helpful. About 70 percent of people with myasthenia improve when given steroids or the drug azathioprine (Imuran). In some cases a procedure called plasmapheresis, in which the antibodies are filtered from the blood, may be used.

See also: **Fatigue; Immune system; Immunosuppressive drugs; Injections; Lymphocytes; Muscles; Nervous system; Thymus; Tiredness; Tumors**

Nails

Questions and Answers

My husband is a mechanic and seems to have oil permanently under his fingernails. Could this be dangerous in any way?

The oil, although unsightly, is not dangerous. However, it can adhere to other dirt particles, and also act as a breeding ground for germs. Try to encourage your husband to keep his nails cut as short as possible and get him a good stiff brush with which to clean his nails after work each day. An orange stick can also be useful to help remove dirt from under his nails.

I caught my finger in the door and have severely bruised the nail. Is it likely to fall off?

Yes, if the nail has been badly damaged it is possible that you will lose it; however, a new nail will grow. This is a slow process and could take a few months.

I have managed to stop my son from sucking his thumb. Now he bites his nails. What can I do?

Your son's nail biting is simply an alternative to thumb sucking, and until you find the cause of his anxiety you will not be able to rid him of such habits, however much you nag and scold. In fact, this may make his nail biting worse. Perhaps your son is having problems at school; or maybe he is jealous of a younger sibling and is seeking attention.

My daughter bites her nails constantly and I am worried that her fingers will become infected. Could this happen?

It could, but such an infection is usually a minor one in the area around the nail. However, infections can lead to dermatitis, flaking, and hardening of the skin, all of which would need treatment.

The condition of the nails can reflect someone's general health. Changes in the appearance of the nails can be due to injury, infection, or disease. Good nail hygiene and care are essential to protect the nails from injury.

Nails are made of dead cells that grow from living skin cells in the tissues of fingers and toes. The part of the nail that shows itself is dead and so will not hurt or bleed when it is cut or if it is damaged—but any injury to the living roots can be painful.

Nails can be an indicator of someone's state of health. For example, a change in the appearance of the nails can indicate a deficiency of iron or cysteine.

Infection can occur in the nails, resulting in conditions such as paronychia, a common complaint among people who frequently immerse their hands in water. Such problems can be prevented by regular, thorough care of the hands and feet and by wearing cotton-lined rubber gloves when the hands have to be in water. It is also important to keep nails clean, because dirt can harbor germs that may spread diseases.

How nails are formed

Each nail is made up of a horny, proteinaceous substance called keratin. The visible part of the nail is called its body. The shape of the body can be determined, at least in part, by genetic factors, so nail shapes tend to run in families. The bottom part of the nail, which is implanted in a groove in the skin, is called the root. Overlapping the root are the cuticles (eponychia). These layers of skin cover the white crescent or lunula found toward the base of the nail. The lunula, usually most clearly visible on the thumb, is slightly thicker than the rest of the nail, and so looks white because it hides the blood vessels beneath.

The lowest layer of cells in the skin composing the nail folds is known as the general matrix. The cells of the matrix divide, and the upper ones become thickened and toughened with keratin. When the cells die they become part of the nail itself. If the matrix is seriously damaged, the whole nail will be lost.

Rates of growth

Nails grow an average of about 0.03 inch (0.5 mm) a week, but the actual rate of growth will vary between individual fingers and toes. Studies of nail growth have shown that growth can be slowed down by a hormonal imbalance, by mineral deficiencies, and even by a psychological

ANATOMY OF A NAIL

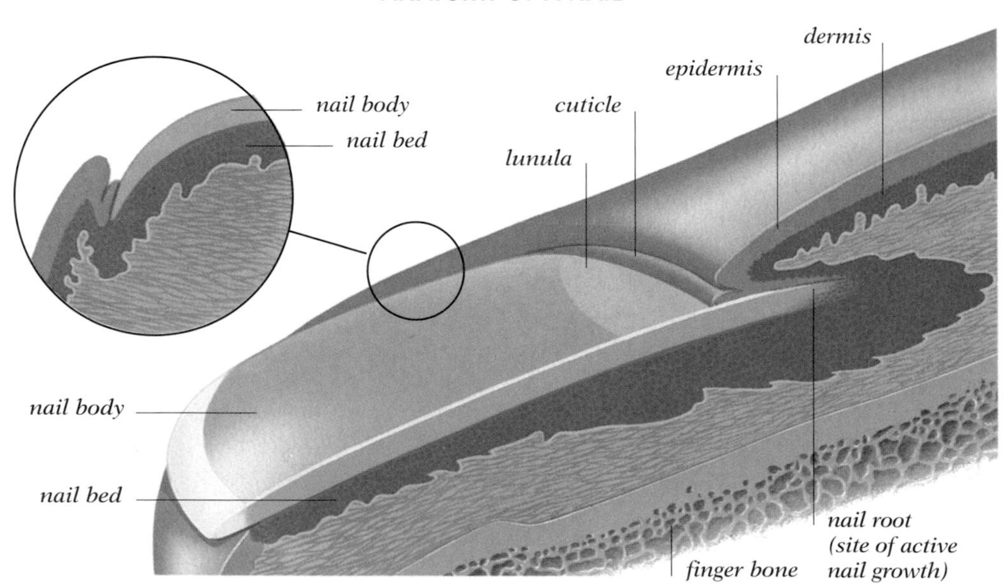

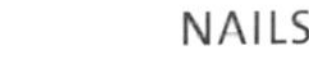

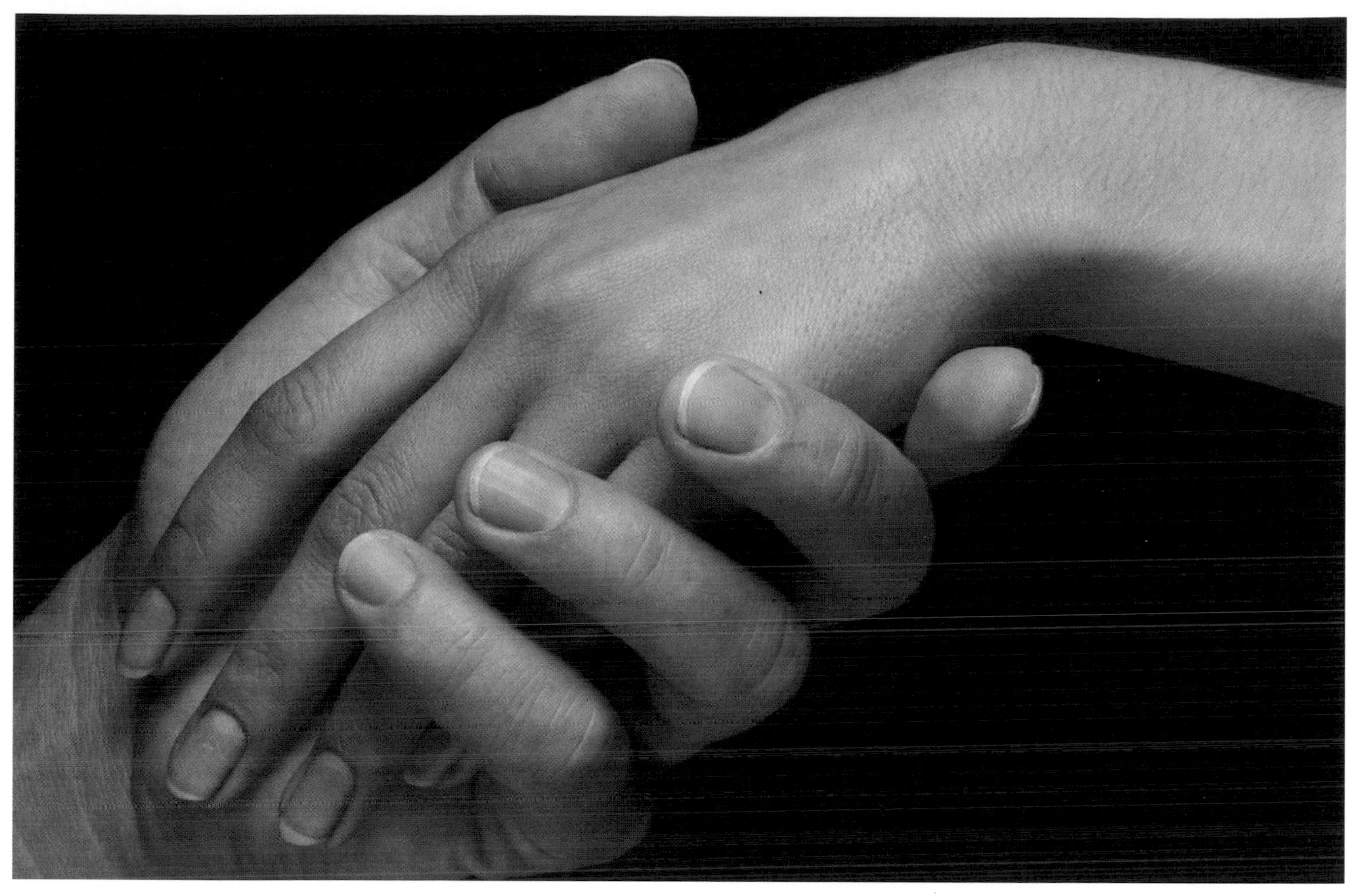

▲ *Dirty, bitten, or ragged nails can become infected. Good hygiene and regular care of the nails will keep them healthy. General care of the hands need take only a few minutes each day and can prevent injury and trauma to the nails.*

disturbance. Poor health is also reflected in the nails, and about 40 different disorders, including anemia, lung disease, heart disease, infection, and hemochromatosis all cause changes in the nails that can help in the diagnosis of disorders.

Functions of the nails

Nails are used mainly to manipulate objects. The living tissue around and beneath them is well supplied with nerve endings, so the nails are also involved in the sense of touch.

Nails also support the tissues of the fingers and toes, particularly when the hands or feet are pressed onto a firm surface when a person is standing and walking.

Nail problems

The most common problem is that the skin around or beneath the nails becomes infected with bacteria. The infection may be caused by incorrect growth of a nail or by a small injury at the side of the fingernail. Acute infections are commonly caused by small pieces of nail, called hangnails, that grow from the side of the nail into the skin, or by bacteria entering skin through minor wounds. This kind of infection, known as paronychia, is easily treated with antibiotics. If pus forms, it may need to be released by surgical means. Another problem that may occur is ringworm. This is caused by a fungal infection but is easily treated with antibiotics.

When nails have split horizontally, they can be very difficult to repair. However, a special glue will hold the nail edges in place until the nail grows enough to be filed down. White spots may be due to minor damage from a knock or blow. Ridges in the nails are common in elderly people and can be a sign of rheumatoid arthritis. Flaky nails are normally too dry; they should be massaged with moisturizing hand cream.

Too little iron tends to make the nails concave. This condition, known as koilonychia, is due to softening and thinning of the nail plate. Everyday splitting of the nails does not seem to have any underlying cause. The nails can be treated with nail hardener, but a well-balanced diet and general care should keep them healthy.

The condition known as ingrown toenail does not always involve nail growth into the tissue as is commonly believed. Infected and inflamed tissue along the nail edge can swell over the edge, causing the typical appearance. It is seldom necessary to remove the whole nail. Treatment is directed at the control of the infection in the surrounding tissues. Sometimes, one or both edges of the nail may have to be cut away.

Nail biting

Nail biting can start at the toddler stage and develop into a habit. In older children and adults, the same habit is probably related to anxiety or boredom. Bitten nails look unattractive and can be a source of infection if they are bitten down to the nail bed or beyond.

Care of nails

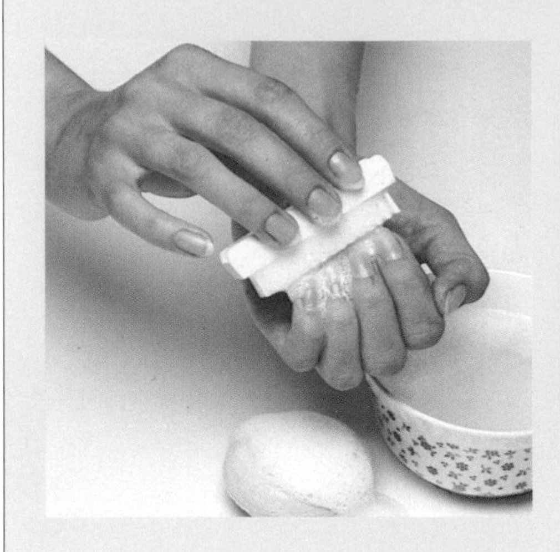

▲ *To clean the nails, gently scrub the tips of the nails using soap on a nail-brush to loosen the dirt. Take care not to damage the cuticles. Rinse well in clean warm water; dry.*

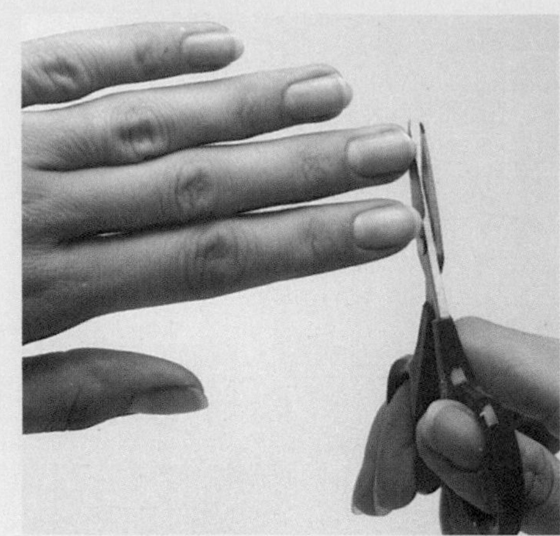

▲ *Cut your nails to the required length with sharp nail scissors. Avoid blunt scissors, because these will tear the nail. Do not poke at your cuticles with scissors, and do not use scissors to dig under the nail.*

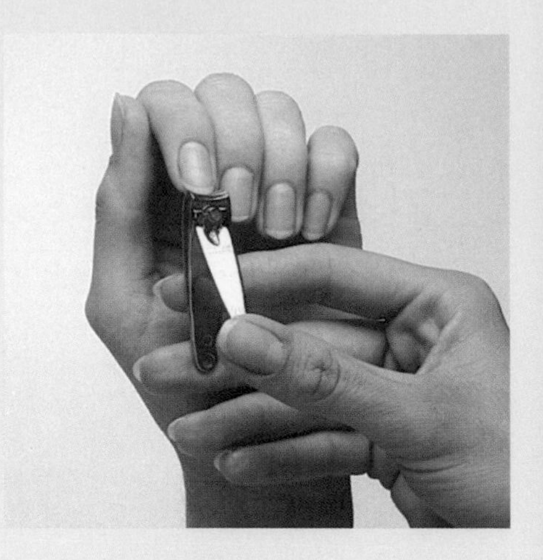

▲ *Nail clippers may be easier to use, especially to clip the right hand if you are right-handed and the left hand if you are left-handed. Make sure you buy a large enough size. Clip off only small amounts of nail.*

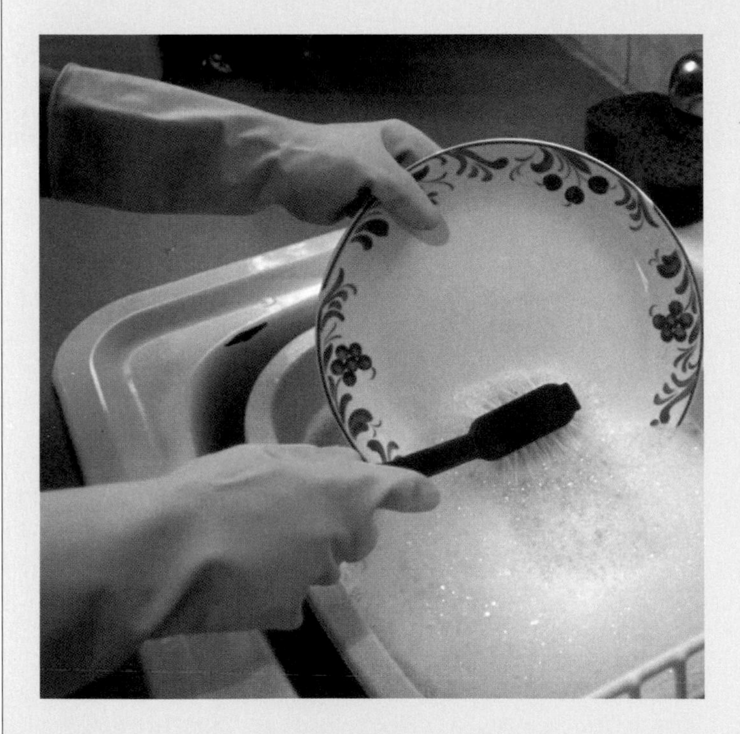

◄ *Cotton-lined rubber gloves will protect the hands when they are exposed to water and prevent conditions such as paronychia. This disorder is caused by repeated immersion of the hands in water, causing swelling and infection around the nail.*

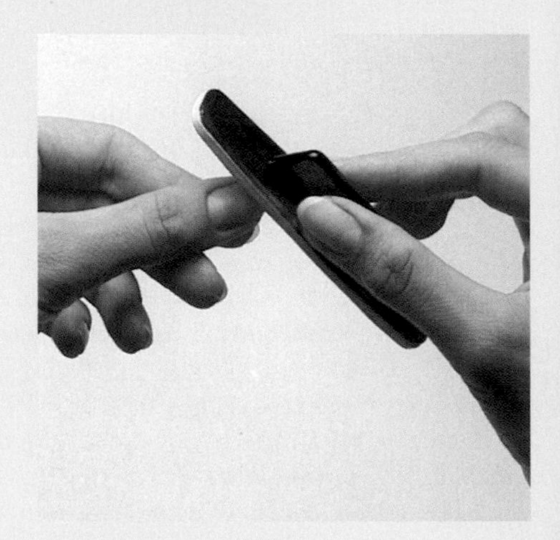

▲ *A buffer—a piece of chamois leather mounted on wood—can be used to give the nails a natural shine. The longer you use the buffer, the more lustrous the sheen will be.*

Strong, attractive nails begin with a good diet. If you eat a balanced diet of meat, fruit, vegetables, and dairy products, your nails, like your general health, will benefit. Unlike bones, nails contain no calcium but are made of a hard protein called keratin; contrary to popular belief, calcium supplements have no effect on the nails.

Nails should be kept scrupulously clean, not only for the sake of appearance, but also because they trap dirt and can spread infection. Protect your hands and nails with rubber gloves if you are going to do really dirty work. Dry your hands and nails thoroughly after immersing them in water.

If a nail snags, do not peel it off; you could end up with a painful tear. Instead, cut off the main part of the nail, then file the rest to shape.

Push cuticles back gently with an orange stick tipped with cotton batting and soaked in cuticle cream. Be sure not to tear the skin, and do not get into the habit of nibbling the skin. Remember to push the cuticle back on each nail every time you dry your hands.

Nail polish will not harm healthy nails; however, be sure to

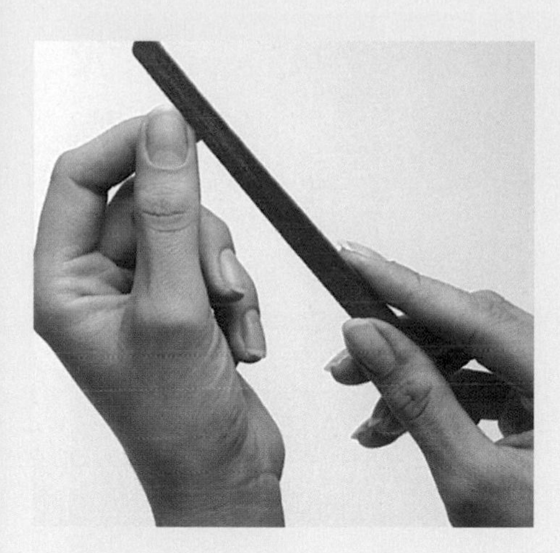

▲ *Emery boards are gentler than metal files. Use the emery board in one direction only to prevent the nail from splitting. Filing the nails to sharp points tends to weaken them.*

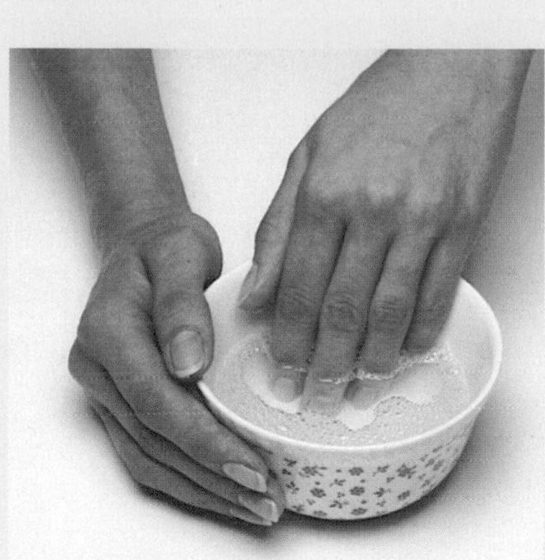

▲ *After you file your nails, the nail area will be rather dry and powdery. Soak your nails in warm soapy water, and rinse and dry them carefully before continuing with the remainder of the manicure.*

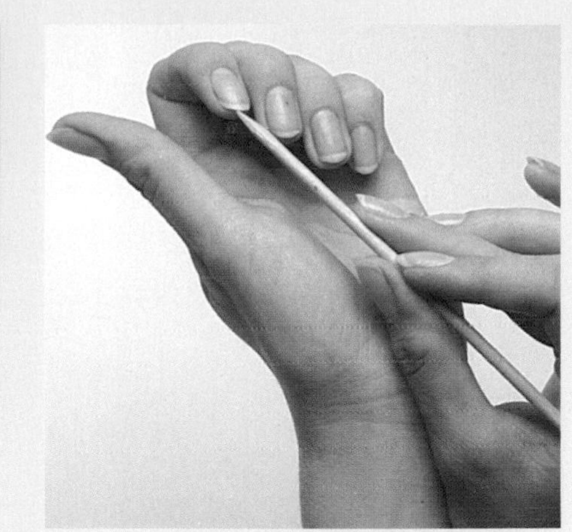

▲ *Gently insert the point of an orange stick under the tip of each nail to clean it thoroughly. Take care that you do not tear the skin. Your nails should now look and feel exceptionally clean.*

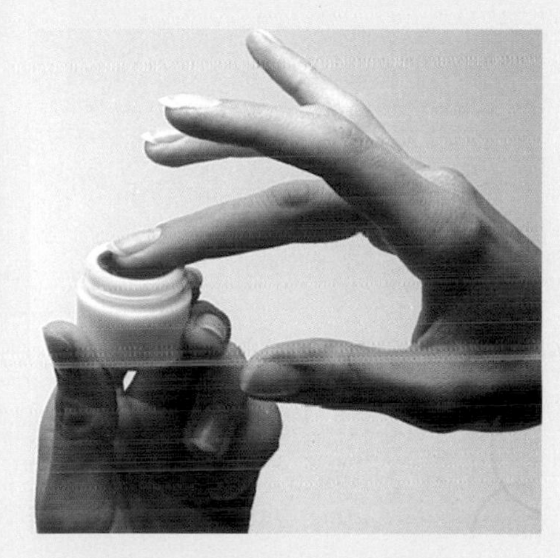

▲ *Rubbing nail cream into your cuticles helps nail growth. When the cuticles are softened by the cream, use the tip of an orange stick wrapped in cotton to push them back gently.*

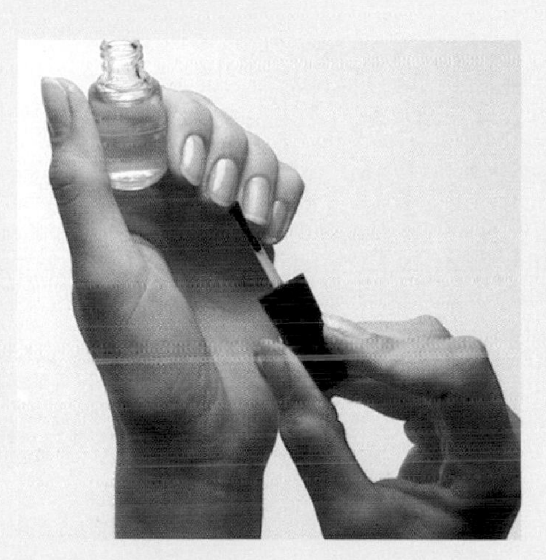

▲ *Colorless nail polish gives a natural sheen. Some people also like to use nail hardener on their nails. Colored nail polish will not damage your nails—but take it off with a good remover.*

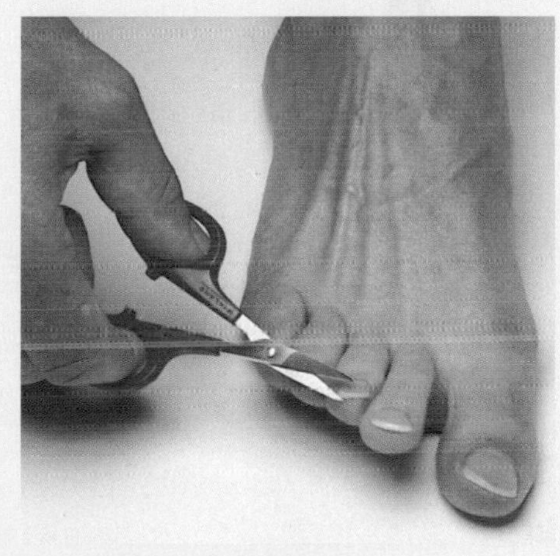

▲ *Toenails may be harder than fingernails and should be cut with scissors or clippers after bathing. Cut toenails straight across because infected skin can grow around short, shaped toenails.*

use a good nail polish remover (with added conditioner). If you want your nails to look longer, paint straight down from the cuticle and leave a thin line at each side of the nail. Do not pick at chipped nail polish—you could pull away flakes of nail. After taking off your nail polish, wash your hands in warm water and treat your nails to a 10-minute soak in warm olive oil.

Toenails tend to be much harder than fingernails, and so it is easier to cut them after taking a bath, which softens the nails. Scrub your toenails while in the bath and press the cuticles back with a towel when you get out. Cut your toenails straight across with a sharp pair of scissors or a nail clipper. File them carefully. Keep a lookout for signs of an ingrown toenail or any other infection. Do not forget to clean beneath the toenails.

Toenails should be dealt with in the same way as fingernails; they benefit from the same moisturizing treatments and care as fingernails.

Hands and feet have to work hard under pressure, so it is beneficial to treat them to an occasional professional manicure or a pedicure.

Questions and Answers

One of my fingernails grows very little, if at all, but the others grow normally. Why does this happen?

The cells that produced this nail have been damaged or even destroyed. As a result, the nail is not being continually renewed as it should be. This is nothing to worry about as long as the nail does not fall off altogether, indicating that the matrix from which the nail grows has been destroyed. If this happens, consult your doctor.

Will my son get ingrown toenails if he wears tight shoes?

Shoes that are too tight are a common cause of ingrown toenails, because the soft tissue is pushed onto the edge of the nail and damaged by the shoe. Badly-fitting shoes can also cause a host of other foot problems, so it is not worth taking the risk of letting your son wear shoes that are too small for him.

I am determined to break my nail-biting habit. How can I do this?

Try painting your nails with white iodine, or use a commercial preparation. You could also try treating yourself to expensive nail polish and telling yourself you will use it when your nails grow to a reasonable length. If neither of these measures works, see your doctor about behavior therapy.

My mother is disgusted by the way my children bite their nails and says the only way to stop it is by making them go to bed wearing gloves that are tied to their wrists. Is this a sensible approach?

Most people now agree that it is best not to make an issue of nail-biting. After all, it is not a major failing. Instead, try to persuade your children to overcome the habit by pointing out how nice unbitten nails look and praising them if they succeed in growing their nails. Whatever you do, do not nag them.

Nail biting

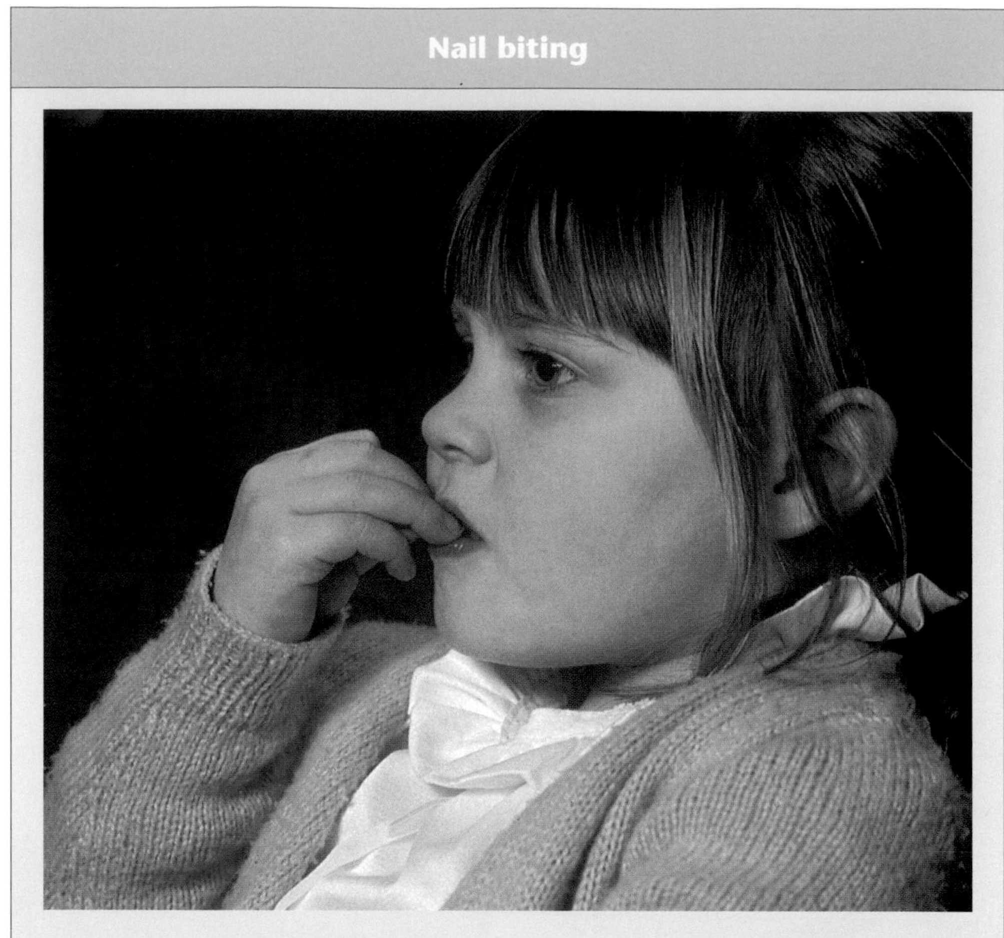

If your child is a persistent nail-biter, he or she may be upset about something. Try to find out if there is unhappiness at school or distress caused by some event in family life such as a new house or a new baby. If it just seems to be a habit, try not to nag—this will only make the problem worse. Try to persuade the child to stop nail biting by the promise of a treat or a reward. A daughter may be encouraged to give up nail biting if you give her her own manicure set.

If everything else fails, there are unpleasant-tasting substances, which you can buy from the drugstore to paint on the nails. However, do not worry too much about this minor habit—most children grow out of it.

Some people bite their nails until they bleed and become sore and infected. It is best to avoid making nail biting an issue with children. If the habit is too difficult to break, commercial preparations are available from drugstores. These can be painted on the nails, and they taste so unpleasant that fingers are usually kept well away from the mouth. Adults may try painting their nails twice a day with white iodine, which is also very unpleasant to taste.

If the habit is very ingrained and commercial preparations are not a deterrent, some doctors may recommend behavior therapy. Therapy involves habit-reversal training, which teaches awareness of the habit, how to relax, how to perform a competing response (see Behavior Therapy), and that motivation can overcome any habit.

Nail care

Nails should be kept clean so that they do not attract bacteria. Nails should never be filed to sharp points, because this shape weakens them and can cause them to break: a gentle oval is better. Colored nail polish should never be used to cover up dirty nails. Massaging cream or warm olive oil rubbed into the cuticles will aid healthy nail growth, but a diet high in protein and rich in vitamins is the best guarantee of healthy nails. Try to protect the nails by avoiding physical trauma to the fingertips.

See also: **Hygiene; Ingrown toenail; Pus; Ringworm; Whitlow**

Narcotics

Questions and Answers

My husband says all narcotics are addictive. Is he right?

Basically yes, if they are taken in uncontrolled doses. Narcotic addiction varies in severity from total addiction to heroin to occasional dependence on synthetic opioids. However, narcotics should always be taken under medical supervision, which lessens any danger of addiction.

Why was I given meperidine hydrochloride instead of morphine when I had my baby?

Both medications have similar effects but meperidine hydrochloride is usually given by intramuscular injection and the effect lasts longer. It also causes less nausea. Both drugs can be given in early labor, but pain relief may not be as effective as that achieved with an epidural: local anesthesia that numbs the nerves to the uterus and birth canal.

Is it dangerous to take medicines containing codeine for a long time?

Codeine is an opium derivative present in many well-known pain-relieving pills, cough syrups, and preparations for diarrhea; it can be habit forming when taken in prolonged and very high doses.

My daughter has made friends with some well-known drug abusers. How can I tell if she has also become addicted to heroin?

If your daughter seems drowsy or appears to be in a stupor, then heroin abuse could be the cause. Look for needle marks on her arms and legs, constricted pupils, or equipment such as a syringe or burned tinfoil. If you discover these signs and your daughter is addicted to heroin, consult your doctor about possible treatment and counseling services.

Narcotics are drugs that relieve pain and also alter a person's mood and behavior significantly. They are derived either from opium or from synthetic substances and can be highly addictive.

Strictly speaking, a narcotic drug is any drug that produces a dulling of consciousness, stupor, and the relief of pain. However, in popular usage, the term "narcotic" has come to mean any drug that is used illegally, such as cocaine—which is actually a stimulant—and a broad spectrum of other drugs that affect the central nervous system, such as the barbiturates. In a medical context, drugs that doctors refer to as narcotics include opium, derivatives of opium, and opium's synthetic relatives.

All narcotic drugs are both physically and psychologically addictive if they are not prescribed in correct amounts, and so they are nearly all under strict control and available only by prescription. The legal and controlled use of narcotics is mainly to relieve severe pain and distress, for example, after surgery or during a very painful illness.

Opiates

Opiates are drugs made from the white milky substance that is obtained from the unripe seed pods of the opium poppy. They include opium, morphine, and codeine. These drugs can be inhaled, ingested, or injected, and they can rapidly cause both psychological and physical addiction.

Pure opium is rarely used medicinally, but its most important derivatives—morphine and codeine—are often prescribed by doctors. Other opium derivatives—such as papaverine, a relaxant of involuntary muscles; and dextromethorphan, a cough suppressant—are also used widely (see Cough Syrup).

Morphine

Morphine is one of the most valuable drugs available to medicine, and it is 10 times stronger than opium. It can be used to control severe pain and will also relieve the fear and distress that are usually associated with such pain. However, because of its addictive properties, doctors usually prescribe morphine for short-term use only—for example, after surgery, or to deal with the pain encountered in terminal cancer.

Morphine has been found to cause constipation and is therefore used to treat diarrhea. It can also be used to suppress coughing.

Morphine is administered as morphine sulfate directly into a vein or muscle; or patients may take it orally. It also occurs as a component in other preparations.

Codeine

Codeine has the advantage of curing moderate pain without being too easily addictive. It also differs from morphine in that it produces excitement in the patient rather than narcosis (drowsy numbness). Codeine is used in many cough syrups, diarrhea medications, and painkillers. It is often used in combination with acetaminophen or aspirin, because it provides relief that cannot be obtained from either of the drugs individually.

► *Narcotics will take effect most rapidly if they are injected directly into a vein with a hypodermic syringe—this is the quickest way of relieving pain.*

Questions and Answers

If narcotics are addictive, why are they used?

Narcotics are addictive only if they are abused. Used properly, under the guidance of a doctor, narcotics are among the most valuable drugs in medicine.

My doctor talks about opiates and opioids. What is the difference?

Opiates are drugs derived from the juice of the white poppy—a natural substance. Opioids are synthetic substances with many of the same properties as opiates, including pain relief.

My son is a heroin addict and is being treated with methadone. How will this help?

Methadone blocks the withdrawal effects of heroin and substitutes itself as the addictive agent; however, it is easier to come off methadone than heroin. Another advantage is that methadone is more effective taken by mouth than by injection—psychologically, this weans the addict away from the ritual of injecting the drug.

My uncle is suffering from cancer and his doctors have prescribed morphine. I know that this drug is addictive, so can't he be given some other kind of pain control?

There are other drugs available for the treatment of cancer, and other methods of pain relief such as electrostimulation or even neurosurgery. However, for pain in the advanced, final stages of cancer, morphine or other opiate derivatives are by far the most effective in controlling both pain and distress.

Do any other illegal drugs have the same effect of extreme delirium as that of LSD?

Marijuana, barbiturates, cocaine, amphetamines, and opiates can all cause delirium, although their effects are not usually as severe as the hallucinations caused by LSD.

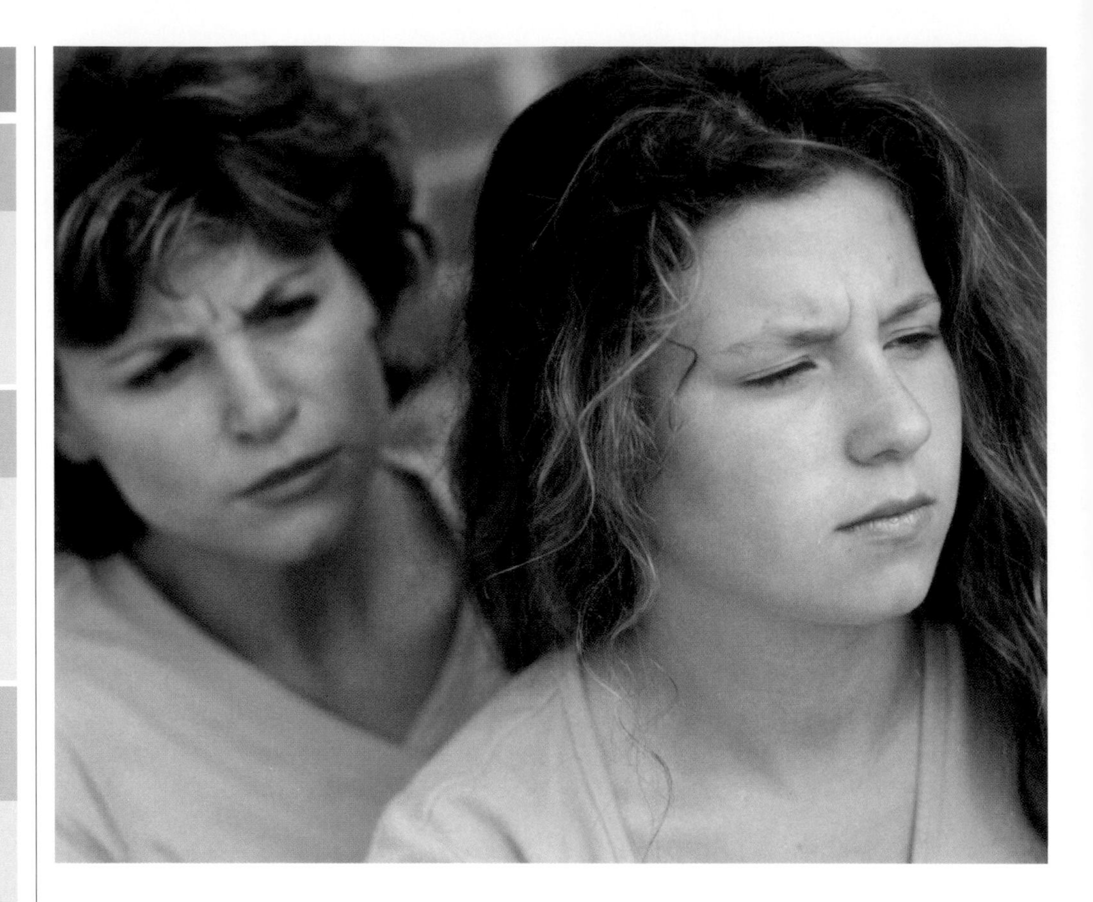

▲ *Parents often react angrily if they discover that their adolescent child has become addicted to narcotics such as heroin. However, understanding and support are vital if they want to get to the root of the problem and help stop the drug abuse.*

Synthetics

Meperidine hydrochloride: Many drugs with actions similar to the natural opiate alkaloids have been manufactured synthetically. These include meperidine hydrochloride (Demerol), which acts to relieve pain.

Heroin: Heroin is the most important drug in the group of synthetic opiates. Heroin is actually no more powerful than morphine and is, in fact, quickly converted to morphine in the body. However, it is much more rapidly assimilated than morphine and seems more powerful as a result. It is for this reason that heroin causes addiction more rapidly than morphine.

Heroin acts as a depressant on the central nervous system and is used as a euphoriant among opiate addicts. It is sold in the form of a white powder that has usually been mixed with comparatively harmless substances such as baking soda or lactose (milk sugar). The narcotic can be smoked or inhaled, but often—in a process known as "mainlining"—addicts liquefy it over a flame and then inject it into the bloodstream directly.

When it is first used, heroin can cause sickness, but otherwise its use results in relief from anxiety and tension, as well as in drowsiness and stupor. Regular use rapidly causes addiction and increased doses are craved not just to repeat the "high" experienced but also to stave off painful withdrawal symptoms. Sometimes unsterilized needles are used by heroin abusers, and these can lead to blood poisoning, hepatitis, and AIDS. Overdose is common and often fatal.

Withdrawal

Withdrawal from heroin can be acutely painful but is never fatal (see Withdrawal Symptoms). The synthetic opiate, methadone, is sometimes substituted for heroin to lessen the withdrawal symptoms and so that gradually reduced oral doses can be measured easily. However, methadone itself is also addictive and the patient must, at some point, withdraw from it. This can be hazardous without the proper supervision of a physician or another informed person.

See also: **Drug abuse; Heroin; LSD; Morphine**

Natural childbirth

The techniques of natural childbirth can help a woman in labor to take a calm, active part in the delivery of her baby. A more relaxed, homelike atmosphere can also help ease the shock of birth for the baby.

There is really no such thing as completely natural childbirth. Human beings are social animals, and even the most primitive cultures have rituals, customs, and taboos surrounding birth—much as they have with death. People grow up strongly influenced by the ideas and expectations about birth that they receive from their respective communities. For example, in the United States, emphasis is placed on the possible difficulties of childbirth. Hospitals provide medical care in the form of drugs and monitoring equipment as a matter of routine before and during childbirth. Indeed, medical intervention is often seen as a necessity in a natural process that still claims many lives in developing countries where medical care is not always available.

However, in recent years many women have become concerned that a natural process has become overmechanized, and that control of birth has been taken away from the mother-to-be. Many types of natural childbirth have been developed—or rediscovered—out of these concerns.

In effect, natural childbirth entails the avoidance of medical intervention as far as possible during labor. Many women are now able to discuss the type of birth they want with their doctor.

▼ *For a mother, holding her baby immediately after birth helps to form a strong bond.*

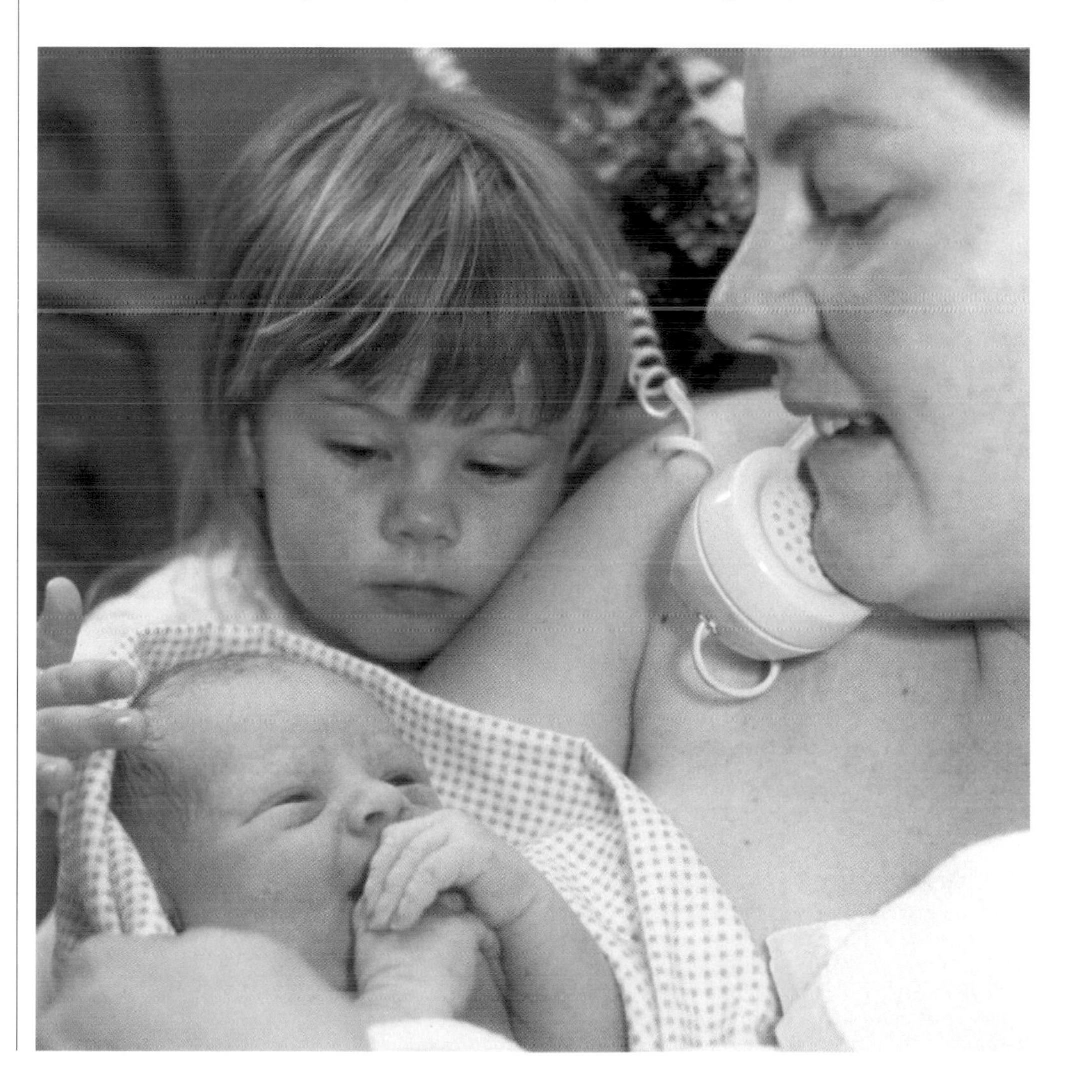

Questions and Answers

A nurse-midwife is going to deliver my baby by natural childbirth in a hospital. If there is any problem, will she be able to cope with it?

In the United States, nurse-midwives are trained to deal with most problems. They can always call the obstetrician on duty in the hospital in an emergency.

Under what circumstances should a woman not have a natural birth?

You should not set your hopes on natural childbirth if you have any condition requiring special medical attention—for example, diabetes, kidney or heart disease, or preeclampsia.

If you are carrying two or more babies or go into premature labor, you may also need skilled medical intervention. Although a baby in the breech position (bottom first) can be delivered naturally, most obstetricians opt for a surgical delivery (cesarean) if they cannot turn the baby in the uterus.

Does natural childbirth mean a pain-free birth?

No. There can be no guarantees about the way in which a woman will experience labor. However, natural childbirth techniques can help her to approach labor and childbirth with confidence.

My wife is having a natural birth. What will my role be?

Your presence and support will be the greatest help of all. During labor your wife will feel very vulnerable and your constant care and reassurance will be invaluable.

On a practical level, if you practice breathing and relaxation exercises or attend classes with her, you will be able to help her to remember what she must do during labor. You might also give her a massage if she wants one.

Questions and Answers

I am having a natural birth. Will my baby be examined before being given to me?

Doctors and nurse-midwives can tell at a glance if a baby is seriously malformed or if he or she appears to be having any breathing difficulties. The nurse-midwife or doctor should be satisfied quickly that there is nothing wrong, and will give you your baby to hold as soon as possible after the birth.

I am just about to have my first child, and I want a natural birth; however, my doctor insists that I have this first baby in the hospital. Why is this?

When a woman is having her first baby, she has no track record, and so she is considered at greater risk. This is because no one can tell how her uterus will behave during labor. However, you may still be able to follow certain natural childbirth techniques in a hospital, and you can request that no drug or intervention is used unless strictly necessary. Some women do have their first babies quite safely by natural childbirth in a nonhospital environment.

A friend has told me that postpartum depression is less common after a natural birth. Is this true?

From the few statistics available, it does appear that women who give birth at home or in a homelike environment are much less likely to suffer from postpartum depression. Some women find hospitals a strange and stressful environment in which to give birth, and this can cause anxiety and depression.

Is it dangerous to have a baby by natural methods?

The risk of complications during childbirth is small if you are a healthy young woman, and if you give birth in a clean environment. Only you can decide the balance of risks and benefits after consultation with a doctor.

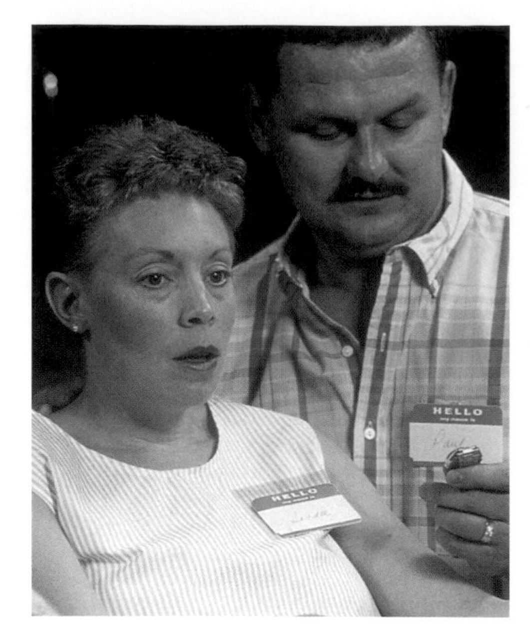

► Prenatal exercises include learning the positions, movements, and techniques of breathing that will help the baby to be born with minimal difficulty.

Standard births

In what is, after all, an understable ambition to make childbirth as safe as possible, hospitals have come to rely increasingly on the use of drugs and complicated machinery. With a normal hospital birth a woman may be offered all or some of the following procedures. Whether she will have any of them is a decision she must make with her obstetrician.

An oxytocin intravenous injection (IV) or pills may be used to induce labor. Oxytocin is a drug that makes the uterus contract. However, the contractions are often stronger, more painful, and closer together than they would be in natural childbirth and are therefore much more difficult for a woman to cope with effectively. Oxytocin is sometimes supplemented with a prostaglandin suppository placed at the top of the vagina; this has the effect of softening the cervix. The membrane may be ruptured, and sometimes all three techniques are used (see Induction of Labor; Prostaglandins).

Electronic fetal monitoring machines are used as a matter of course by most maternity units. They are used to monitor both the mother's contractions and the fetal heartbeat. One type measures contractions externally: it is strapped around the woman's abdomen, has a knob at the top, and is attached by wires to a machine that records the length and strength of contractions. The other type is an internal monitor consisting of a small clip that is attached to the baby's scalp; wires from this come down the vagina to a machine that records the baby's heartbeat.

A procedure that may be performed at the point of childbirth is an episiotomy. During the birth the doctor may make a cut in the perineum (the stretch of skin between the vagina and the anus) to make it quicker and easier for the baby's head to be born.

Doctors say that episiotomies are also done to prevent the perineum from tearing and to prevent stretching of perineal muscles, although this is debatable. It is not painful when the cut is made; however, the stitches can be painful afterward and may affect the woman's sex life for a time when she returns home. Episiotomies are not performed routinely anymore, and a woman is less likely to be offered one (see Episiotomy).

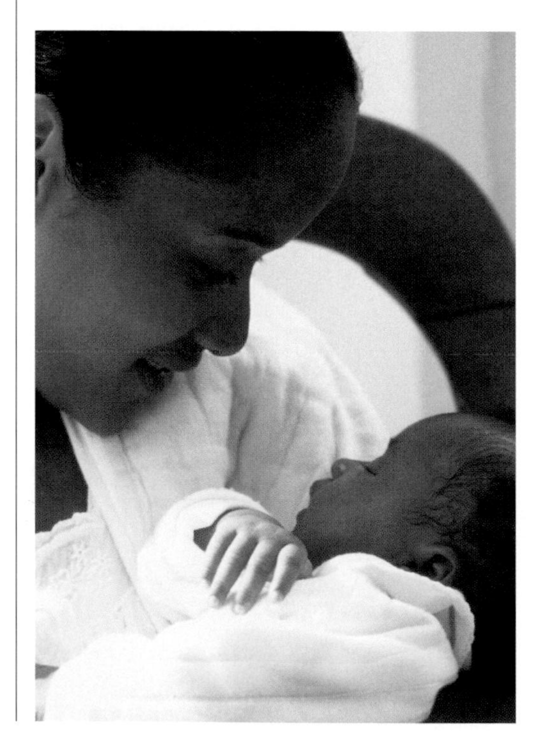

Emotional support

Being alone and in labor in an unfamiliar environment such as a hospital can be a frightening experience for a vulnerable mother-to-be. Most hospitals now recognize that a woman in labor needs emotional support from her partner or from a close friend or relative. It is important that the woman should discuss what is expected with the appropriate friend or loved one during the

◄ If the woman is able to give birth with her family around her, she benefits from their loving support. They can participate in the happiness of welcoming the new baby to the family.

Methods of natural childbirth

PSYCHOPROPHYLAXIS (LAMAZE)

The most widely used and popular method of natural childbirth, Lamaze involves learning to use the mind to control the sensations of the body. The word "psychoprophylaxis" is formed from the prefix "psycho," meaning "mind"; and "prophylaxia," meaning "preventive treatment." It consists of two main techniques, as follows.

Breathing: If a woman in labor synchronizes her breathing with her contractions, she feels more in control of what is happening. In prenatal classes she will learn four different levels of breathing for use during labor, from deep breathing for the weaker contractions to very shallow breathing, when the lips blow rapidly against the index finger, for the strongest contractions.

Relaxation and dissociation: Exercises aim to teach the woman what a tight muscle feels like and how to relax it. This is easy in pregnancy because all the muscles can be relaxed. However, during labor a woman needs to relax all her other muscles while one of the most powerful, the uterus, is becoming very tense (a situation that is not under her voluntary control—any voluntary expulsive force she applies comes from the abdominal wall muscles when she bears down). The exercises need to be practiced regularly until they become second nature. They include learning about the position and breathing that will help to push the baby out with the minimum of difficulty. Meanwhile the woman's partner can learn to use massage on her to ease the pain.

THE PSYCHOSEXUAL METHOD

This is based on the view that birth is something that a woman should be free to experience with her entire personality. Its techniques—much the same as those of psychoprophylaxis but applied in a less mechanical way—emphasize the need for women to recognize and understand their feelings about birth and about their bodies.

THE CROUCHING METHOD

This is, in fact, a birth position. Women in the most primitive societies give birth sitting, squatting, or standing, simply because gravity makes the process quicker and easier. Tearing is less likely if a woman gives birth squatting, but anyone unused to the position should lean against a wall or use some other support, such as a bed or the support of her partner.

LEBOYER METHOD

The gentle childbirth method was developed by a French doctor, Charles Leboyer, whose aim was to reduce the pain and shock of birth for the baby. The delivery room is very quiet and dimly lit, and there may be music playing softly in the background. The child is not held up in the air by the feet. Before the umbilical cord is cut, the baby rests on the mother's stomach for a few minutes and is gently massaged. When the cord is cut, the baby is put first into a basin of warm water to re-create the atmosphere of the womb and then weighed later.

BIRTH IN WATER

More and more hospitals are making this method available in the West, but it was originally pioneered in the former Soviet Union. The baby is born in water warmed to body temperature. There is greater relaxation during the first stage of labor, and because the mother is relieved of the distraction of pain, she can help her child to come into the world more quickly and easily. By re-creating for the baby the conditions of the womb, birth in water softens the shock of entering the world.

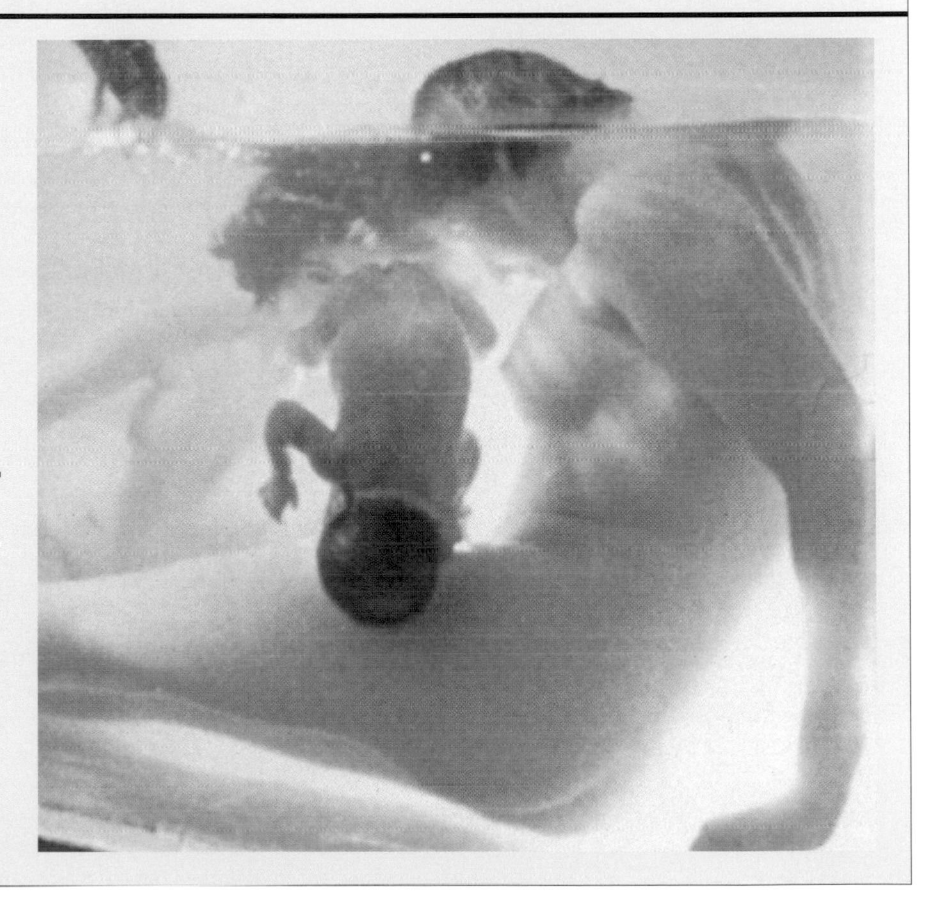

Questions and Answers

I've heard that in some hospitals women in labor are given episiotomies as a matter of course. Is an episiotomy necessary, even in natural childbirth?

It shouldn't be, especially if the woman gives birth in the squatting position. If the baby's head is allowed to appear slowly and gently, the perineum should stretch without tearing. However, some doctors do perform episiotomies as a matter of routine, so you should make your wishes known to your doctor.

When I had my first baby, I wanted to move around a great deal, but the obstetrician kept trying to persuade me to lie down. Why was this?

It is easier for a doctor or a nurse to check what is happening and to monitor the contractions and the baby's heartbeat if the woman in labor is lying on her back.

However, research has shown that other positions can be more helpful to the mother and baby. One study found that the weight of a full-term baby could provide a large part of the force that would expel the child if the mother was upright, since the pull of gravity goes on working, even if the womb's contractions slacken.

For the mother and child, achieving a balance between safety and treating normal labor as an instinctive act is usually most helpful.

Two of my friends and I became pregnant at about the same time, and we would like to practice our natural childbirth exercises together with the help of our partners. Is this a good idea?

Yes, it is. Talk to the person who runs your prenatal classes and make sure that he or she can provide you with the simple aids that you will need: a chart to follow for the breathing exercises; a foam wedge to go behind your knees in relaxation exercises; two pillows or cushions; and a bolster (this can easily be made out of a long oblong of foam rubber).

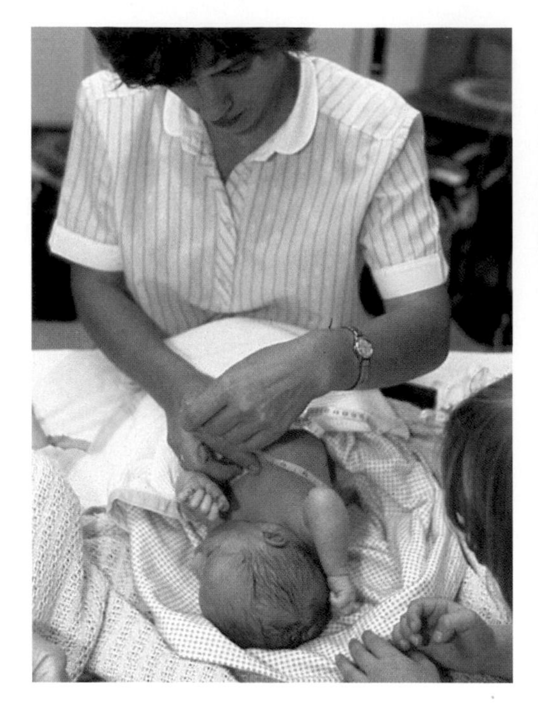

► *One of the advantages of a birth in a home birthing center is that the mother and child have the undivided attention of a particular nurse-midwife. Checking the baby's measurements after he or she is born helps to make sure that all is well.*

period of prenatal care so that when the moment arrives, everyone involved will be relaxed and prepared for the birth itself.

Some doctors recognize that lying flat or even propped up in a hospital bed is often an uncomfortable and unnatural position for a woman in labor; they may also be happy for her to walk around because they recognize that gravity can actually help to speed the birth. Moving around also helps to take the woman's mind off the next contraction until it comes. Most women prefer to be as mobile as possible until the very end of their labor.

Cuddling the baby immediately after the birth is crucial. Research has shown that there is a period for human mothers immediately after the birth of the child when they will accept and love their babies more readily if they are allowed to hold and feed them. If the baby is not given to his or her mother immediately, she may find it more difficult to form that bond later on. Most doctors and nurse-midwives understand this, but women should check their local hospital's policy on this matter.

About pain

Medical science is still trying to help women deal with the pain of childbirth. Drugs can often alleviate this pain, although sometimes at the expense of a degree of sensation and the woman's ability to go through the second stage of labor (bearing down) unassisted (see Local Anesthetics). Some women prefer not to use any drugs and opt instead for natural childbirth. The advocates of natural childbirth do not claim that it is pain-free. What this method does try to provide is a means for a woman to cope with the sensations she experiences without feeling overwhelmed by them. Once she understands how her body is working and is in tune with the pattern and rhythm of the contractions, the pain becomes less frightening and more bearable. Also, if she can relax the rest of her body during the period of time that the uterus is contracting, she removes the additional pain caused by physical stress and tension.

Home births and birthing centers

Planned home birth in the United States is rare, and in some states it is even illegal. Most doctors prefer babies to be born in a hospital. This is because hospital is a safer place for both mother and baby if there are any unexpected complications. However, women who feel that birth is a natural event that should take place in a family atmosphere can find birthing centers (some in hospitals) that are set up to feel more like a home. One of the advantages of having this type of natural birth is that the woman is in a more familiar setting and feels more relaxed. Also, she will not be separated from her partner or children, and she will have the sole attention of a nurse-midwife—who ideally will have been in charge of her prenatal care. The mother-to-be will be much freer to choose the kind of birth she wants. One disadvantage of a home birth is that the nurse-midwife may not have all the painkilling drugs that are available at a hospital. However, the main disadvantage of such a birth, or of one that takes place in a birthing center that is not attached to a hospital, is that if anything were to go wrong, the necessary facilities may not be on hand. The mother would then be dependent on being able to get to a hospital as quickly as possible.

Complications

If a complication does develop during the course of natural childbirth, the way it is dealt with will depend a great deal on the nature of the complication and on where the baby is being born.

BREATHING TECHNIQUES IN NATURAL CHILDBIRTH

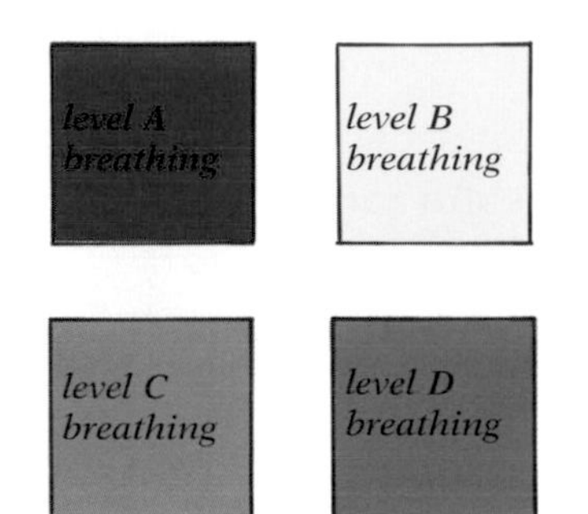

Level A: Breathe in deeply with mouth open. Hold and blow out through mouth.
Level B: Mouth open. Emphasize out breath slightly. Shallower than level A.
Level C: Almost allow air to flow into lungs of its own accord. Say "Out" on out breath. Shallower still than level B.
Level D: Shallow, natural breathing. Choose a song and mime it as you tap the rhythm on your lips with your finger.

Blowing: Sit upright as you breathe in and mouth "One, two, one, two." Blow out and let your whole body sag.
Block and push: Breathe in and hold. Lie on your back, legs apart, and pull your knees toward your chest. Bear down, then breathe out.
Panting: Give a small push and then pant, with the tongue out and the mouth open.

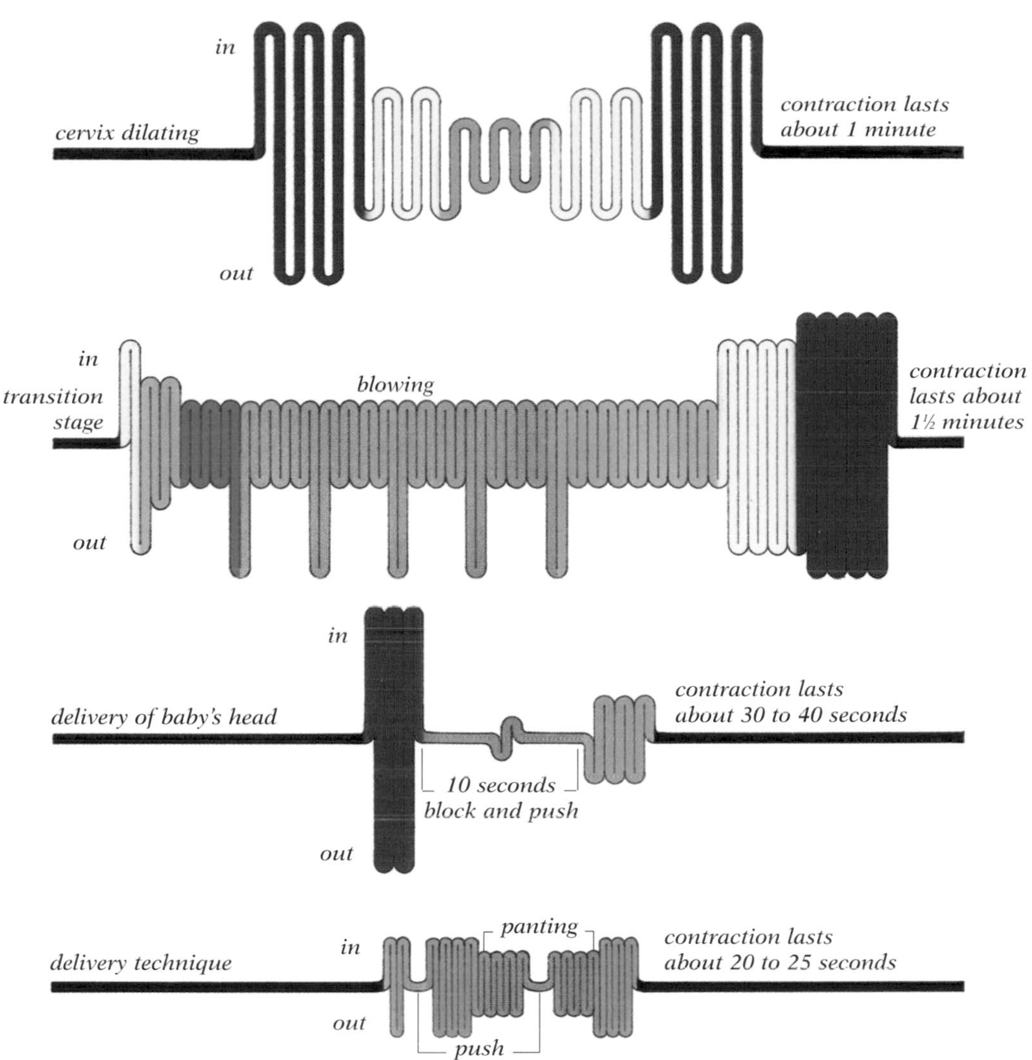

▲ *Illustrated above are some of the breathing techniques a mother-to-be learns in Lamaze classes. These will help her to synchronize her breathing with her contractions, so that she can feel in harmony with what is taking place in her body and will be able, to a great extent, to control it. It is helpful for women to practice the various kinds of breathing with the help of someone reading out the instructions and timing each imaginary contraction. Deep, level A breaths come from the diaphragm. Level B breaths rise from the lower rib cage. Shallower, level C breaths rise from the area of the breastbone. The fourth level, D, is almost in the throat, so that there is practically no effort involved in the actual breathing.*

For example, if the birth is taking place in a hospital, doctors and the necessary equipment will be on hand to deal with any problems that do arise. However, if, for example, the birth is taking place at a home birthing center, emergency medical services should be called, and the nurse-midwife should handle the immediate complication until the local mobile emergency medical unit arrives.

Birth plan

Any woman who wants to have her baby by a natural childbirth method should discuss the matter with her doctor, who will help her decide on an appropriate birth plan, and whether she should have her baby at home, in a birthing center, or in hospital. If a woman decides on a birth plan against her doctor's advice, and if the doctor feels unable to be responsible for her, she should contact her hospital or the American College of Nurse-Midwives, 1522 K Street NW, Suite 1120, Washington, D.C. 20005, who will be able to advise her.

The aim of natural childbirth

The aim of natural childbirth is to provide more options for mothers. It means avoiding unnecessary medical intervention, and using relaxation techniques to cope with the pain.

Women should be made aware of the changes that occur during and after pregnancy and during and after birth. Childbirth classes are now offered to all women and their birthing partners so that they can acquire this knowledge. An informed woman is better able to decide whether to use drugs or breathing and relaxation to alleviate her pain. Giving birth is a unique experience and one that should be as joyful as possible. What affects the mother inevitably affects the baby. If a woman is frightened and tense, the birth can be much slower and more difficult and may negatively affect the baby.

See also Birth; Obstetrics; Pregnancy; Prenatal care

Naturopathy

Questions and Answers

Is naturopathy the same thing as homeopathy?

No. Naturopathy is an overall philosophy of life and a system of health care that relies on the body's inherent ability to heal itself. Various treatments may be used, but they must follow the naturopathic philosophy of helping the body to restore its own balance, rather than simply masking symptoms, as many conventional drug treatments do.

Homeopathy is a particular method of treatment based on the principle that substances which cause symptoms similar to those of a disease can—provided that they are sufficiently diluted—help the body to heal itself. Your naturopathic doctor can explain what this treatment entails in your particular case, or he or she can refer you to a homeopath.

I was told that raw foods, such as fresh fruit and vegetables, are better for you than cooked foods and are recommended as part of a naturopathic diet. Is this true?

The idea behind eating raw foods is that the body absorbs more essential nutrients from food in this form that it would from cooked or processed food, in which some elements may be changed during the prolonged high temperatures used in cooking. In addition, raw and whole foods contain more fiber, which is important for digestion.

However, you needn't live on salads alone. Lightly steamed or stir-fried vegetables also provide a healthy choice. In fact, some nutritionists believe that the body can absorb nutrients from these foods more easily, because the nutrients have been partially released by small doses of heat. In general, the closer food is to its natural state—as fresh as possible with minimal preparation—the more of its original nutritional value is retained.

Naturopathy, or "nature cure," is a holistic system of health care that relies on the body's innate power to resist and conquer illness. Nutrition and modified lifestyle are used to help the body keep its own healthy balance.

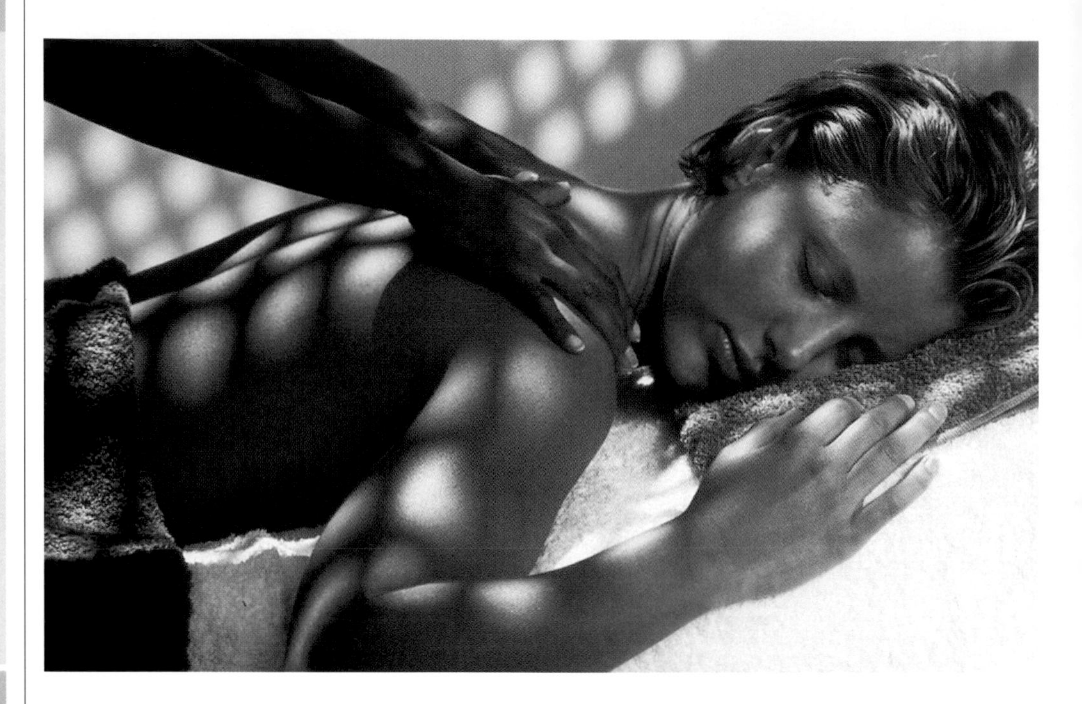

▲ *Naturopathic treatments—such as massage, which releases stress and tension—are designed to restore the body's balance.*

Naturopathy is a system of healing that stresses the importance of health maintenance in the prevention of disease, and a reliance on the human body's ability to restore its own balance and thereby heal itself.

The term "naturopathy" was first coined in the late 19th century, but its roots can be traced back to around 400 B.C.E. when Hippocrates, called the "father of medicine" by historians, began to develop a system of treating patients according to natural laws.

Some of Hippocrates' basic principles, which naturopathic practitioners believe to be the self-evident laws of health, are that the body will heal itself if it is given the chance to do so; that food is medicine and what a person chooses to eat has a major effect on his or her system (that is, "you are what you eat"); and that disease is the body's way of ridding itself of toxins—in other words, disease provides a method of purification so that a healthy balance can be restored. Modern medical scientists, however, reject the toxin theory as inadequate.

Philosophy

There are three basic principles based on Hippocrates' ideas that combine to make up the philosophy of naturopathy as it is practiced today. However, these views are not shared by orthodox medical scientists.

First, the body possesses the power to heal itself through internal knowledge and energy; followers of naturopathy believe in the healing power of nature first over any form of drug or invasive treatments.

Second, disease is an expression of the body's vital energy to remove obstructions to the normal functioning of tissues and organs. An imbalance in the body can stem from many causes—whether chemical, mechanical, or psychological—and the naturopathic doctor strives to discover and remove these causes.

For example, imbalances in the body's chemistry may be caused by an improper diet. They may stem from the retention of waste products due to the inefficient functioning of organs such as the kidneys, intestines, lungs, and respiratory system (see Excretory Systems); or they may be the result of poor functioning of the circulatory system. Examples of mechanical malfunctioning of the body include muscular tension (due to stress or injury), stiff joints, strained ligaments, poor posture, and spinal misalignment. Such factors can impair the proper working of the nervous system and musculoskeletal system. Psychological factors include worries, phobias, anxieties, and pressures at work or home; all of these elements can become major causes of stress-related malfunctioning.

The third basic principle is that naturopathy takes into account the mind, body, and spirit of the individual; that is, it is a holistic approach to health. The body or diseased organ is never treated in isolation by a naturopath, because each person is made up of a combination of his or her mind, body, and spirit. In addition, each person has a unique response to his or her own environment, with individual sensitivities, needs, and inherited tendencies.

Naturopathic techniques

At the first consultation, a naturopathic doctor will talk to a patient and help him or her to understand the basic laws of health as they relate to relaxation, nutrition, exercise, and lifestyle. The naturopath will probably ask many questions about the patient's habits and his or her likes and dislikes, and will try to discover which inherited family tendencies may take effect in the future. The patient will also be encouraged to take more responsibility for his or her own health, because maintaining or improving health and fitness is a major factor in the prevention of disease.

The therapist may also carry out a physical examination. He or she will measure the patient's blood pressure and pulse rate and will also look at the patient's posture and the condition of his or her skin, hair, nails, and tongue. Some naturopaths recommend blood tests, urine analysis, X rays, or mineral analysis of the patient's hair.

Many different natural therapies or techniques may be employed in naturopathy. When treating a patient, the naturopath will consider which will be the most appropriate and effective treatment for any specific condition he or she has.

Nutrition and diet

The naturopathic treatment of all diseases tends to stress the importance of a wholesome and balanced diet. Controlled diets will also be used by therapists in certain cases to treat more specific conditions. For example, a low-salt diet may be appropriate for people who are suffering from high blood pressure, and a low-fat diet can be used to treat obesity.

Fasting

Fasting may be recommended in some cases. Contrary to popular belief, a fast is not a period of starvation. A person can fast on fruit juice, fruit, or plain brown rice. This form of therapy gives the overworked digestive organs a rest, and the energy that would normally be used for digestion can be channeled into the healing process. Some people claim that the temporary lack of food boosts the immune system. Others claim that it works as a basic purification of the body. It may be used in the treatment of high blood pressure, obesity, some allergies, arthritis, and rheumatism.

Botanical medicine

Plants have been used throughout history for their medicinal value. Although the general popularity of herbal remedies has declined in the past 100 years in the West—as a result of the rise of the modern drugs industry—herbal medicines are still used by the majority of people in the developing world. It is also estimated that about 25 percent of all commercial drugs are still manufactured from substances derived from plants (see Herbs and Herbalism).

Certified naturopathic doctors must train as herbalists and must have a thorough knowledge of the traditional uses of plants, as well as the use of plant substances in modern drugs. They may prescribe botanicals to be used in preparations such as teas, tinctures, massage oils and bath oils, and poultices; or some herbs may be added directly to food, such as garlic, which has antibiotic properties, and ginger, which stimulates the circulation and aids digestion.

Naturopathic dietary guidelines
Instead of insisting on a strict diet that may be difficult for a patient to follow, naturopaths usually suggest guidelines. They believe that a person should eat healthfully from the foods that he or she likes, rather than completely cutting out certain foods. In this way the patient can build a diet of healthy foods that he or she not only will enjoy but will continue to eat as part of a nutritious daily diet.
Eat as much food as necessary for yourself as an individual, but do not exceed this amount.
Fats and oils should not make up more than 30 percent of your daily caloric intake.
Protein—whether from plant or animal sources, or both—should make up only about 10 percent of your daily intake.
Unrefined carbohydrates—for example, whole wheat bread and brown rice—should make up 60 percent of your daily intake of food.
Fiber should be increased in your diet whenever it can be increased.
Fresh—preferably organic—fruit and vegetables should be chosen; these should be eaten raw or lightly steamed or stir-fried whenever possible.
Drink plenty of water—preferably spring or filtered water.
Consumption of refined sugar, salt, and caffeine should be reduced to the lowest possible level.
Food should be eaten only when you are hungry; chew all food thoroughly.
Make enough time for eating properly, and above all, enjoy your food.

Questions and Answers

I work as a waitress five nights a week and often feel exhausted. Is there a naturopathic technique that will restore my energy?

Hydrotherapy (water treatment) may be the answer. One of the best ways to restore energy is simply to take a bath, adding a few drops of peppermint oil, which stimulates the system.

My sister lives in the country and has a naturopathic doctor who says that she should eat only organic foods if possible. Why?

Organic foods are grown on farms that are certified as organic— that is, the farmer must prove that pesticides have not been used for at least three years on the fields where crops are grown. Crops grown in this soil are not contaminated by pesticides, which contain poisons that can build up in the body. It is thought that this accumulation can lead to illnesses such as cancer. It therefore makes sense to buy organic vegetables and fruits, even though they are more expensive.

Naturopaths believe that organic produce is important to good health. If you cannot find or afford organic produce, be sure to wash all produce before you eat or cook it.

Is it a good idea for me to take antioxidant vitamins to counteract the effects of air pollution?

Research has shown that the antioxidant vitamins—A, C, and E, plus selenium—can combat the effects of free radicals. These substances, which accumulate in the body as a result of pollution and cigarette smoking, are thought to lead to an increased risk of conditions such as cancer and coronary disease.

Vegetables, nuts, fruits, seeds, and cold-pressed oils are good sources of antioxidants, and if your diet contains plenty of these, you are probably getting enough. If you live in or near a polluted city or industrial plant, you may want to try taking supplements.

Hydrotherapy

Water has been used as a treatment for many centuries, both internally and externally (see Hydrotherapy). It may be used to treat injuries, reduce fevers, and relieve aches and pains; and it can act as both a stimulant and a relaxant. Hot and cold baths, steam baths, compresses, sprays, spa and hot tubs, saunas, and showers are all forms of water treatment. Drinking plenty of filtered water or mineral water is also recommended by naturopaths to cleanse the system of toxins.

Air and sunlight

Spending as much time as possible in the fresh air is good for both the mind and the body. A naturopath may advise a patient to take air baths. This involves walking about for a few minutes without wearing clothes, so that the skin can breathe. Naturopaths also believe in the benefits of ionization, and a therapist may advise a person to take a vacation in a spa resort or a mountainous area with a large number of waterfalls.

Physical medicine

Therapies include various forms of structural manipulation, such as osteopathy, chiropractic, postural reeducation, neuromuscular techniques, and therapeutic exercises. Physical therapy equipment, such as ultrasound and other electromagnetic techniques, may be used.

Acupuncture

An ancient Chinese system of medicine involves the stimulation of certain points on the body to control the flow of chi (vital energy) along its meridians (pathways) to balance the yin and yang (female and male) energies. The acupuncture points are stimulated by inserting tiny needles, moxibustion (the application of heat), laser or electrical means, massage, or a combination of these methods (see Acupuncture).

Lifestyle modification

Because naturopathy is a holistic system of medicine, practitioners are trained to be counselors so that they can help their patients to better understand their lifestyle and patterns of behavior. A naturopath will use active listening skills and will assess body language when diagnosing

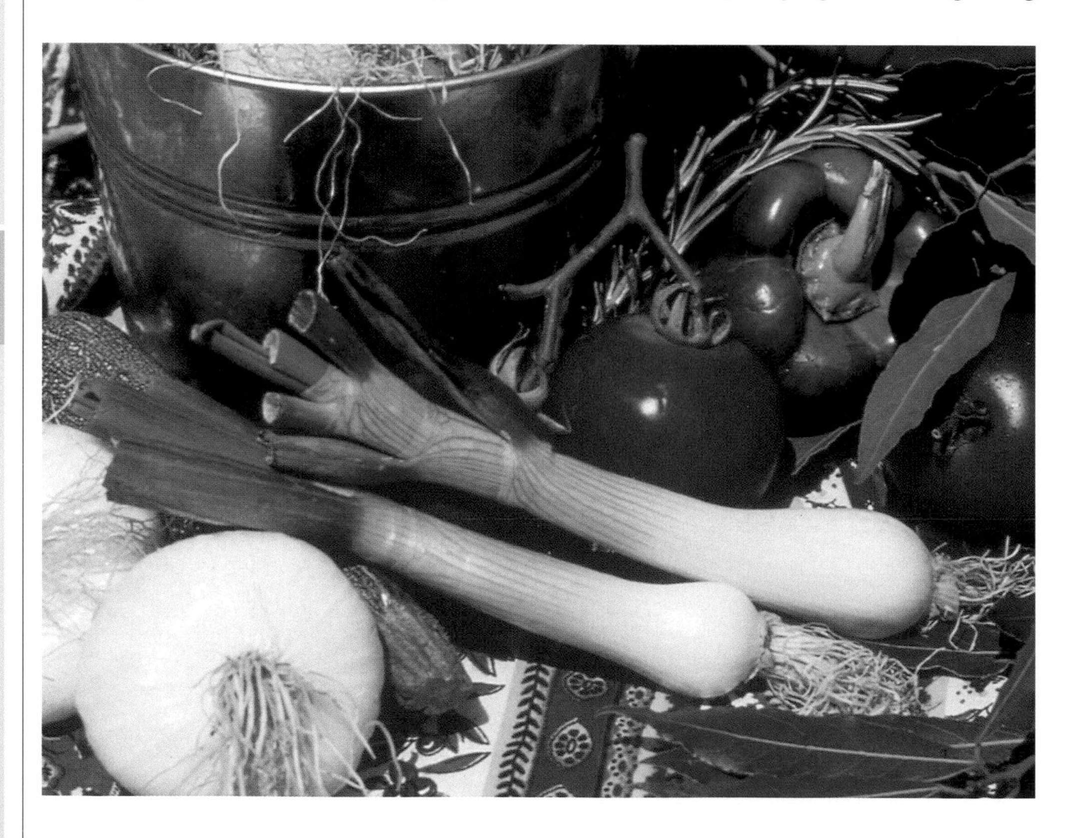

▲ *Naturopaths usually recommend a diet that contains plenty of fresh fruit and vegetables. People are encouraged to eat organic produce when they can.*

Botanical plants used in naturopathic medicine

NAME	LATIN NAME	USES
Garlic	*Allium sativum*	Can lower blood pressure if taken over a period of time; reduces cholesterol; decreases the tendency of blood to clot. Antibiotic; acts on bacteria, fungi, viruses, and parasites. Cautions: high sulfur content—do not use if you have a peptic ulcer or an inflammatory bowel disorder, since garlic can irritate tissues.
Peppermint	*Mentha piperita*	Aids digestion and relieves nausea, colic, and flatulence; can benefit ulcerative colitis. Baths containing a few drops of peppermint oil can relieve rheumatic and muscular pain.
Ginger	*Zingiber officinalis*	Stimulates circulation; improves digestion; reduces flatulence. Helps rid the body of toxins, and cools fevers. Chewing on a small piece reduces travel sickness. Cautions: those prone to migraines should avoid ginger; strong ginger tea may cause headaches. Do not place near eyes, as it will cause irritation.
Lemon balm	*Melissa officinalis*	Taken as a tea, lemon balm is used as a remedy for fevers, sore throats, and coughs. Useful for nervous conditions, tension headaches, indigestion, colic, and flatulence. Crushed leaves soothe cuts, grazes, and insect bites.
Rosemary	*Rosmarinus officinalis*	Traditionally thought to strengthen memory and focus the mind. Good for headaches and mild depression. Stimulates circulation; aids digestion. Oil used for prevention and reduction of hair loss; as a massage oil, relieves joint and muscular pain.
Fennel	*Foeniculum vulgare*	Soothing effect on digestion—improves digestion of fatty foods; eases flatulence and colic. Traditionally said to increase flow of milk in nursing mothers. Can be taken during pregnancy. Use seed or fresh vegetable.
Aloe	*Aloe vera*	Helps to heal all burns, grazes, scratches, sunburn, and bruises. Helps prevent scarring. Break open fresh cactus and apply directly to skin; or use pure aloe vera gel purchased from health food shops (although this is slightly less effective).

▲ *Naturopaths are great believers in the beneficial properties of fresh air, and this can be combined with stimulating exercise.*

patients' conditions. In addition, he or she will be able to recognize psychological problems such as abnormal behavior, addictions, and stress. He or she may use treatment techniques including hypnosis, visualization, and family counseling when appropriate.

Other therapies

Other complementary therapies that follow naturopathic principles may also be recommended to patients. These include herbalism, relaxation techniques, and nutritional biochemistry.

Steps to recovery

Certain phenomena are recognized when a patient undergoes naturopathy and is on the road to recovery. These include a progressive improvement in his or her general health; the return of old symptoms in the reverse order from which they first occurred, especially with symptoms that have been repressed, possibly through the masking effects of conventional drugs; and a movement of the disease from the deeper tissues of the body to those closer to the surface.

The ideal is for the patient to gradually come to the point where he or she no longer needs any therapy and can maintain his or her health with fresh air, wholesome food, positive thinking, and plenty of exercise. However, people who are elderly, or terminally ill or who have congenital weaknesses may need continued treatment.

Outlook

Although in the past conventional medicine has looked upon naturopathy with suspicion and even scorn, many of its principles are now beginning to be embraced by the profession. Stress reduction, lifestyle modification, exercise, and a diet that includes a high fiber content have been recognized as key factors in maintaining good health.

Some advances in conventional medicine are claimed to be naturopathic in philosophy, for example, the use of genetically engineered substances. These substances include human growth hormone to treat growth hormone deficiency; monoclonal antibodies to combat tumor antigens; and antiviral substances and those that enhance the body's natural immune system, such as interferon and interleukin, both of which are used to fight acquired immunodeficiency syndrome (see AIDS).

See also: **Alternative medicine; Chiropractic; Diet; Exercise; Holistic medicine; Massage; Nutrition; Osteopathy; Relaxation; Stress**

Nausea

Questions and Answers

My daughter often vomits in the car, and none of the pills seem to work. What else can we try?

Any motion sickness drugs should be given about an hour before a journey starts. Also, children with motion sickness are less likely to be ill if they are distracted. A good view should get her attention, so sit her high up in the seat looking ahead through the front window. This will minimize the effect of the car's motion. However, do ensure that her seat belt is fastened safely.

My uncle says he feels nauseated all the time and has lost weight. Is this serious?

Yes. He should see his doctor immediately. Constant nausea with other important symptoms such as weight loss or pain is a sign of several serious conditions.

I worry constantly about little things and worry even more that I will vomit. Is this normal?

You are probably suffering from severe tension. Learning how to relax may help. Once you know you will not vomit, you may still be anxious; however, you will be less distressed by these feelings.

If I feel nauseated after a meal should I make myself vomit?

If you feel nauseated after a large meal, either you are overeating or you have a stomach problem. If you get nauseated and vomit after a small meal, see a doctor. Making yourself vomit is not a good idea.

My mother's pills make her feel nauseated. How can she improve her appetite?

She should discuss this with her doctor. There are many drugs that are effective in suppressing nausea.

Feeling nauseated at some time or other is common and usually no cause for alarm. However, anyone who suffers frequent or repeated episodes of nausea without an obvious cause should seek medical advice.

Nausea is an unpleasant feeling of imminent vomiting. It may be associated with sweating, increased salivation, skin pallor, and rhythmical contraction of the muscles of the abdominal wall. Vomiting, which commonly follows nausea, is the involuntary, and often forceful, expulsion of the contents of the stomach. It occurs when the sphincter muscle at the lower end of the esophagus relaxes and the abdominal wall muscles suddenly tighten to compress the stomach.

Nausea is produced by the stimulation of a collection of nerve cells in the brain, called the vomiting center. If the stimulation is severe enough, the nausea is followed by actual vomiting.

In most instances of occasional nausea, little or no treatment is required. However, if nausea persists or is accompanied by other symptoms such as pain or weight loss, it is important for the sufferer to consult a doctor. It is also important to discover the cause of nausea and vomiting if they occur repeatedly. In many cases, such as in pregnancy or motion sickness, the cause is obvious. However, there are other possible reasons for frequent nausea. Most of these causes

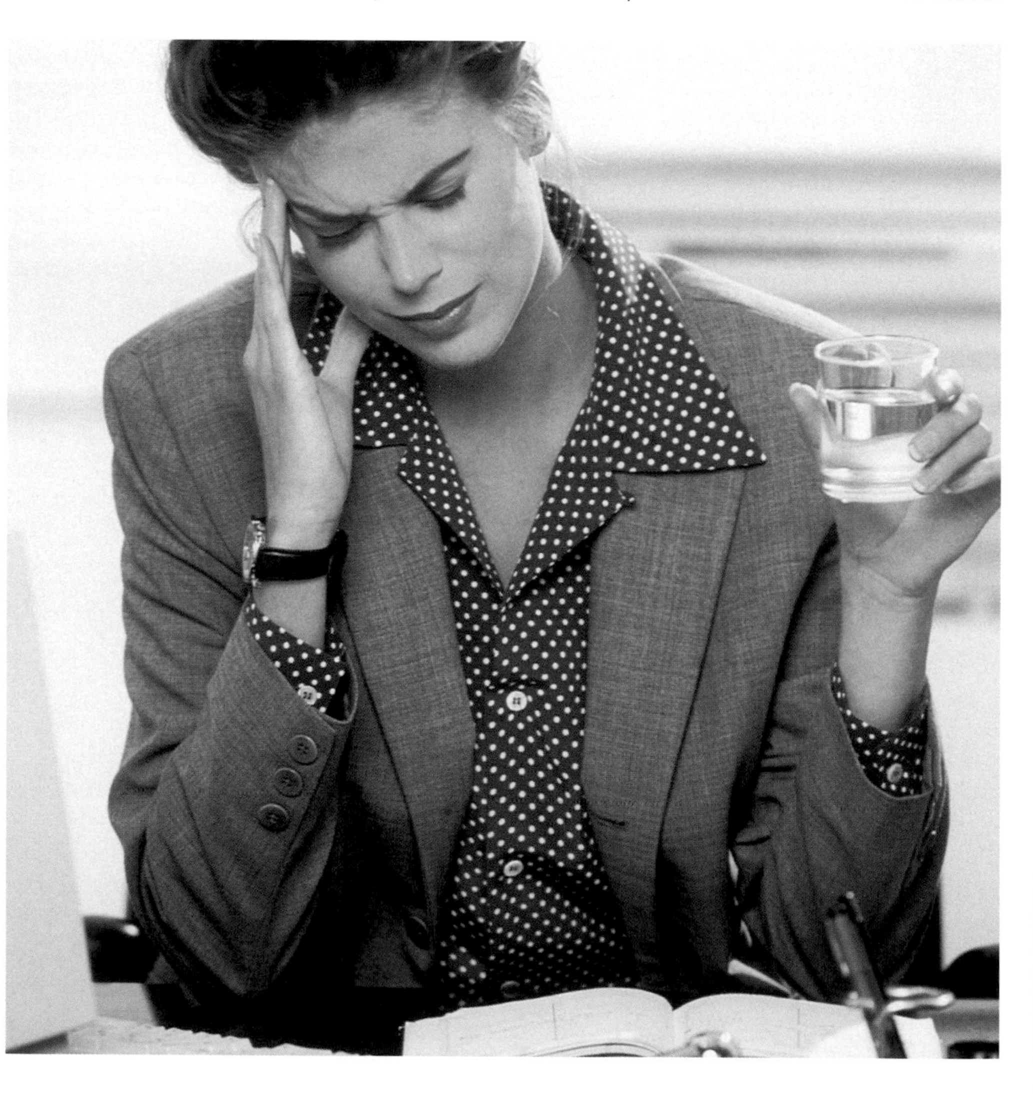

▲ *The stress of working life can manifest itself in uncomfortable feelings of nausea—sometimes followed by actual vomiting. Learning to relax can alleviate these feelings.*

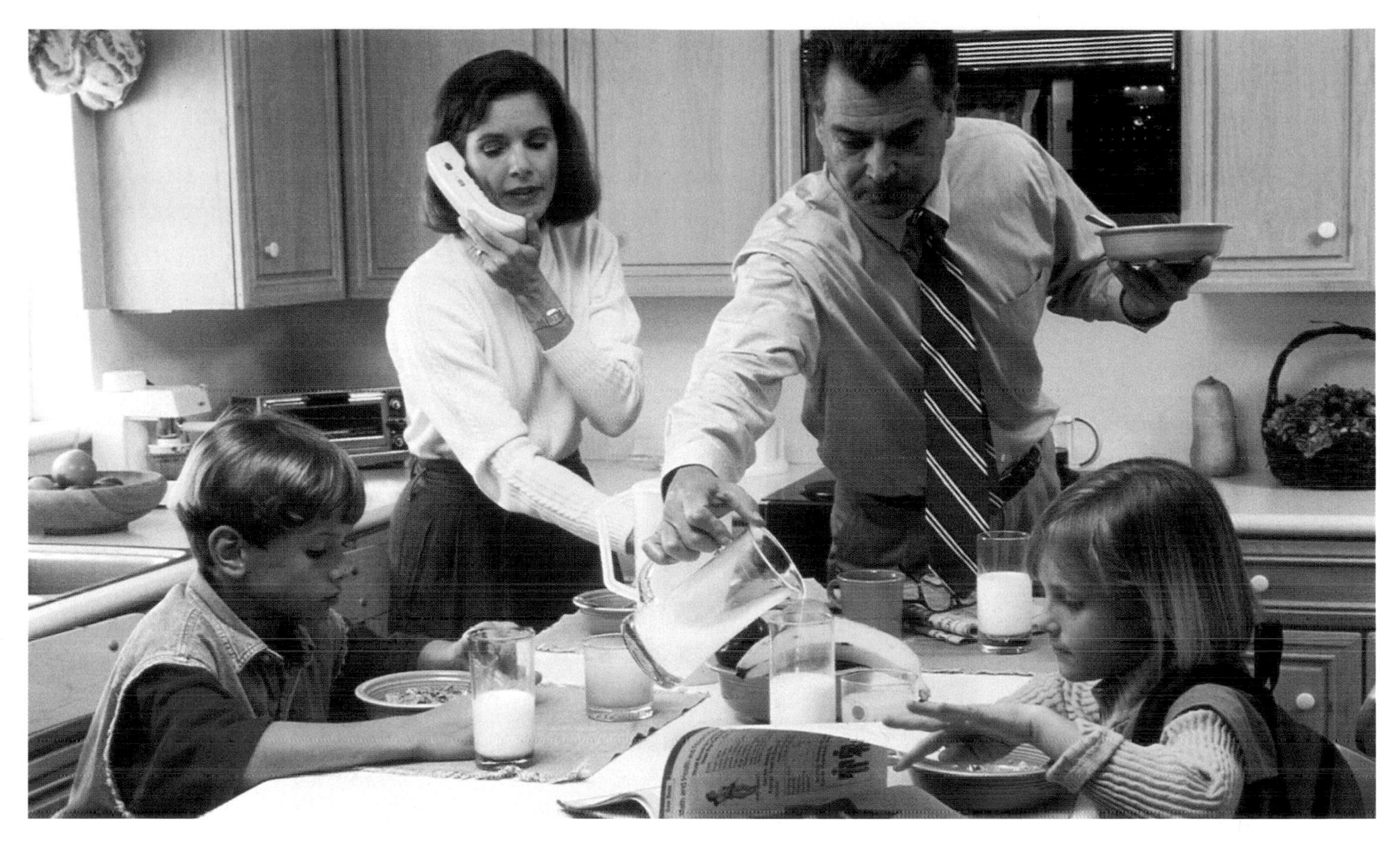

▲ *Indigestion is a common problem caused by overeating or by eating too quickly. Take the time to enjoy your food—mealtimes are one of the most important parts of the day.*

require medical attention, and many are serious. Sometimes nausea is the only immediate indication of a potentially dangerous condition.

Principal causes

A number of conditions that affect the digestive system can produce nausea, one of the most common being indigestion from overeating. Similarly, people feel sick when they have a fever, since any food in the stomach becomes difficult to digest as blood is directed elsewhere in the body. Another common cause of nausea is a virus infection of the gut; this also gives rise to vomiting and diarrhea. During such an attack, the patient appears pale, may sweat profusely, and feels dizzy.

Nausea precedes motion sickness, which occurs when the balance organs are disturbed. It also precedes morning sickness, which is probably prompted by the increased hormonal activity of pregnancy.

In serious stomach conditions, such as gastric ulcer or cancer, nausea is nearly always accompanied by other, more serious symptoms such as black stools or weight loss. Patients with severe liver or kidney failure may feel constantly nauseated, and may lose weight through loss of appetite. In the case of a brain tumor or meningitis, nausea results from a buildup of pressure in the fluid around the brain.

Other causes

Nausea and vomiting need not be of an organic or toxic origin. Self-induced nausea and vomiting may occur in various psychiatric conditions such as anorexia nervosa, bulimia, or hysteria.

Psychogenic vomiting is fairly common and may be either self-induced or the result of situations that are considered threatening, unpleasant, or distasteful. However, psychogenic nausea should not be assumed until the patient's doctor has eliminated all possible organic causes. There are numerous organic causes of nausea, including alcohol abuse, food poisoning, the side effects of taking medication (such as anticancer drugs), intestinal gas, premenstrual syndrome, middle- and inner-ear diseases, appendicitis, and malignancy. Less frequent causes of nausea include septic shock, food allergies, worm infestation, and foreign bodies in the intestine.

Treatment

Ideally, nausea should be treated by removing the cause rather than by giving antiemetics (drugs that prevent or relieve the symptoms of nausea and vomiting). Nausea that accompanies an upset stomach or an illness such as influenza is best treated by plenty of fluids, antacids, and rest. With a child it is best to provide comfort and keep a bowl handy for him or her to use if vomiting.

Except in the most serious cases of morning sickness, drugs are best avoided in pregnancy. Medication can, however, provide relief in travel sickness and for nausea that accompanies cancer or results from radiotherapy. Nausea and vomiting associated with anticancer drugs can often be relieved by cannabis (see Marijuana). There is, however, resistance to the drug's legalization for medical purposes. All treatments for nausea should be given under medical supervision. A doctor should be consulted in cases where nausea recurs or persists, or occurs with other symptoms.

See also: **Cancer; Indigestion; Morning sickness; Motion sickness; Vomiting**

Neck

Questions and Answers

My son's Adam's apple sticks out a long way at the front of his neck. Is this a symptom of some disease?

Almost certainly not. The Adam's apple is a piece of cartilage that supports the vocal cords. It can be any size, in the same way that ears and noses vary in size and shape.

My wife is having her thyroid gland removed. Why is this being done?

If her thyroid is overactive, the body's metabolic rate may increase, causing heart problems, weight loss, and hyperactivity. Sometimes an overactive thyroid responds to drugs; in other cases surgery is necessary to remove part of it and reduce its action.

My friend broke his neck in a car crash. Will he die?

The extent to which the fracture affects the spinal cord is very important. Severe damage can cause paralysis. If the top part of the cord is torn, death will result. Other fractures of the bones in the neck may be no more serious than any other broken bone.

Can a stiff neck be the sign of a serious disorder?

Perhaps. If the stiffness persists for longer than a week and does not respond to warmth, massage, and rest, consult your doctor. The stiffness may indicate a reaction to the infection of the lymph glands, a crack in one of the vertebrae, or osteoarthritis.

My newborn baby does not seem able to lift her head. Is this normal?

Yes. A newborn baby's neck always needs support, but nerve and muscle control develops quickly. She will be able to lift her head by three or four months of age.

The neck not only supports the skull but also contains life-supporting parts of the human body—the vital windpipe, the spinal cord, and important veins and arteries.

The neck connects the chest with the skull. It runs from above the clavicles, or collarbones, upward to the lower jaw at the front and the base of the skull at the back. The neck is built around the seven cervical vertebrae of the spinal cord and has powerful muscles at the back that support and move the head.

At the front of the neck is the cavity that contains the throat, leading downward to the trachea (windpipe) for the intake of air to the lungs. Also in the throat are the esophagus, which takes food down into the stomach; the thyroid gland; four parathyroid glands; the vocal cords; the thyroid cartilage, or Adam's apple; a collection of lymph glands; and the major blood vessels that supply and drain the whole head including the brain—the carotid arteries and the jugular veins. At birth, the neck also contains the thymus, but this gradually shrinks after puberty.

Seven cervical vertebrae are found in all mammals (even giraffes, despite their long necks), and the upper two are the most mobile of those found in the spinal column. The topmost vertebra is called the atlas and joins the skull. It allows the head to nod. The second vertebra is called the axis and allows the head to rotate. The mobility of the head is extremely important.

Humans rely greatly on their hands and feet, coordinated by highly developed binocular vision. It is important, therefore, to be able to move the head without having to make exaggerated movements of the whole body. People who have suffered from a stiff neck know how apparently simple actions such as crossing the road become difficult when they have to change the whole body position quickly.

SKELETON AND MAJOR BLOOD VESSELS OF THE NECK

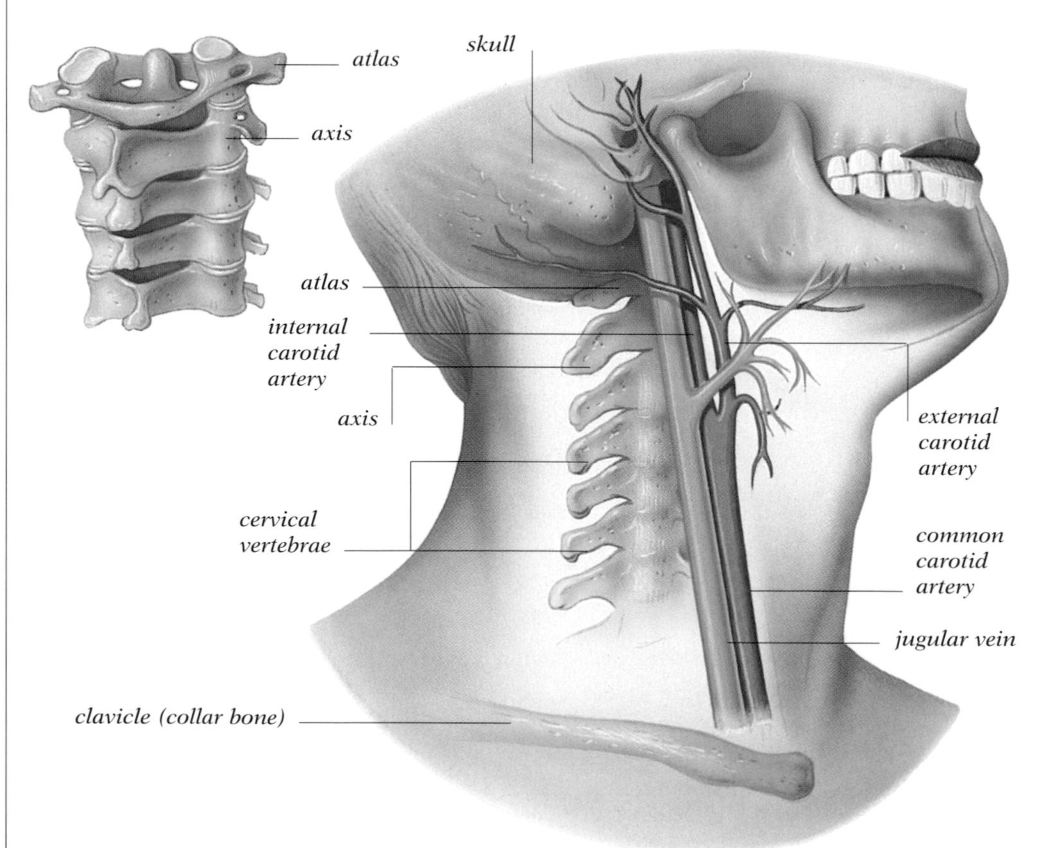

IMPORTANT MUSCLES AND NERVE SUPPLY OF THE NECK

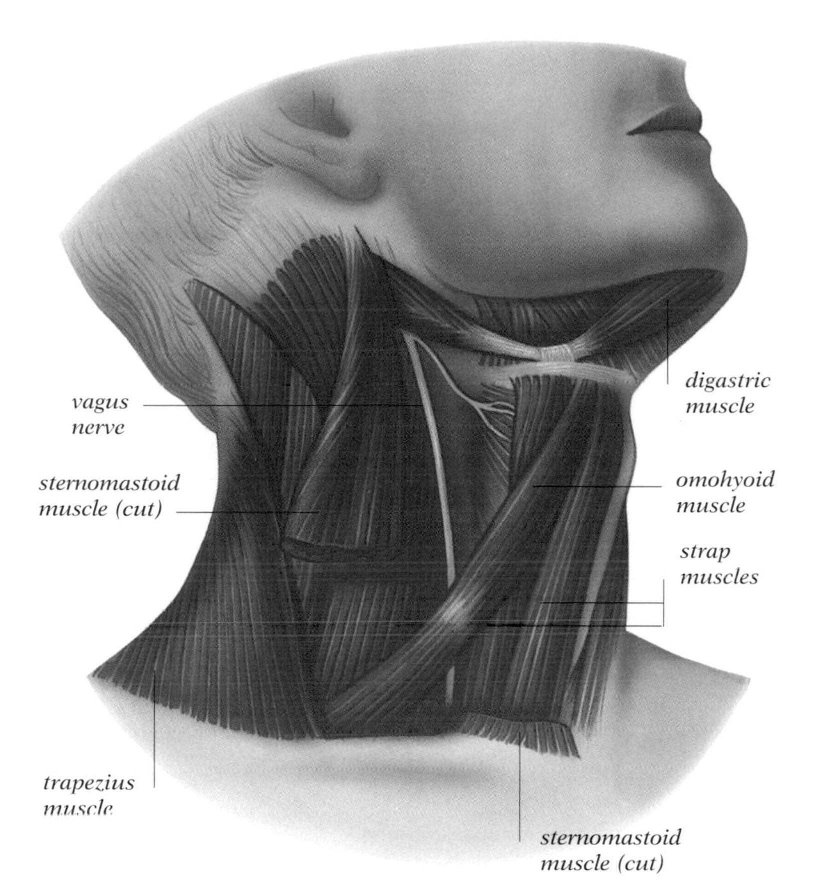

The front of the neck is extremely vulnerable, since it contains so many important organs. The trachea, or windpipe, is at the front of the throat and consists of hoops of cartilage that hold open elastic tissue. It is easy to feel the trachea with the fingers through the skin at the base of the neck. At the upper part of the neck, the windpipe is covered by the thyroid cartilage, or Adam's apple.

Above the trachea lies the larynx, the narrowest part of the windpipe (see Larynx and Laryngitis). If the larynx becomes blocked, air cannot get into the lungs, and an operation called a tracheotomy may need to be performed. This procedure involves inserting a pipe into the trachea to let air into the lungs and suck fluid out of the lungs. After the obstruction has been removed, the opening heals (see Tracheostomy).

Not much can go wrong with the trachea, because it is lined with a mucous membrane that contains cells with tiny hairs called cilia, which waft invading germs and dust back up into the throat to be swallowed. If there is an infection of the tracheal membrane (tracheitis), it is usually part of a general infection of the respiratory tract and often accompanies bronchitis.

The vocal cords

At the top of the trachea is the larynx, or voice box, which contains the vocal cords that allow humans to speak. The box comprises a series of cartilages—the thyroid cartilage at the front; a ring of cartilage that forms the top of the trachea at the bottom; and finally, a pair of movable cartilages, the arytenoids.

The vocal cords are stretched across from the thyroid cartilage to the arytenoids, which can move apart to open or close the cords. The vocal cords are generally kept apart, but when a person swallows food they close, and a flap of tissue, the epiglottis, covers the entrance.

CONTENTS OF THE THROAT

CROSS SECTION OF THE THROAT

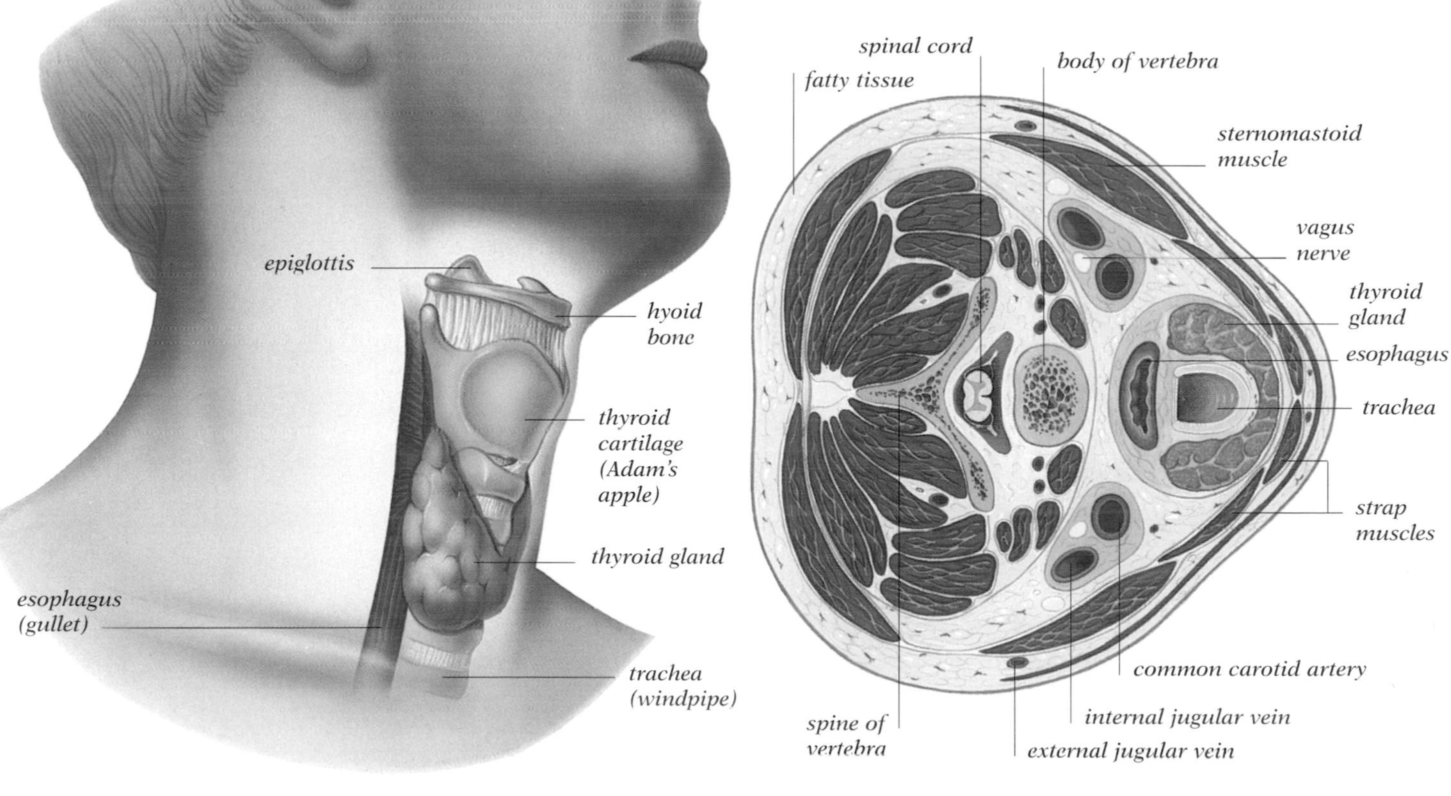

Questions and Answers

Why do people who live in certain geographical areas seem particularly prone to goiter?

A goiter is a swelling of the thyroid gland. This gland needs a supply of iodine from food or water to produce its hormone, thyroxine. If there is a deficiency of iodine, the thyroid swells up. Certain areas of the world, particularly inland mountain regions, lack iodine in the soil and water, so the inhabitants lack iodine too. In such areas one must use iodized table salt. This type of goiter is called endemic goiter and is five times more common among women than men.

I hurt my neck in an accident and was told that this was a whiplash injury. What is that?

A whiplash injury occurs when the head is suddenly jerked, much as a whip is cracked. This may happen when an automobile suddenly collides with something just in front of it. Even if they are wearing seat belts, passengers' heads are still violently jerked. The injuries sustained may range from two or three days' pain from strained muscles and ligaments to much more serious damage involving the vertebrae and the spinal cord.

Can people lose their voices through shock?

Yes. This is possible in two ways. You may be so taken by surprise by something that you cannot collect your thoughts and thus "lose your voice"; or a longer period of muteness may follow a profound emotional disturbance. This is a psychological problem, like the loss of memory that may occur in similar circumstances.

Why do some people have longer necks than others?

Simply because they have inherited a long neck. We all have the same number of vertebrae in our necks—some are just longer than others.

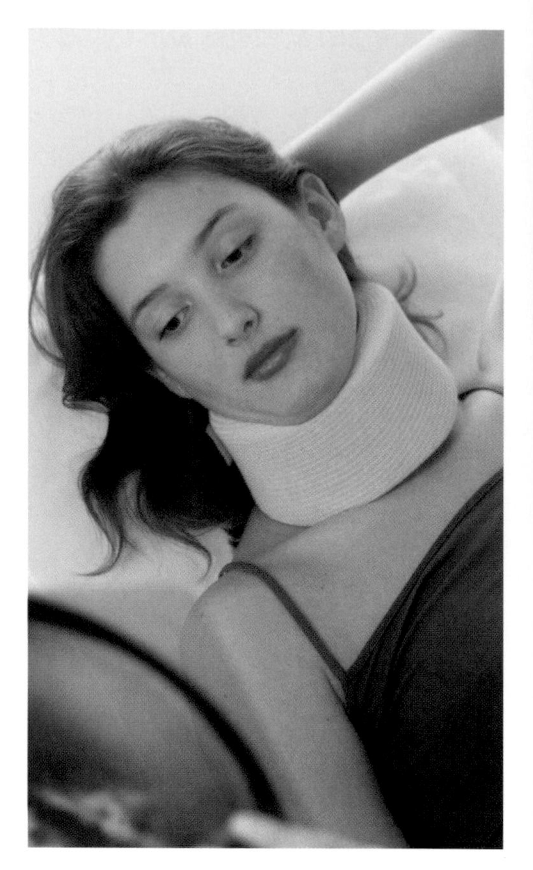

► *An adjustable cervical collar is used in all cervical fractures to ensure that the neck is kept stretched while it is healing.*

For speaking the cords are closed but the epiglottis is open and air is passed over them to create speech. Varying the tension in the cords changes the pitch of the voice; the amount of air pushed up from the lungs determines the amount of sound that is made; and intonation, or the sound of the words, is created by the nose and adjusted by the shape of the mouth.

Swallowing

The esophagus lies behind the trachea and is a muscular tube that conveys food from the throat to the stomach. When it is empty it lies flat, but when food passes through it the muscles force the ball of food downward. Food usually passes through in only about five seconds. When vomiting takes place the muscular contractions that force the food down are reversed and food is brought up instead (see Vomiting).

Glands of the neck

People are born with two glands in the neck—the thyroid gland and a set of four parathyroids.

The thyroid is found just below the level of the larynx and can be seen or felt just like the Adam's apple. It has two lobes and is shaped like a butterfly. The two lobes lie just in front and at either side of the windpipe, or trachea, as it passes down the front of the neck. The two lobes are connected by a small bridge of tissue. In an adult the gland will weigh about 0.66 ounce (19 g).

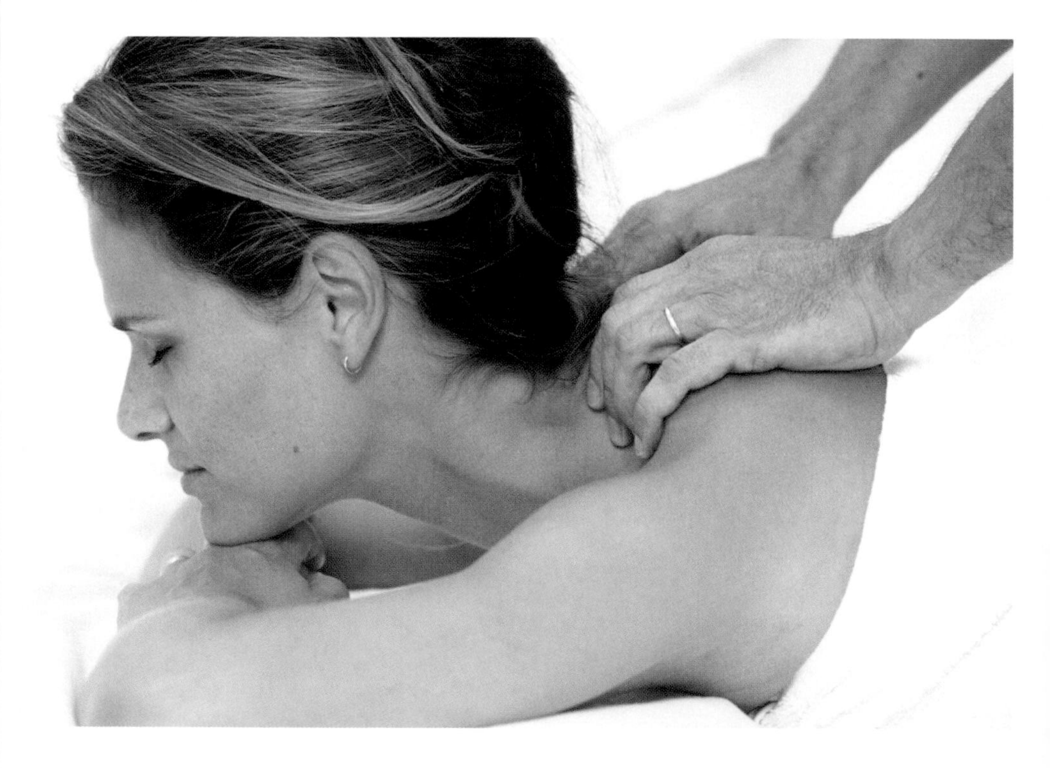

▲ *The muscles in the neck and shoulders can retain a lot of tension and become very stiff and sore. Regular massage can help relax these muscles and release the tension.*

The hormone thyroxine is made and secreted by the thyroid gland. The thyroid requires iodine to function; it is the only organ of the body that requires iodine. Since it is vital for activity, the thyroid is very efficient at trapping all available iodine from the blood. The four parathyroid glands lie behind the thyroid and have one function—the production of a hormone called parathormone, which regulates the concentration of calcium in the blood (see Calcium).

Besides containing particular organs, the neck has important jugular veins and the carotid arteries passing through it that convey blood to and from the brain. The vagus nerve, which is an important part of the parasympathetic nervous system that controls unconscious actions such as breathing, runs close to the internal jugular vein.

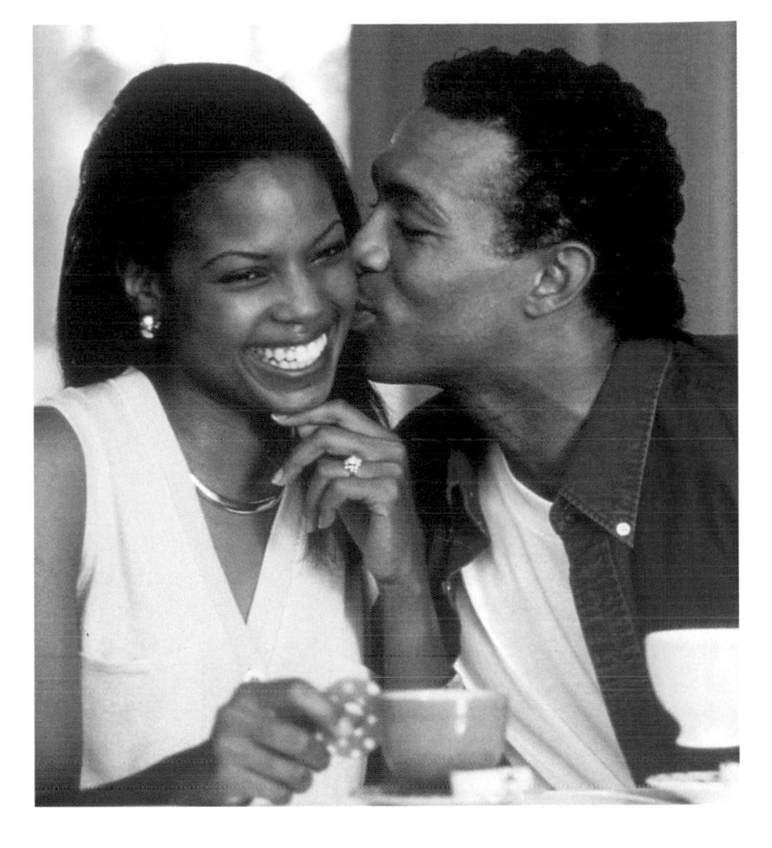

▲ *Men tend to have larger Adam's apples than women. This photograph shows the characteristic shape—but its size can vary considerably between men.*

Neck problems

Stiffness of the neck can occur after sleeping in a cramped position or in a cold draft, or after some unaccustomed exercise, such as playing tennis or digging in the yard or garden. The pain will often disappear on its own: otherwise two days of rest, massage, keeping the neck warm, and taking painkillers such as acetominophen or aspirin should clear up the trouble (see Stiffness).

Other causes of a stiff neck may be the swelling of the lymph nodes that drain the neck, and this probably has its source in an infection of the throat or ears, which should be treated. Pain and difficulty in moving the neck also result from arthritis of the joints between the vertebrae (see Arthritis). This effect can occur with rheumatoid arthritis or, more commonly, with osteoarthritis. The arthritic process may cause pressure on the nerves leaving the spinal cord and produce numbness or paralysis in the hands, which are controlled by these nerves.

The voice can be lost by damaging the vocal cords. This can happen after a long bout of shouting—for example, at a football game—or after a long singing session. Trauma of this kind can cause a small swelling or polyp. Professional singers sometimes suffer from polyps, but these can usually be easily removed without any permanent damage (see Polyps).

Cancer can affect the larynx and cause hoarseness. Eventually an operation is needed to remove cancerous cells. Sometimes the whole larynx must be removed, but it is possible to learn to speak by using a different method. One way is by swallowing air and releasing it in small bursts to create enough sound to be heard. Almost all cases of cancer of the larynx are caused by smoking.

Laryngitis is an inflammation of the throat that is caused either by a virus or by the inhalation of harmful chemicals. Sometimes inflammation may be a symptom of tuberculosis.

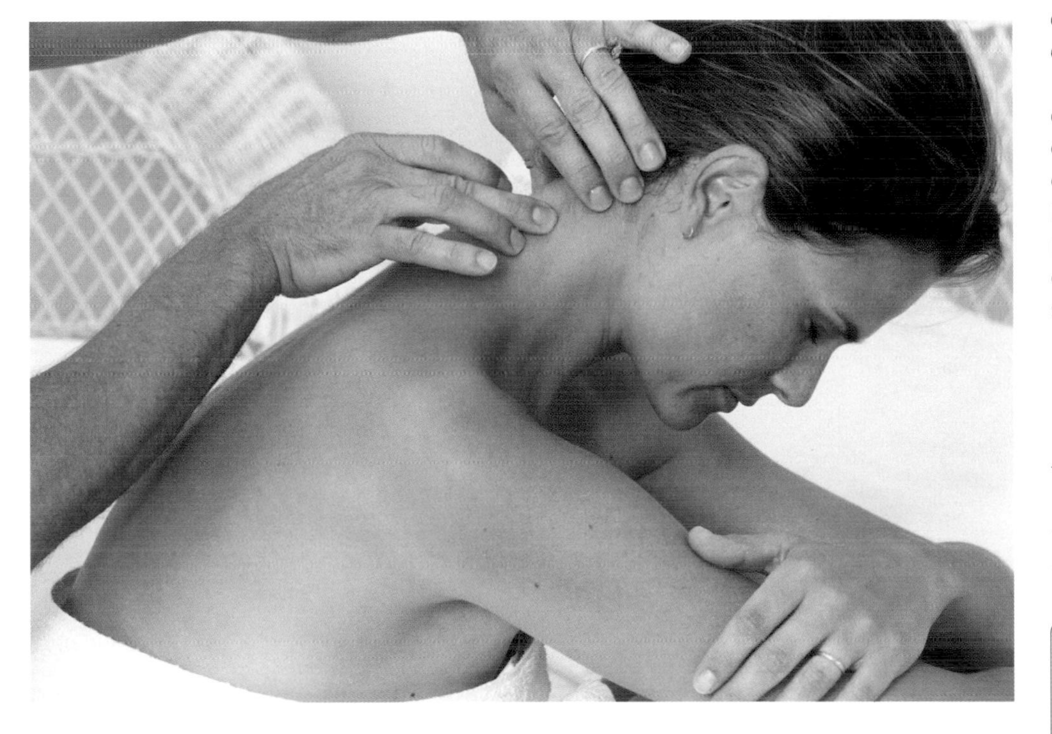

▲ *The neck consists of seven cervical vertebrae. Damage to any of these vertebrae, as through a whiplash injury, can cause neck pain that will require treatment.*

See also: **Goiter; Lymphatic system; Osteoarthritis; Parathyroid glands; Spinal cord; Throat; Thymus; Thyroid; Vocal cords; Whiplash injury**

Neonatal intensive care unit

Over the previous century, great strides have been made in the field of neonatal care. The creation of neonatal intensive care units with incubators and other equipment for babies born prematurely or with diseases or difficulties that need immediate treatment has helped decrease mortality rates among newborns.

Of the four million babies born annually in the United States, about 10 percent require care in a specialist neonatal intensive care unit (NICU). Dedicated to the care of sick newborns, babies stay an average of 15 days in the units. Some babies are treated for minor illnesses and others for life-threatening diseases or defects. There are 3,700 board-certified neonatologists in the United States, who practice at more than 1,500 NICUs throughout the country. The increase in NICUs over the last 20 years has had a dramatic impact on the infant mortality rate: in 2002, 90 percent of babies born weighing between 2 pounds 7 ounces and 3 pounds 3 ounces (1.25–1.5 kg) were expected to survive. Of babies born weighing between 1 pound 7 ounces and 2 pounds 2 ounces (0.75–1 kg), 80 percent survived, mostly without handicaps.

Why are babies admitted to the NICU?

Although most pregnancies are uneventful, some infants are born into a medical emergency. This may be because the baby was delivered early owing to a problem during the pregnancy, or because of problems during the birth. Some babies stay for months in the NICUs, and others may

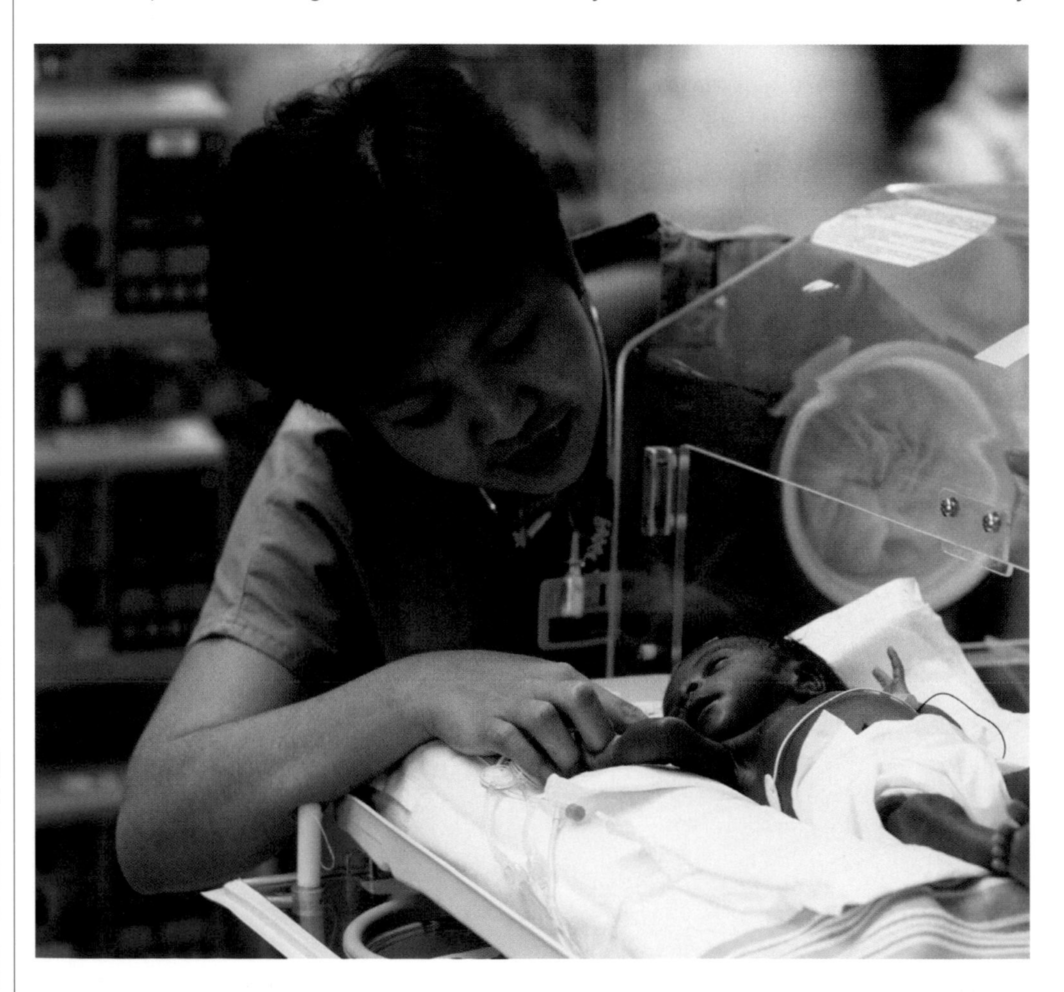

▲ *A nurse tends to a premature baby in a neonatal intensive care unit. Studies show that babies are more likely to survive in NICUs where the nurse-to-baby ratio is highest.*

Questions and Answers

Can neonatal care sometimes create problems?

The impact of neonatal intensive care on long-term outcomes for low-birth-weight infants is complex. A study published in 1997 by the Office of Technology stated that the large decline in mortality among very low-weight infants over the previous century had been accompanied by a rise in seriously handicapped, as well as normal, survivors. The decline of mortality has been accompanied by a moderate increase in the prevalence of cerebral palsy, which can cause both mental and physical problems and other adverse health effects in such infants. Some people argue that the medical costs of this increase, and the strain it places on families, should be considered in any evaluation of neonatal intensive care.

When is a baby considered to be "viable"?

There is much debate about when very young infants are considered viable. Some studies have shown that babies who have reached a gestational limit of 24 weeks do much better than babies with a lower gestational limit, and that very few babies under 22 weeks survive without brain injury. In the United States, health professionals and babies' families discuss treatment for babies with a gestational limit of 22 to 24 weeks. Questions about gestational limits are likely to become more prevalent as health resources become more scarce.

What are the main problems that lead to mortality in neonatal intensive care units (NICUs)?

The three main reasons for infant deaths in NICUs are prematurity, birth defects, and intrauterine growth restriction (IUGR) of the fetus in mothers.

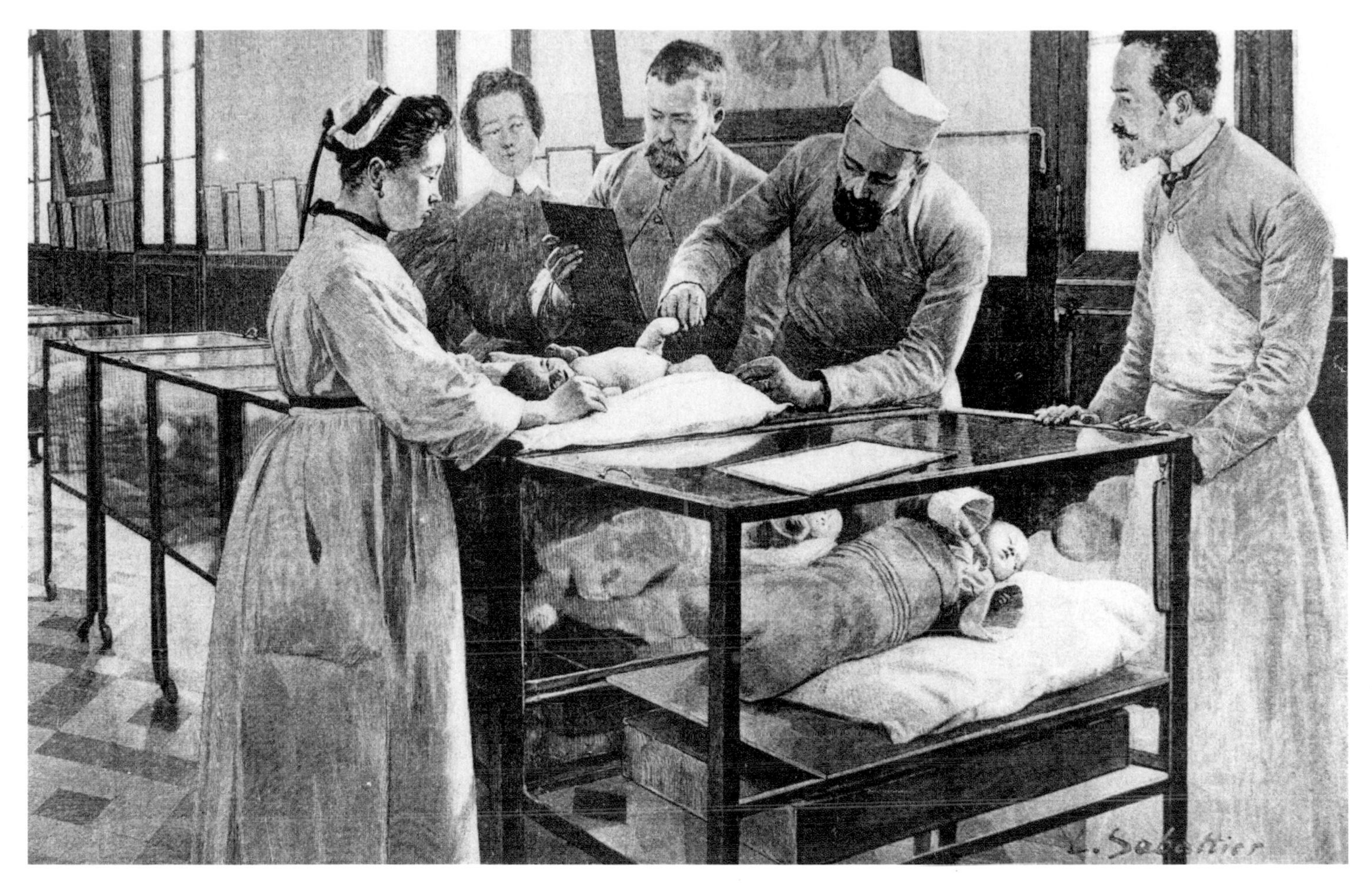

▲ *This illustration of a maternity hospital ward in Paris, France, in 1885 shows some of the first incubators—originally referred to as "hatching cradles"—that were invented to treat "weakly born" babies.*

be discharged after only a few days. The most common problems seen in the NICU are due to prematurity and breathing or heart conditions, but many other problems such as infection, malformations, or surgical issues may also be involved.

The most common functions of the NICU are assisting the babies with breathing, supporting their circulatory systems or regulating their temperature, and helping them to feed. Most babies improve over time.

Who works in the NICU?

The NICU staff is a multidisciplinary team of specialists, usually headed by the primary attending physician—a specialist who directs the team caring for the baby. A consulting physician may also offer advice if the baby has a particular disease that would benefit from specialized knowledge and expertise. The nursing staff includes neonatal nurse practitioners, who have advanced training to deal with newborn babies; and bedside nurses, who provide round-the-clock care for sick infants. Lactation specialists are nurses with special training to assist breast-feeding mothers to nurse their babies (see Breast-Feeding). Social workers are often on hand to help families. The staff may also include developmental specialists, who help the family to adjust to having a sick baby and monitor the baby's development, and a neonatologist—a pediatrician with special training in the care of sick infants. Many NICUs now also have a perinatologist, who monitors the development of the fetus during the last trimester of pregnancy.

Equipment in the neonatal intensive care unit

Modern NICUs are equipped with high-tech equipment to give babies the best chance of survival and recovery. These often include high-frequency ventilators that can "breathe" for babies at 900 breaths per minute so as not to damage their fragile lungs; blood-gas analyzers, which continuously monitor the level of oxygen, carbon dioxide, and blood acid; and a heart-lung bypass system that allows babies' hearts and lungs to recover after surgery or serious illness. The units also have neonatal incubators designed to improve the physical and neurological development of premature infants: babies born prematurely at 28 weeks or before have a less developed cerebral cortex and therefore poor sensory development, which may lead to problems in later life. Keeping noise and light to a minimum, the special incubators mimic life in the womb and help the infants to develop as they would naturally. Babies are rotated by a special item of equipment called a "baby Susan" so that their sleep is not disturbed. Equipment that can regulate the temperature and humidity to protect a baby's skin can be built into the incubators.

History

The first specialist NICU was opened in 1960, but doctors were developing methods to care for newborns more than a century ago. The first incubators for infants were modeled on incubators for chicks and were developed in France at the end of the 19th century.

Questions and Answers

Does neonatal care differ depending on the size of the baby?

Yes. Doctors now know that infants have different needs depending on their weights. What is appropriate for an infant weighing 3 lbs. 5 oz. (1.5 kg) may not be right for a infant weighing less than 2 lbs. 3 oz. (1 kg). For example, infants of various gestational ages show different fluid loss through the skin, and while fluid restriction in a larger infant is appropriate during the first 12 to 48 hours, this would lead to severe dehydration in an infant at 26 weeks of gestation. Also, techniques to ventilate a larger baby with, say, pulmonary hypertension (when the pressure in the lung blood vessels is abnormally high) would have adverse effects on a 28-week-old baby with immature lungs.

Do doctors have any way to predict a baby's chance of survival in a neonatal intensive care unit?

Yes. A scoring system called the Clinical Risk Index for Babies (CRIB) was developed by the International Neonatal Network to predict the mortality risk for infants weighing 3 lbs. 5 oz. (1.5 kg) or less. The score is based on birth weight, gestational age, maximum and minimum fraction of inspired oxygen, and the presence of congenital malformations. It is taken from information compiled within 12 hours of the baby's admission to the unit. Doctors estimate the baby's chances of survival based on its CRIB score, which is far more accurate than judging by the birth weight alone.

Do babies in NICUs feel pain? If so, are they given medication for it?

Yes. Scientists used to believe that the nervous system of newborns was too immature to sense pain, but new research has disproved the theory. Pain in infants can be measured by observing changes in facial expression, crying, heart rate, blood pressure, and hormones. NICU babies in pain may be given anesthetics, sedatives, or various other types of painkillers.

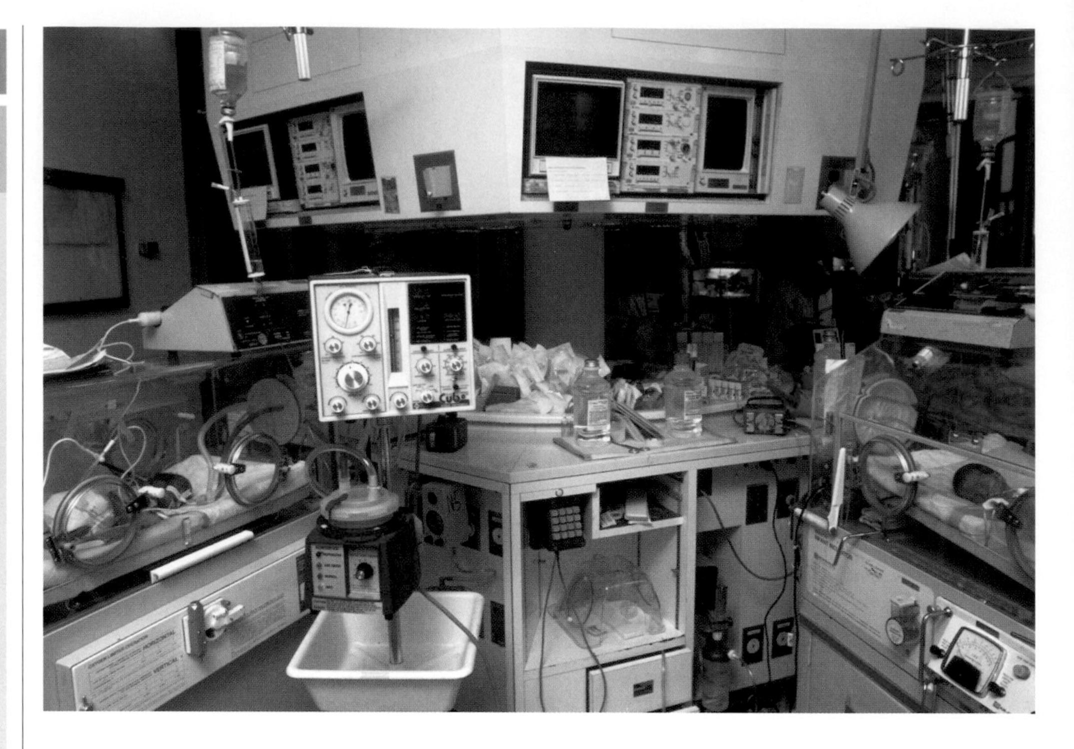

▲ *Equipment found in NICUs today include a ventilator (bottom left), intravenous fluid dispensers (top left and right), monitors (top center), and incubators (far left and right).*

An incubator station for newborns was developed in 1899 at the Chicago lying-in station, and ideas about the care of newborns began to take hold in the first half of the 20th century. The first specialist intensive care unit for babies was opened in October 1960 at Yale New Haven Hospital. At that time equipment and methods of assessing unborn babies were limited: weight was assessed by palpation (lifting the baby), and X rays determined size or maturity. Prior to 1960, laws in the United States prohibited mixing healthy and sick babies, premature and term babies, and babies needing medical or surgical treatment. This prohibition was due to fears about the spread of *Staphylococcus aureus* infection, which was common at the time. The opening of the first NICU followed studies by scientists at Stanford University, which developed ways to stop the spread of such infections. The first NICUs were equipped with incubators augmented with infrared heat. Babies were helped to breathe by adult ventilators, and EKG machines were used as heart monitors. Eventually, large numbers of infants were put together in the same room, and each infant's station was set up separately with supplies.

Outlook

Several studies have indicated the significance of NICUs in reducing the infant mortality rate in the United States. As technology and education have increased, so has the likelihood of survival for most premature babies. Doctors working in the field of neonatal medicine point to the need to improve survival and recovery rates for infants born weighing less than 1 pound 7 ounces (0.75 kg), of whom only 50 percent survive. They stress the importance of reducing the incidence of premature births with better monitoring during pregnancy. Although the number of neonatal units throughout the United States has risen in the last 20 years, these are distributed unevenly. In a study in 1995, researchers at Dartmouth College in New Hampshire reviewed birth and death records to correlate infant mortality with the number of NICUs. They found that areas with a low supply of neonatologists—2.7 per 10,000 births—had a 7 percent higher mortality rate than areas that had 4.3 neonatologists per 10,000 births, also considered a low supply. However, once the number of neonatologists rose to 5.9 there was no further benefit. According to the report, the distribution of NICUs needs to be investigated further to determine whether more resources would lead to better newborn outcomes.

See also: **Birth defects; Fetus; Hospitals; Incubation; Intensive care unit; Pregnancy; Premature babies**

Nephrectomy

Questions and Answers

I have been told that I will have a a drainage tube and a catheter after surgery to have my kidney removed. What does this mean?

All surgery requires a tube to drain pus and excess fluids. Some surgeons insert a tube into the bladder (a catheter) as well so that they can measure the amount of urine being excreted from the remaining kidney for the first day or two after surgery.

Is a kidney removed only if the other one can function normally?

Not always. In certain cases a kidney may be removed when the other kidney is not normal. If this happens, then the patient may experience chronic renal failure, or long-term failure of the kidneys.

If both kidneys are removed or fail completely, the patient must be treated with dialysis or have a kidney transplant.

After a nephrectomy, are there any fluids or foods that I must avoid?

If your other kidney is normal, you will have no dietary restrictions. However, the disease that was affecting the kidney that was removed may be affecting the remaining one, and you may have to decrease the amount of salt and protein in your diet.

Will the operation to remove one of my kidneys leave a scar?

There will be a noticeable scar at first, but it should fade to a white line after a year or so.

Is it true that after I have my kidney removed, I will be more prone to high blood pressure?

If the remaining kidney is normal, there is no increased risk of developing high blood pressure.

In most cases the removal of a kidney—a nephrectomy—is not dangerous and has no ill effects on a person. However, the operation is carried out only when all other treatments have failed or are not possible.

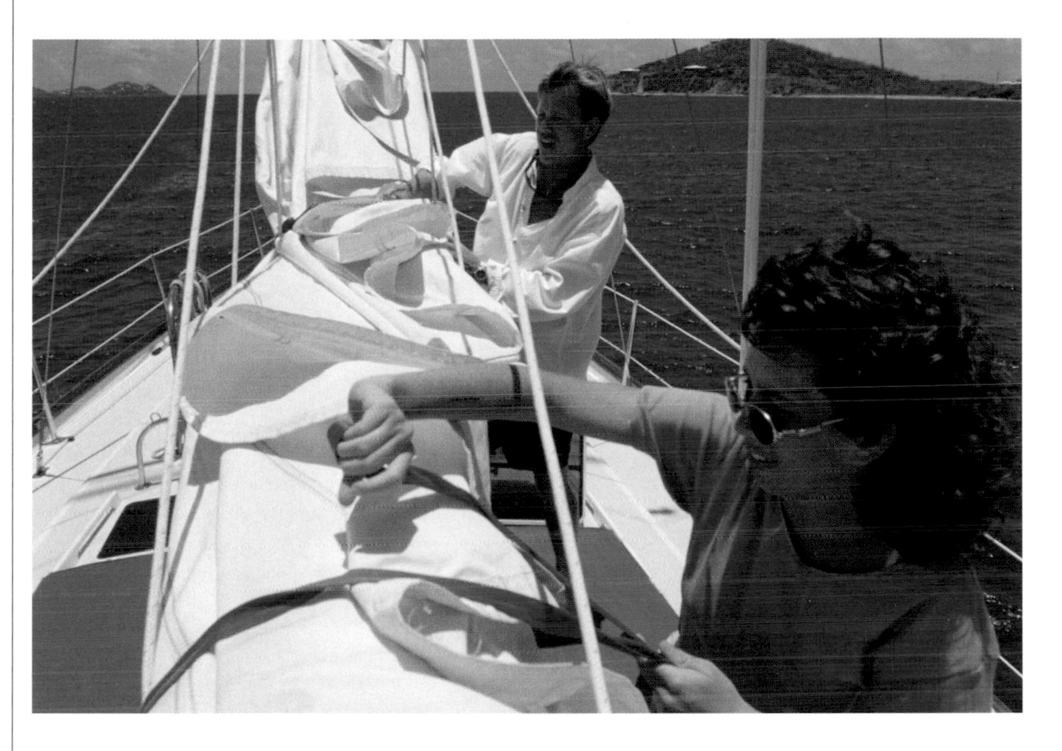

▲ *Most people are able to lead a normal, active life after having had a kidney removed.*

Functional redundancy is a feature of all human body systems. Therefore, if a person has to have one kidney removed, the other kidney (provided it is healthy) will take over the work of the first.

There are various reasons for a nephrectomy. Some people are born with a congenital abnormality of the kidney—one that has not formed properly and does not function. If a kidney is severely damaged—for example, in an automobile accident—it may have to be removed to prevent the patient from losing too much blood. The presence of a tumor in a kidney may also necessitate a nephrectomy to prevent the tumor from spreading to other parts of the body.

When a kidney is blocked by a kidney stone or other matter, the whole organ may become infected and may have to be removed. On the rare occasion that a stone blocks a renal artery, it lowers the blood pressure to the kidney. The kidneys respond by releasing the hormone renin; this raises the blood pressure in the entire body and requires immediate treatment.

The operation

Nephrectomy is performed with the patient lying on his or her side, with the kidney to be removed uppermost. The operating table is bent upward in the middle so the space between the ribs and the pelvis is opened up. The surgeon makes an oblique cut, which passes over the lower ribs in the back toward the front of the abdomen. The kidney is then cut free until it is attached only by its artery, vein, and ureter; each is tied carefully. A tube may be inserted so that any blood that collects inside the wound can be drained, and the wound is closed with suture stitches.

There may be pain from the incision and on movement for a few days, but drugs can help. Most patients notice a patch of numbness on the skin below the incision, but this may eventually disappear completely. The patient can usually walk around the next day.

See also: Kidneys and kidney diseases

Nervous breakdown

Questions and Answers

I know two people who have had nervous breakdowns. One is well, but the other is in a psychiatric facility. How do you explain this?

"Nervous breakdown" is not a medical term. It is a colloquial expression used by nonmedical people to refer to a psychological disturbance—however mild or serious that disturbance may be.

I have heard my doctor use the term "nervous breakdown." Does it have some medical meaning?

Doctors, especially older doctors, often use euphemisms such as this, perhaps to avoid worrying their patients or to avoid disclosing a more precise, upsetting diagnosis.

Can the nervous system recover after a nervous breakdown?

The term "nervous breakdown" is misleading. Whatever form of psychological disturbance it refers to, there is no actual structural change in the nervous system.

What actually happens in a nervous breakdown?

Psychiatric disorders are related to changes in the nervous system, but these are subtle changes in function, often mediated by alterations in chemical substances called neurotransmitters. Many of the drugs used to treat psychiatric disorders affect the functioning of these neurotransmitters.

Is a nervous breakdown a result of chemical changes?

It might be, but psychological disorders also spring from genetic factors and from environmental pressures or deficiencies. Early childhood experiences are obviously important in analyzing any psychological problem.

This vague term is no longer used by the medical profession. It was introduced many years ago to describe any one of a wide range of emotional and psychiatric disturbances but is now used only in nonmedical circles.

Some doctors still find the term "nervous breakdown" convenient when talking colloquially to patients; however, in a strictly medical context it has no precise meaning. Its origin dated back to the time when little was known about the nature and cause of psychiatric disturbance or about the physiology of the nervous system. As a result, any psychological upset was assumed to be some kind of breakdown in the nerves—possibly some kind of a structural change. Such changes do occur in specific nerve diseases, but these do not generally give rise to psychiatric disturbance.

When the phrase "nervous breakdown" is used, however, it may be applied with equal validity to any kind of emotional or psychiatric disorder, or any disturbance ranging from a minor, and very brief, hysterical attack to the most profound and serious form of psychotic illness. Therefore, the duration of a nervous breakdown may range from a few minutes to a large part of a lifetime. The designation is most likely to be applied to a patient when the onset of a condition occurs acutely and is associated with a sudden inability to perform the normal functions of living.

The following is a review of the conditions that may be associated with a nervous breakdown.

Neurosis and psychosis

The term "neurosis" is less popular among psychiatrists than it used to be, mainly because the word has acquired a disparaging quality. Because of this, and because it is now universally recognized that most neurotic disorders involve anxiety, the tendency is to avoid it and to use more specific terms that indicate the form of anxiety involved (see Anxiety). Hence psychiatrists are more likely to refer to panic disorder, hypochondriacal anxiety, obsessive-compulsive anxiety, phobic anxiety, and so on.

Psychiatrists always make a clear distinction between the whole class of neurotic disorders and the various psychotic conditions. Neurotic disorders, however severe they may be, do not involve any loss of contact with reality. Nor do they feature severe thought disturbance, irrational beliefs (delusions), disturbance of sensory perception (hallucinations), or grossly abnormal behavior. These elements are the characteristics of the psychoses—the much more severe class of psychiatric disorder that includes bipolar (manic-depressive) psychotic, schizophrenic, and paranoid states.

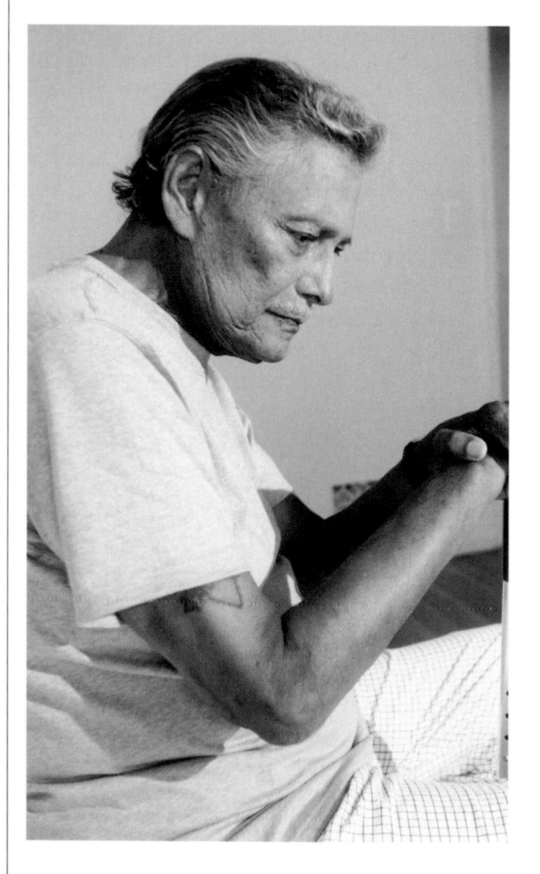

▲ *What many people consider to be a nervous breakdown is usually the onset of a neurotic or psychotic disorder.*

Hysteria

A term that has also fallen into disfavor in medical circles because of its defamatory quality, "hysteria" tends to be replaced by the term "conversion disorder." "Hysteria" is, however, still used, especially in a nonmedical context, to refer to dramatic, histrionic behavior that appears to be designed to attract attention and perhaps elicit sympathy, or to achieve some other desired purpose.

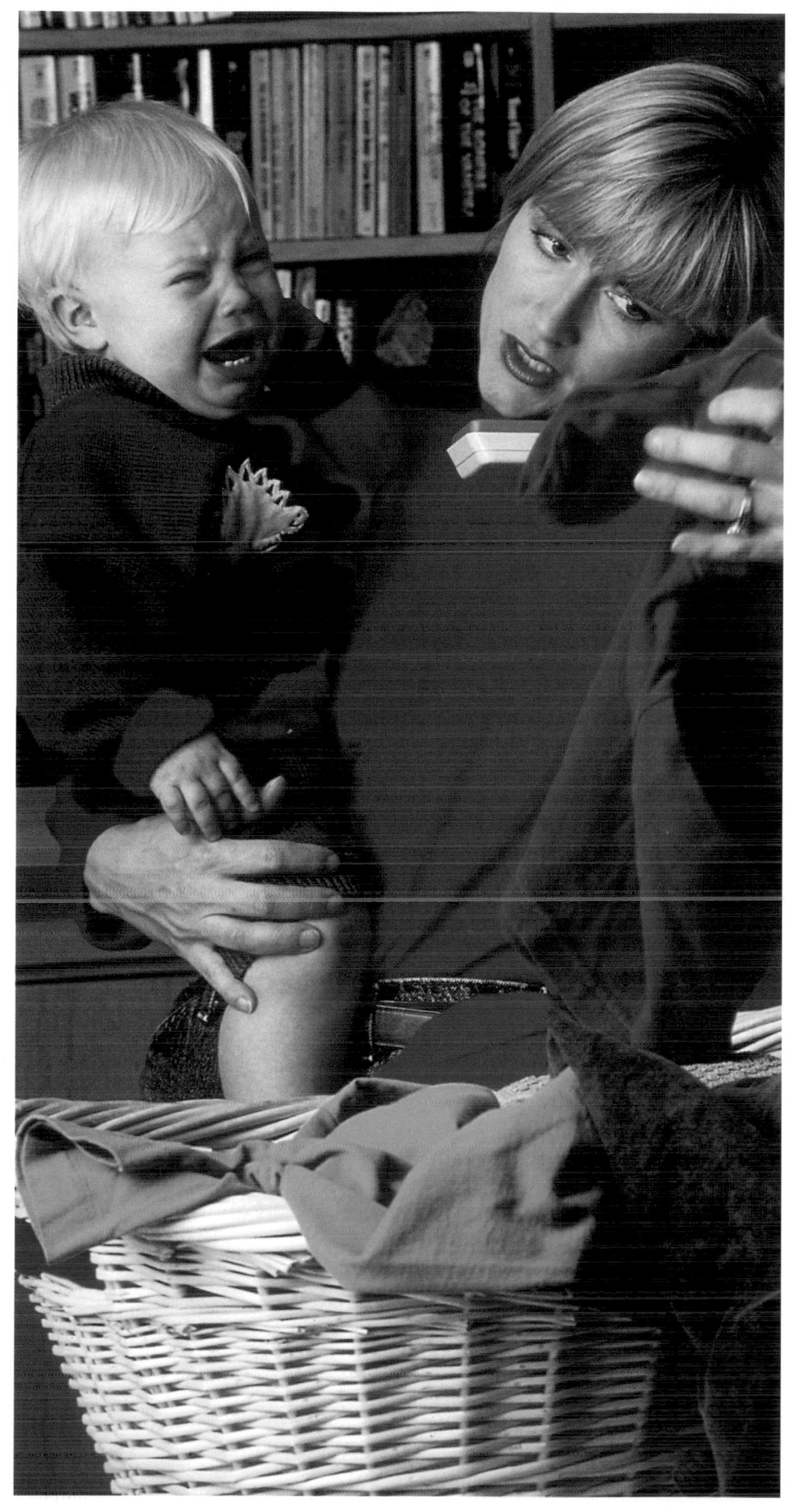

Symptoms of disorders
The symptoms vary depending on the psychological condition that produces them. Most disorders can be classed as neurotic or psychotic.
Extreme and often undefined anxiety.
Reluctance to act for fear of imagined consequences.
Tearfulness.
Shaking or trembling.
Heart palpitations.
Excessive mood swings.
Hysterical outbursts.
Unshakable depression.
Disturbance of thought processes.
Hallucinations such as hearing voices.
Delusions.
Illogicality or confusion of speech.
Convictions of persecution (paranoia).

However, true hysteria is more likely to be characterized by apparent indifference rather than high emotional levels. Its hallmark is a seemingly unexplained loss of function of some kind—such as paralysis, sensory loss, blindness, or an inability to walk—which cannot be accounted for by an organic disease or any other physical cause (see Hysteria).

Anxiety disorders

Anxiety disorders include most of the range of conditions that were formerly described by psychiatrists as neuroses. Anxiety is by far the most common manifestation of psychological disturbance. If a person has a generalized anxiety disorder, he or she will

◄ *Coping with a baby on top of other demands such as work and running a home can trigger severe depression.*

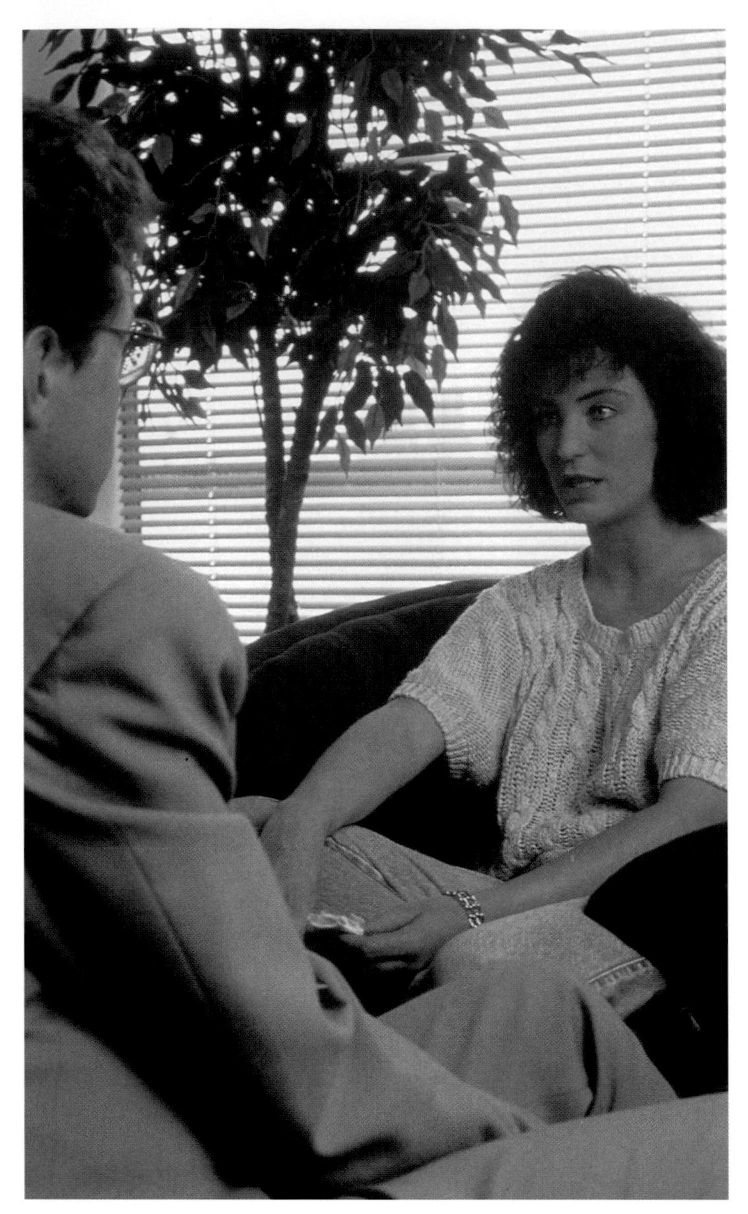

▲ *Therapy, counseling, and the appropriate use of drugs can do much to cure—or at least control—most psychiatric disorders that might be called nervous breakdowns.*

experience an inappropriately excessive level of apprehensive anticipation and worry about one or more of life's everyday circumstances. Such a disorder lasts for six months or longer. The anxiety may relate to money, children's safety, educational attainment, personal attractiveness, or other matters. The worry is present on most days and causes physical changes in the sufferer such as trembling, restlessness, sweating, palpitations, dry mouth, lump in the throat, and butterflies in the stomach.

Free-floating anxiety is different. This is a pervasive feeling of anxiety that is not attached to any particular idea or object. It is a constant, undefined nervous apprehension.

Hypochondriacal anxiety occurs when a person is worried about the physical functioning of his or her body, and about the possibility that some serious illness is present. Severe hypochondriacal anxiety can be significantly disabling, as the problem tends to dominate the thoughts of the person concerned. It leads to constant, fruitless visits to doctors and repeated, expensive medical investigation. Sometimes the focus of the anxiety shifts from one fancied disorder to another; sometimes it remains fixed on one suspected condition.

Obsessive-compulsive anxiety is characterized by a recurrent or almost constantly present thought or feeling, or an uncontrollable need to perform a purposeless action. This action is commonly hand-washing or repetitive checking connected with domestic security. In such cases the obsessive element relates to fear of contamination or infection and to fear of trespassers or burglars.

Phobic anxiety relates to an unreasoning fear of some particular event, activity, experience, or object. It commonly takes the form of a social phobia such as fear of public speaking or even of eating in public. Agoraphobia, fear of wide open spaces; claustrophobia, fear of being enclosed; and animal phobias such as arachnophobia, fear of spiders, are also common forms of phobic anxiety.

Closely associated with phobic anxiety are panic disorders. These are episodes of acute confusional distress and often a sense of impending death. Panic may be associated with uncontrollable overbreathing (hyperventilation), which can make the situation worse.

Any of these anxiety disorders is more likely to be described as a nervous breakdown if the more dramatic aspects are prominent.

Mood disorders

These are more serious conditions that fall into the category of the psychoses. They may be characterized by pure depression or bipolar disorder—a condition in which both depression and abnormal elation occur at different times. The episodes of depression are often profound, and there is always a danger of suicide (see Depression).

In bipolar mood disorder (formerly called manic depression), the affected person will also, at some stage, have an episode or episodes of extreme euphoria, excitement, and irritability in which all mental and physical activity is markedly accelerated. Manic episodes commonly involve excessive drinking, thoughtless overspending, gambling, expensive phone calls, dangerous driving, and sometimes complex delusions.

Schizophrenia

A severe psychiatric disorder, schizophrenia characteristically starts in adolescence or early adult life. It was formerly called dementia praecox, but only the second half of this term is valid; it is not a dementia. The features of the condition include bizarre delusions; prominent hallucinations, such as hearing nonexistent voices; the belief that one is being controlled by the thoughts of other people; inappropriate emotional reactions or flattening of the emotions; social isolation or withdrawal; loss of motivation; deterioration in personal hygiene and grooming; and eccentric beliefs.

Paranoid schizophrenia is the form in which the delusions are prominent and usually of a persecutory nature. Schizophrenia is a fairly common disorder that affects about one young person in 100 and causes total disruption of normal living—not only for the victim, but often for his or her family as well. Once established, it is usually permanent. However, nearly all symptoms can be abolished, or at least controlled adequately, by medication and therapy. The sudden and acute onset of this condition is often called a nervous breakdown.

See also: **Bipolar disorder; Hypochondria; Obsessive-compulsive disorder; Phobias; Psychiatry; Schizophrenia**

Nervous system

Every time a person does anything—literally anything at all—the nervous system is intimately involved at every stage. The nervous system is the body's most complex and important network of control and communication.

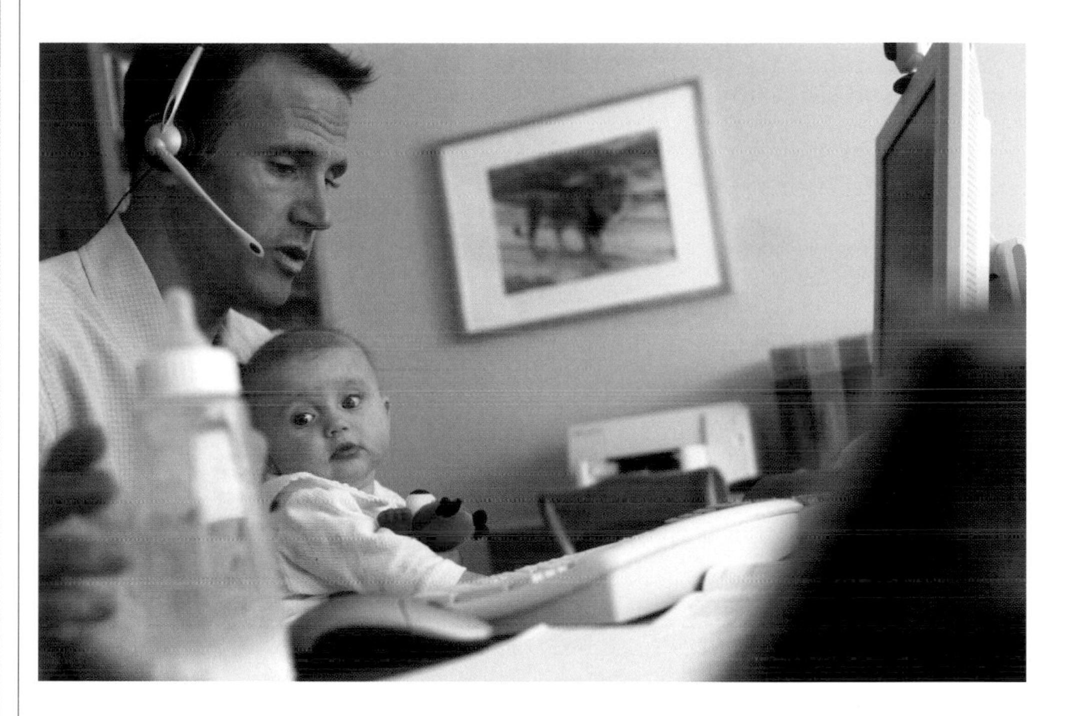

▲ *The action of the nervous system allows several activities to be carried out at the same time. This man is using his cell phone and his computer, as well as feeding a baby.*

The nervous system is essential to sight and hearing; the perception of pain and pleasure; the control of movements; the regulation of bodily functions, such as digestion and breathing; and the development of thought, language, memory, and decision making. Basically, the nervous system collects and receives information from the outside world and uses it to frame the body's response.

The working parts of the nervous system include millions of interconnected cells called neurons. Their function is similar to the wires in a complex electrical machine: they pick up signals in one part of the nervous system and carry them to another; here the signals may be relayed to other neurons, or they may initiate some action, such as the contraction of muscle fibers.

Neurons are delicate cells that are damaged easily or may be destroyed by injury, infection, pressure, chemical disturbances, or lack of oxygen. Since neurons cannot be replaced after they have been destroyed, any damage to them tends to have serious consequences.

The nervous system has two interdependent parts. One of them, the central nervous system, consists of the brain and spinal cord. The other, the peripheral nervous system, consists of all the nerve tissue outside the central nervous system. The central and peripheral nervous systems are each further divided into a number of components.

Peripheral nervous system

The peripheral nervous system has two main divisions: an outer system called the somatic nervous system and an inner one—the autonomic nervous system.

The somatic system has a dual role: first, it collects information from the body's sense organs and conveys this information to the central nervous system; and second, it transmits signals from the central nervous system to the skeletal muscles, thus initiating movement.

The autonomic nervous system is concerned with the regulation of the internal organs and glands, such as the heart, stomach, kidneys, and pancreas.

Questions and Answers

My friend says I'm a nervous wreck. Might I have a nervous system disturbance or problem?

This is unlikely—although there are a few physical illnesses that can lead to generalized anxiety.

Your nervousness is probably caused by fear. This may be unconscious—for example, a fear that you are about to lose your job. Being anxious is a normal response to such stresses and need be a cause for concern only if the nervousness is ever present.

Many forms of anxiety can be relieved by, for example, changing your job, living conditions, or lifestyle, or by seeking medical help or therapy. However, first you may have to identify exactly what it is you are worried about.

Do "pins and needles" have anything to do with nerves?

Yes. If a nerve containing sensory fibers is slightly compressed, its individual fibers may fire off a number of random signals; these signals are perceived by the brain as a tingling sensation.

For example, pressure on the nerves running from your foot up the back of the thigh—perhaps caused by sitting cross-legged—may be felt as the familiar pins and needles in the foot. Continued compression may prevent the nerve fibers from transmitting signals altogether, resulting in a loss of sensation, or numbness.

Can heavy drinking damage nerves?

Yes. Heavy drinking over many years may cause a permanent disturbance in the conduction of signals by nerve cells. It can also speed up the rate at which nerve cells in the brain die, causing mental deterioration. Alcoholics often have vitamin B1 deficiency, too, because of poor diet, and this also disturbs nerve functioning.

Questions and Answers

What is it about the "funny bone" that causes such a strange and painful sensation if I knock it?

The sensation you describe has nothing to do with bone but is due to the ulnar nerve. This passes behind the elbow on its way to the forearm and is prone to injury here. A slight knock can cause a volley of signals in the nerve's sensory fibers, and these can be excruciatingly painful.

A friend said the pain I have in my hands and arms could be caused by a pinched nerve. What is this?

At some point along their length, many nerves have to pass through a restricted space—especially near joints. Any displacement or swelling in this space may squeeze or pinch the nerve, causing pain, muscle weakness, numbness, or a tingling sensation.

The median nerve running through the wrist is the nerve most often affected. It may be squeezed between the ligaments and tendons in the wrist and wrist bones, causing numbness and tingling in the index finger, middle finger, and ring finger; pain in the hand and forearm; and weakness in the thumb. The condition, called carpal tunnel syndrome, can affect people who use keyboards frequently. If you have any of these symptoms, you should see your doctor—an operation to free the nerve may be necessary.

Two months ago I had a foot amputated. Why do I still feel that the foot is there and even have pain from the missing toes?

Although your foot has been amputated, the sensory fibers that used to send messages from the foot to the brain are still present in the remaining part of your leg and have their endings in the stump. If these endings are stimulated, the fibers send messages via the spinal cord to the brain, which from past experience interprets the message as having come from the foot. It takes some time for the brain to realize that the foot is not there.

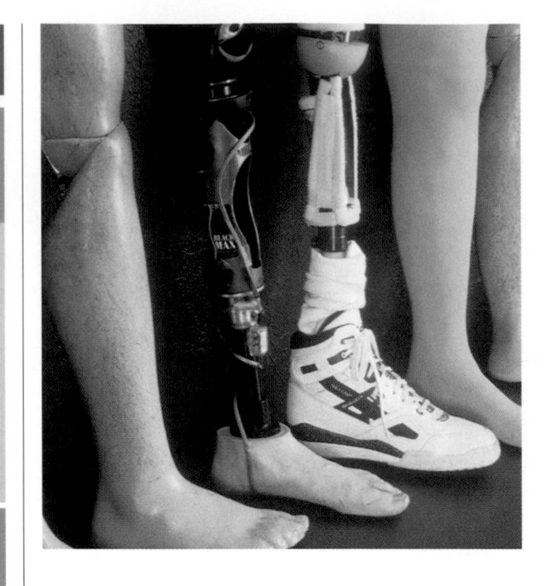

◄ *People with artificial limbs can be trained to use them skillfully. However, they may sometimes experience phantom pain—pain that seems to come from the lost limb.*

The somatic nervous system has two main components: the sensory and motor systems. Information is picked up by sensory organs such as the eyes, which contain receptor cells. There are similar cells for hearing, taste, smell, pain, touch, and skin temperature.

Signals from the receptor cells are carried toward the central nervous system in the sensory nerve fibers. The pattern of signaling in these fibers, which may amount to millions of impulses every second, gives the body and mind essential data about the outside world. Just as the sensory fibers carry information toward the central nervous system, so the motor fibers transmit signals away from the central nervous system toward the skeletal muscles.

Both sensory and motor fibers are themselves part of the sensory and motor neurons. All neurons have a cell body, as well as a number of projecting fibers. The motor and sensory fibers of the peripheral nervous system, called axons, are merely the longest fibers of their respective neurons. The sensory fibers have their cell bodies just outside, and the motor neurons have theirs inside, the brain or spinal cord. An axon may be 10,000 times the length of the nerve cell body.

The motor and sensory fibers that carry messages to and from a particular body organ or area are gathered together in a bundle called a nerve. Different nerves are said to supply a particular area or organ. All together, 43 pairs of nerves emerge from the central nervous system: 12 pairs of cranial nerves from the brain and 31 pairs of spinal nerves from either side of the spinal cord.

The cranial nerves mainly supply sense organs and muscles in the head, although a very important cranial nerve—the vagus—supplies the digestive organs, heart, and air passages in the lungs. Some cranial nerves, such as the optic nerve to the eye, contain only sensory fibers.

The spinal nerves emerge at intervals from the spinal cord and always contain both motor and sensory fibers. They supply all areas of the body below the neck. Each spinal nerve is attached to the spinal cord by means of two roots, one of which carries motor fibers and the other sensory fibers. At a short distance from the spinal cord, each spinal nerve splits into a number of branches.

In effect, the peripheral nervous system acts only to relay sensory and motor messages between the central nervous system and the body's muscles, glands, and sense organs. It plays almost no part in the actual analysis of those sensory signals or the initiation of motor signals. Both of these activities, and much in between, occur in the central nervous system.

The central nervous system

The brain and spinal cord form the nervous system's central processing unit. They receive messages via the sensory fibers from the sense organs and receptors, filter and analyze them, and then send out signals along the motor fibers that produce an appropriate response in the muscles and glands. The analytical, or processing, aspect may be relatively simple for certain functions performed in the spinal cord; however, analysis in the brain is usually a highly complex process that involves thousands of different neurons.

The spinal cord

The spinal cord itself is a roughly cylindrical column of nerve tissues about 16 inches (40 cm) long, which runs inside the backbone from the brain to the lower back. It has two main functions. First, it acts as a two-way conduction system between the brain and the peripheral nervous system. This action is achieved by means of sensory and motor neurons, whose fibers extend in long bundles from parts of the brain. They run varying distances down the spinal cord, and at the ends that are farthest from the brain they come into contact with the fibers or cell bodies of sensory and motor neurons that belong to the peripheral nervous system. Messages can be transmitted across the gaps—called synapses—between the peripheral neurons and the spinal neurons.

LAYOUT OF THE NERVOUS SYSTEM

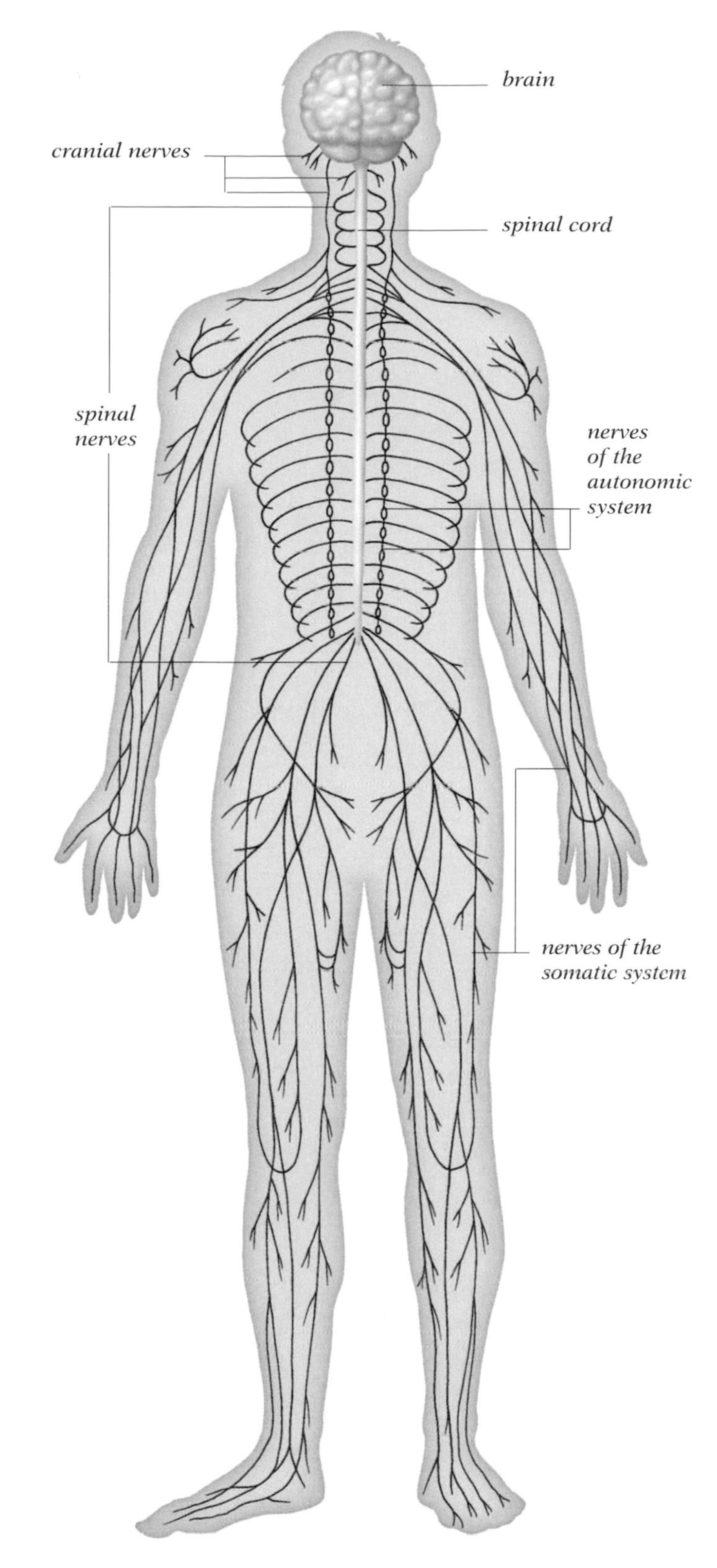

▲ *From the central nervous system (spinal cord and brain), pairs of nerves radiate all over the body to form the peripheral nervous system. This in turn has two main subdivisions: the autonomic system, responsible for unconscious control of functions such as breathing; and the somatic system, responsible for conscious control.*

The second function of the spinal cord is to control simple reflex actions; this control is achieved by neurons whose fibers extend short distances along the spinal cord, and by interneurons, which relay messages directly between the sensory neurons and motor neurons.

If a person accidentally puts his or her hand on a hot stove, pain receptors in the skin send messages along sensory fibers to the spinal cord. Some of these messages are relayed immediately by neurons to motor neurons that control the movements of the arm and hand muscles, and the hand is quickly and automatically withdrawn. At the same time, other messages travel up the spinal cord and are relayed by interneurons to motor neurons that control the neck's movements. In this way, the head is automatically turned toward the source of the pain. Further messages are carried all the way up to the brain and cause the conscious sensation of heat and pain.

The brain

The brain has three main parts. The stalk (brain stem) is a continuation of the spinal cord and supports the brain's large cap—the cerebrum. Below the cerebrum is the cerebellum. Although many sensory neurons terminate, and many motor neurons originate, in the brain, the majority of the brain's neurons are interneurons, whose job it is to filter, analyze, and store information.

One of the brain's most important functions is to memorize information from the sense organs. Later that information may be recalled and used in decision making. For example, when a person touches a hot stove, the pain is memorized; that memory will affect the decision whether or not to touch other hot stoves in the future.

Most of the conscious activities of the brain take place in the upper part of the cerebrum, the cerebral cortex. Some parts of the cortex are involved in the perception of sensations such as hearing, sight, taste, and smell. Others are involved in speech and language, and yet more are the starting point of motor pathways and govern the movements of muscle. Between the motor, sensory, and language areas of the cortex are associated areas that consist of millions of interconnected neurons. These neurons are associated with reasoning, the emotions, and decision making.

The cerebellum is attached to the brain stem just below the cerebrum and is concerned mainly with motor activities. Its job is to send out signals, which produce unconscious movements in muscles so as to maintain posture and balance. It also acts in concert with the motor areas of the cerebrum in order to coordinate body movements.

The brain stem contains different structures with a variety of roles. By far the most important of these structures are the centers that control the lungs, heart, and blood vessels. Functions such as blinking and vomiting are also controlled here. Other centers are concerned with the perception of sensations such as pain, or act as relay stations for messages that arrive from the spinal cord or cranial nerves.

One of the smallest parts of the brain stem, the hypothalamus, controls the body's chemical, hormonal, and temperature balance.

The neurons

Neurons are central to the working of the whole nervous system. However, they are not the only type of cell to be found in the nervous system; another type, called the neuroglias—literally "nerve glue"—are present in large numbers. Their job is to bind, protect, nourish, and provide support for the neurons.

Neurons come in various shapes and sizes; however, they all have the same basic structure. They have a nucleus, or center, which is

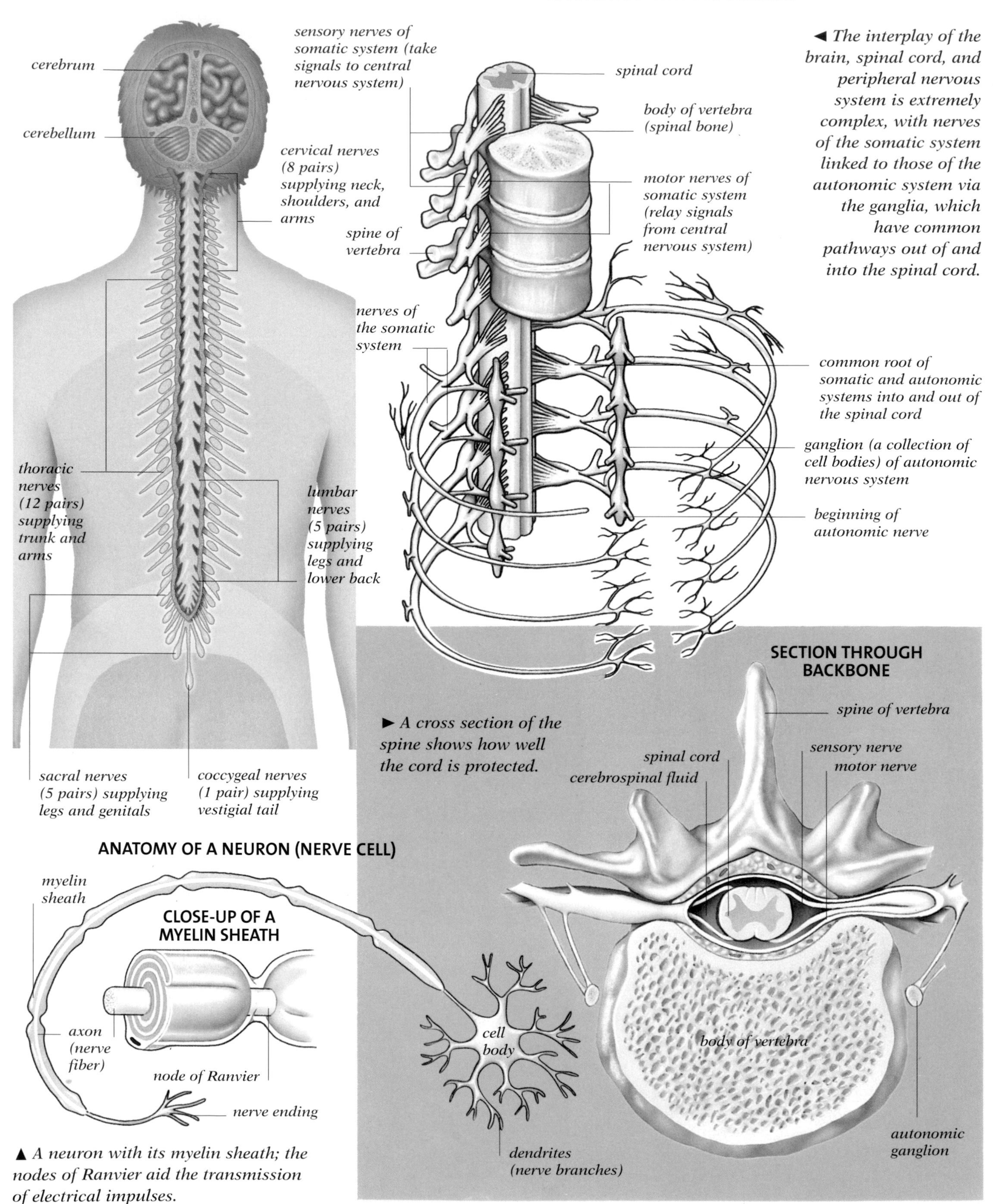

◄ *The interplay of the brain, spinal cord, and peripheral nervous system is extremely complex, with nerves of the somatic system linked to those of the autonomic system via the ganglia, which have common pathways out of and into the spinal cord.*

► *A cross section of the spine shows how well the cord is protected.*

▲ *A neuron with its myelin sheath; the nodes of Ranvier aid the transmission of electrical impulses.*

Common diseases of the nervous system

DISEASE	SYMPTOMS	TREATMENT
Brain tumor	Severe headaches; projectile vomiting; neck pain; fits; odd behavior; personality changes; progressive paralysis.	Surgical excision of tumor; radiotherapy.
Dementia	Memory loss; inability to concentrate; confusion; loss of interest; untidiness.	No cure except when a specific cause is known. Vitamin therapy sometimes helps.
Epilepsy	Convulsive fits or temporary loss of consciousness.	Anticonvulsant drugs.
Ménière's disease	Ringing in ear; giddiness; nausea; vomiting.	Antinausea drugs.
Meningitis	Fevers; headaches; neck and back muscle spasms; intolerance of bright lights; convulsions; vomiting.	Antibiotic drugs.
Multiple sclerosis	Weakness in one or more limbs; numbness; pins and needles; visual disturbances; walking difficulties. Symptoms vary; may improve for a time, then reappear.	No cure. Various drugs may bring about a temporary recovery.
Neuropathy	Muscle weakness; numbness; pain; pins and needles.	Underlying cause treated.
Parkinson's disease	Tremors; uncoordinated movements; facial rigidity.	Anti-Parkinsonian drugs.
Poliomyelitis	Headaches; spinal pains; stiff neck, followed by fever, muscle weakness, and paralysis.	Prevention through vaccination during childhood.
Sciatica	Back and leg pain along path of sciatic nerve.	Bed rest; painkilling drugs.
Shingles	Fevers; pain; skin blistering along the course of affected nerve fibers.	Oral Zovirax (aciclovir) taken early; analgesic drugs for pain and fever.
Spastic paralysis	Spasms; partial paralysis; lack of coordination; uncontrolled movements.	No cure; special education to make best use of unaffected areas of brain.
Stroke	Effects depend on area of brain affected: partial paralysis; speech impairment; severe headaches; visual disturbances; deafness. Sometimes fatal.	Anticoagulants to help prevent blood clotting. Surgery to close off leaking brain artery aneurysms.
Trigeminal neuralgia	Severe pain in the side of face lasting for about a minute. Recurs every few hours, days, or weeks.	Injection of alcohol into nerve; drugs; surgery to allow more room for nerve.
Vestibular neuronitis	Vertigo; vomiting; uncontrolled eye movements.	Treatment with drugs.

contained in a roughly spherical part of the neuron called the cell body. In addition, a number of fine, rootlike fibers project from the cell body. These are called dendrites. Also projecting from the cell is a single, long fiber called the axon. At its far end, the axon divides into a number of branches, each of which ends in a number of tiny knobs.

Each knob is in close proximity to, though not actually touching, a dendrite from another neuron. The gap between the two is known as a synapse, and messages are transmitted across it by chemicals called nerve transmitter substances.

Each neuron is bounded by a a thin, semipermeable wall, and this membrane plays an important part in the transmission of signals. The signals are always started by the excitation of one or more of the dendrites and are first carried toward the cell body. They are then transmitted away from the cell body along the membrane of the axon.

When a signal reaches the knobs at the end of the axon, under certain circumstances it may jump across the synapse to the dendrite of an adjacent neuron and so continue its journey.

To speed up the transmission of these signals, there is a covering along many axons—like insulation on electrical wires—called myelin. The areas of the brain and spinal cord that are insulated in this way are called white matter; the remainder is known as gray matter.

The central nervous system is maintained with a plentiful supply of blood, which provides oxygen and nutrients. The system is also protected by two kinds of covering. The first is bone and consists of the skull, which encloses the brain; and the backbone, which encloses the spinal cord. The second covering consists of three membranes of fibrous tissue: the meninges. These cover the whole of the brain and the spinal cord. Fluid circulates through the brain and the spinal cord and acts as a shock absorber. The cerebrospinal fluid contains nutrients and also white blood cells, which fight infection.

See also: **Autonomic nervous system; Brain; Hypothalamus; Memory; Mind; Movement; Reflexes; Spinal cord**

Neuralgia

Questions and Answers

I get persistent neuralgia over my right eye. What can I do?

If any pain lasts for more than a few days, you should always see a doctor. Neuralgia in one side of the forehead may indicate either the onset of shingles or the start of trigeminal neuralgia.

I sometimes have severe neuralgic pain in my left cheek, but it has recently begun to occur more often. What could be the cause?

It may be that you are in the early stages of facial neuralgia, or perhaps you have a chronic infection in a tooth or sinus. You should see your doctor so that the cause can be established and treatment started promptly.

I have been getting severe neuralgia for several years now as the result of a fracture. Is there any way I can obtain permanent relief?

It is not uncommon for pain to occur along nerves that have been involved in a bad fracture. Often it disappears as the fracture heals, but sometimes the pain persists. Cutting the nerve, or removing a section of it, is likely to eliminate the pain but will also take away all of the feeling from the whole area that is supplied by the nerve.

My elderly grandmother has had facial neuralgia for years. Sometimes it is so severe that she cannot sleep. She won't go to the doctor because she is sure that nothing can be done. Is she right?

A few years ago she would have been correct, but now there are several drugs that can alleviate the condition. A very simple operation can also be performed. If your grandmother talks to her doctor she might take advantage of one of these treatments.

Once applied to all sorts of aches and soreness, the term "neuralgia" really refers to a specific type of pain that is triggered in the nervous system. Such pain can be caused by a variety of conditions.

The term neuralgia means "nerve pain." It is not a disease in itself but a condition that occurs in several diseases that all give rise to sensations of pain along the paths of particular nerves.

Neuralgia is not a general overall pain; it is felt in a specific area of the body. It is also usually a severe, nagging pain that can interfere with sleep or concentration. Sometimes the sensation can be sharp and intense with waves of pain shooting down the affected nerve; it may cause the sufferer to wince or, in some cases, writhe in agony.

Causes

Neuralgia is caused by the irritation of a nerve and interference with its normal function. It can be brought about by neuritis (inflammation of a nerve); a common example of this is the form of neuralgia that often accompanies shingles. It may also be caused by an area of infection or an abscess close to a nerve, such as a tooth abscess that causes severe toothache.

FACIAL (TRIGEMINAL) NEURALGIA

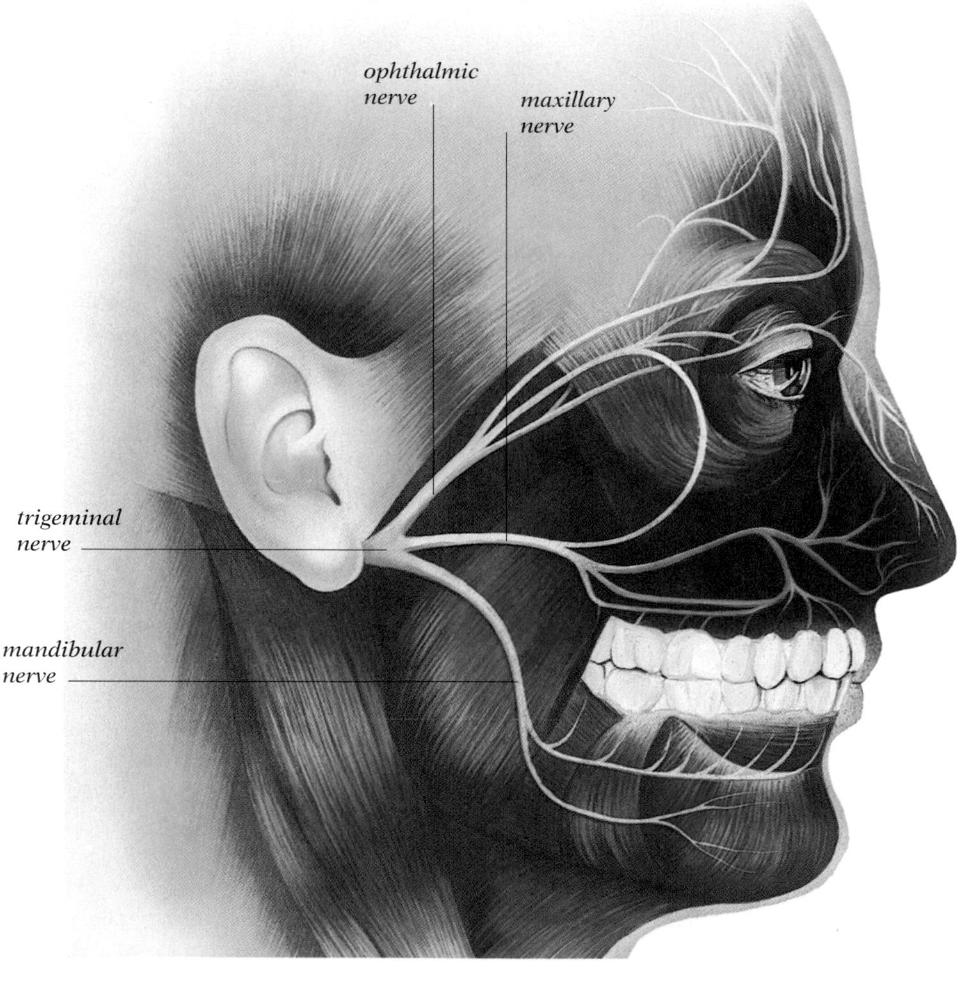

▲ *In facial neuralgia, the three main branches of the trigeminal nerve are affected—often on one side of the face only. The pink area shows where pain has spread from the cheek. This pain may cause the facial muscles to contract in spasm.*

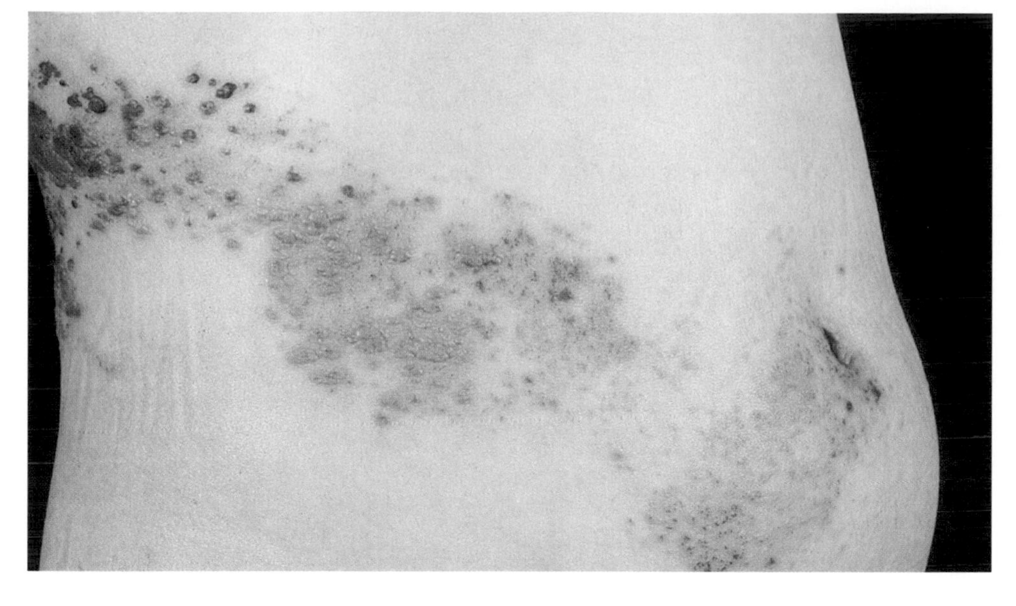

▲ *With shingles, the blisters trace the path of the affected nerves, in this case running from the spine to the abdomen.*

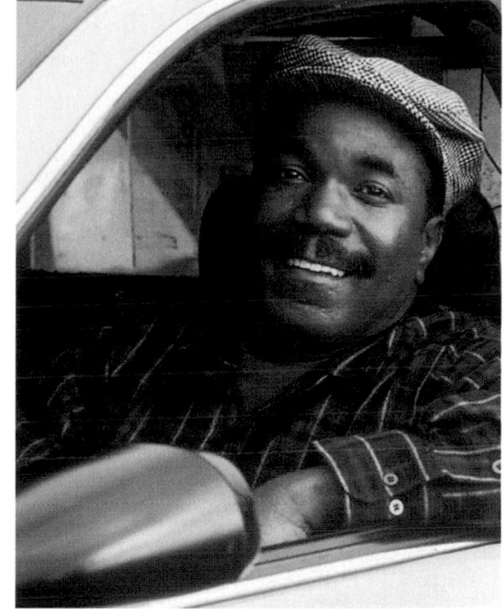

▲ *A person may suffer facial neuralgia as the result of frequently sitting in a draft coming into an automobile window. Such attacks tend to occur more often with time, but modern drugs provide considerable relief.*

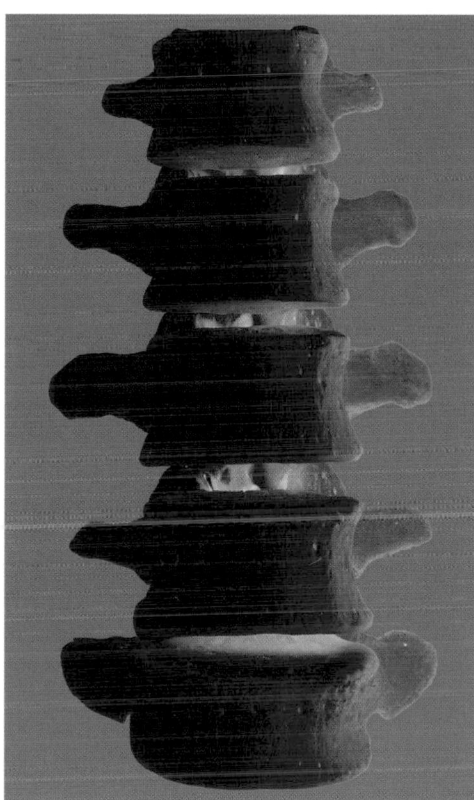

► *Cartilage disks cushion the vertebrae of the backbone. If a damaged disk protrudes, it can can cause neuralgia by pressing on the sciatic nerve.*

If something presses on a nerve, this pressure will also give rise to pain. Examples of this type of neuralgia include a broken or displaced bone, an area of bleeding or swelling in a confined space, and the growth of a tumor. Sciatica occurs when one of the disks of cartilage between the vertebrae in the lower back "slips" and presses on the roots of the sciatic nerve in the spine (see Sciatica).

Most people experience mild neuralgia at some time in their life. The pain may be triggered by twisting some part of the body abruptly and thus stretching or trapping a nerve tract, or it may be the result of an inflammation caused by a cold draft. Such mild instances require no treatment aside from pain relief and usually last for only a day or two. If the pain persists longer, the person should see a doctor.

Symptoms

Facial neuralgia is very common, especially in elderly people, and the severe pain causes a quick spasmodic contraction of the muscles of the face. This pain occurs in spasms that usually last less than a minute. The forehead, cheeks, lips, and jaw can be affected—usually on one side of the face only. Attacks may be triggered by action such as blowing the nose, chewing, or washing the face; or by a draft.

Severe neuralgia is a feature of advanced syphilis. The pain—called lightning pain—is sudden and sharp and is usually felt in the legs, chest, or abdomen; in some cases the sensation of pain may resemble a heart attack or abdominal emergency (see Syphilis).

The most common form of the condition is probably neuralgia that is experienced by patients suffering from shingles. The pain usually occurs a few days before the appearance of the redness and blisters that are typical of shingles. These symptoms usually develop in a band along the path of the affected nerve. Any of the major face, neck, chest, or lumbar nerves may be affected. The victim may continue to suffer severe neuralgia after the shingles has cleared, especially in the facial area.

Treatment

Doctors will often prescribe the drugs phenytoin and carbamazepine to provide relief from neuralgia. However, if they are not effective, it may be necessary to put the nerve out of action. This can be done by the injection of alcohol or by cutting the nerve surgically under a general anesthetic. Surgery is a last resort, because it leaves the affected part permanently numb (see Numbness).

Vitamin B12 injections, antibiotics, and carbamazepine pills may be given to relieve the pain associated with advanced syphilis.

If there is something pressing on a nerve—a slipped disk, for example—the pressure has to be relieved by rest, manipulation, physical therapy, or surgery. Acetaminophen, aspirin (for adults only), or a stronger, prescribed painkiller should also help to alleviate this pain.

See also: **Nervous system; Pain; Pain management; Shingles**

Neural tube defect

"Neural tube defect" is the term for a failure of normal development of the part of the early embryo that forms the central nervous system. The result may range from a minor defect in the newborn baby to a devastating abnormality. However, neural tube defects can usually be avoided.

Neural tube defects have their origin very early in the pregnancy. By the third week a longitudinal groove has formed along the back of the embryo. This groove sinks in and the edges become raised folds—the neural folds—which come together and fuse so that a tube is formed. It is essential for future normality that this tube should form completely. If it fails to do so at the posterior end, spina bifida will result. If tube formation fails at the anterior end, even more serious abnormalities such as absence of the brain (anencephaly) may result.

Failure of closure of the primary neural tube causes open defects so that parts of the nervous system are exposed to the exterior. Failure of development at a later stage, after the tube has closed, produces closed defects in which, although the nervous tissue is covered by skin, it is not covered normally by bone.

How common is neural tube defect?

This condition is becoming less common in the United States. Since 1998, the incidence of neural tube defects has fallen by nearly 20 percent because of the mandatory addition of folic acid to bread and pasta. Cases of spina bifida dropped by 23 percent. The highest incidence is in Appalachia, where the current number is one per 1,000 live births. The incidence is higher in the eastern United States than on the West Coast. Worldwide, the highest reported incidence is in China, where neural tube defects occur in 4 to 6 percent of babies born each year.

Types of neural tube defect

Babies with the most severe type of neural tube defect—anencephaly—cannot survive and usually die within a few hours of birth. Rarely, they may live for about two days. The most common

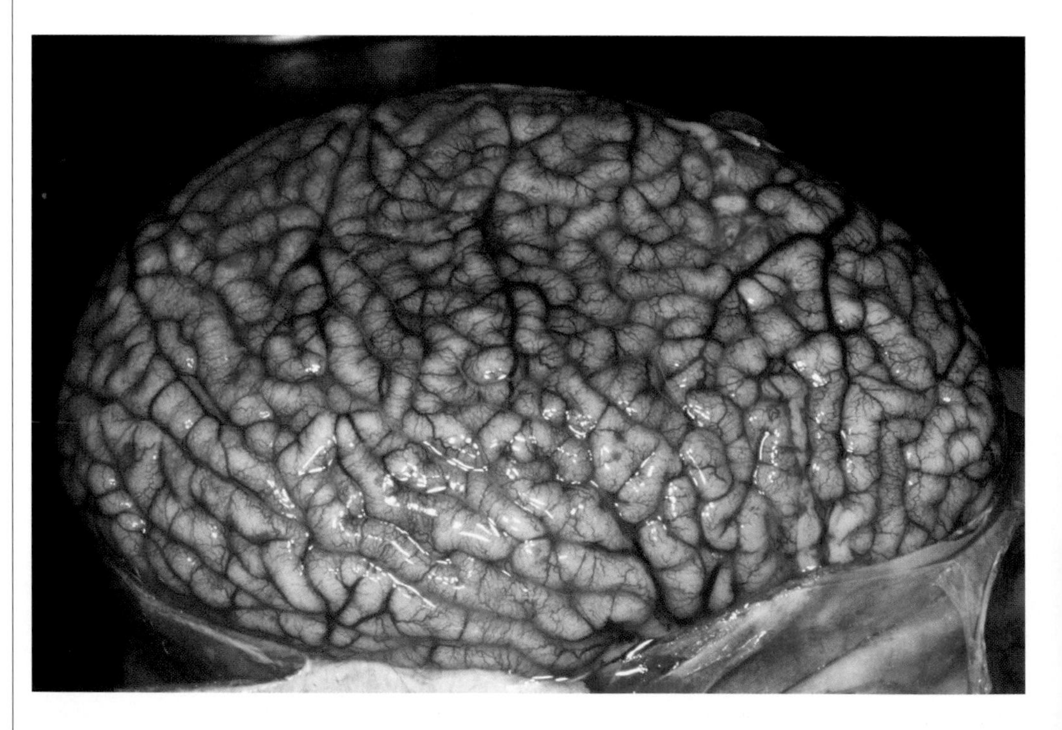

▲ *This brain of a 3½-month child with congenital hydrocephalus shows the enlargement and widening of the small cavities in the brain caused by an abnormal buildup of fluid.*

Questions and Answers

My cousin's left leg has a slightly thinner calf than her right, and her left foot takes a smaller shoe size. No one has ever explained this, and she certainly didn't have polio. Could this possibly be due to a neural tube defect?

There are several possible causes for this problem, and a minor degree of closed neural tube defect is one of them. An X ray would probably confirm the diagnosis, but if she has no other effects, there is no need for her to worry.

Does race affect the chances of having a neural tube defect?

This is uncertain. Before prenatal screening and folic acid supplementation were common, neural tube defects were higher in white European people than in black people. In the United States the risk was three times as high in the Hispanic population as in non-Hispanic white people. Today in the United States there is little racial difference in the risk.

Can neural tube defect be detected before birth?

Yes. Amniocentesis tests and ultrasound examination can detect the more obvious neural tube defects well before the birth.

My first baby had a neural tube defect and is now unable to walk and has recurrent urinary tract infections. I want to have another baby, but is it likely that he or she may be affected in the same way? If so, what can I do to prevent it?

It has been estimated that the risk of a second baby's being affected by neural tube defect is about one in 20. However, if you take folic acid for a month before you become pregnant and throughout pregnancy, the chances of having a perfectly normal child are high.

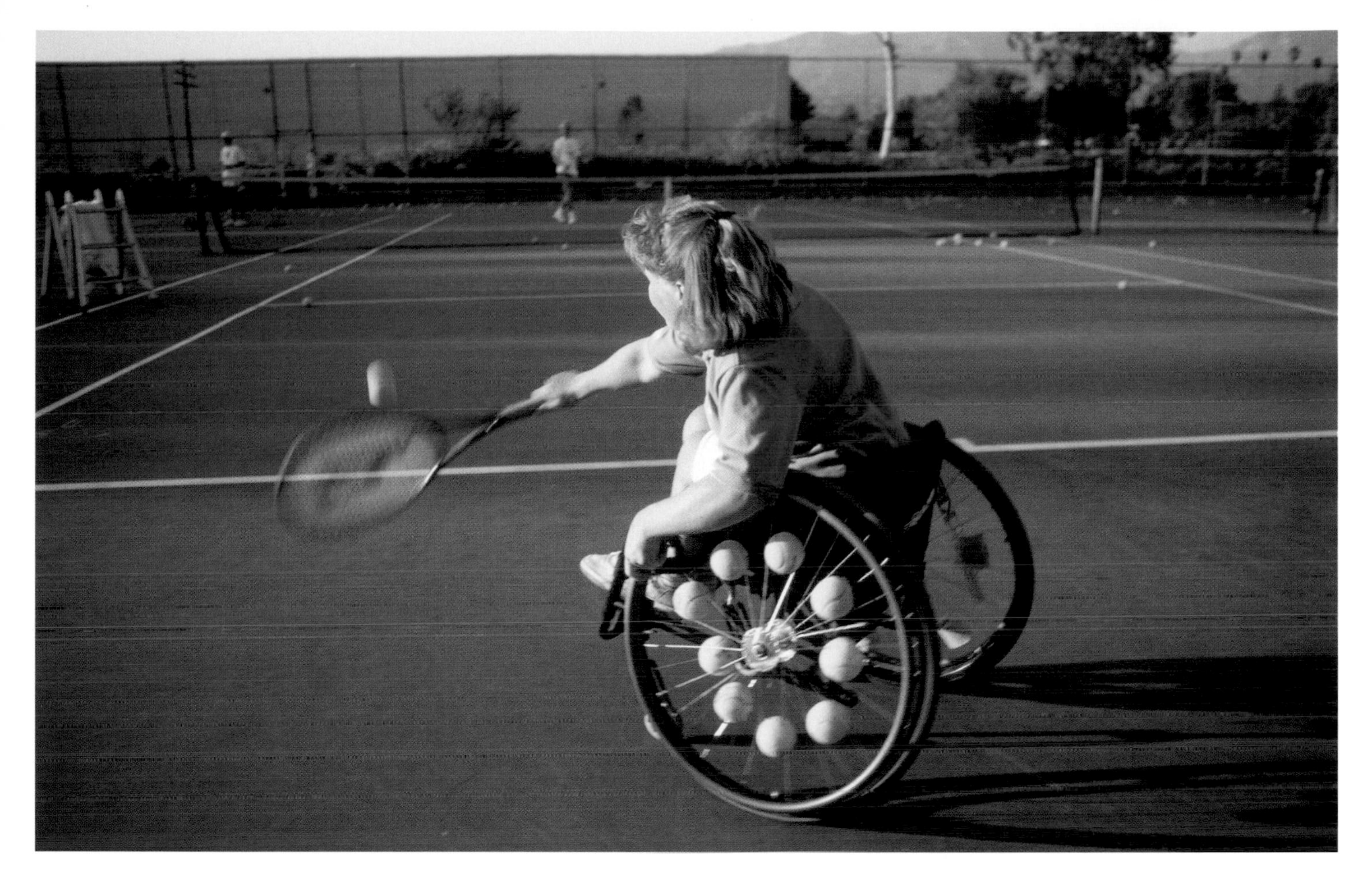

▲ *Victims of less serious neural tube defects such as spina bifida can still achieve much in life. For example, Gina Jalbert has managed to become an expert tennis player, despite being confined to a wheelchair by spina bifida.*

neural tube defect compatible with life is called myelomeningocele. In this condition there is a bony defect in the back of the lower part of the spine (spina bifida) through which a part of the spinal cord, with the membranes that normally cover it (the meninges), bulges out to form a visible sac. This is the myelomeningocele. If only the meninges protrude but the nervous tissue remains in its normal position, the condition is called a meningocele. Myelomeningocele is always more serious than meningocele.

The least serious form of neural tube defect is a spina bifida that is completely covered. Although there is a bony defect in the spinal column, the nerve tissue and its meningeal coverings are intact and in place. This is called spina bifida occulta and is detectable only on X-ray examination (see X Rays).

Neural tube defect is commonly characterized by a blockage of the normal circulation of the fluid that bathes the brain and spinal cord—the cerebrospinal fluid. This result is a rise in the pressure in the fluid and the condition called hydrocephalus.

Symptoms

These vary greatly depending on the type of defect and its severity. When there is a myelomeningocele there is often paralysis of the legs and loss of sensation in the lower part of the body. In the worst cases there may be total paralysis of the lower part of the body (paraplegia) and incontinence. Repeated urinary tract infections can lead to kidney damage, and hydrocephalus can damage the brain, producing, in the worst cases, epilepsy, spastic paralysis, and mental retardation.

About 10 percent of the 6,000 to 11,000 babies born with myelomeningocele in the United States each year suffer severe mental retardation, and about 15 percent of children with myelomeningocele die before reaching the first grade in school. The great majority reach adult life, however, and have an almost normal life expectancy.

Prevention

Since the late 1980s, it has been known that a small daily intake of folic acid, taken before conception and during the early weeks of pregnancy, while the neural tube is forming, will greatly reduce the risk of neural tube defect. A dose of 400 micrograms (0.4 mg) per day—the amount commonly found in over-the-counter multivitamin preparations—is probably enough, and the vitamin should be taken for 28 days before and after conception (see Vitamin B). In 1998 it became a legal requirement in the United States to fortify bread, pasta, and rice with folic acid. Since then the incidence of neural tube defects in the United States has declined by almost 20 percent. Research has shown that such folic acid supplements do not increase the risk of miscarriage.

See also: **Congenital disorders; Fetus; Hydrocephalus; Nervous system; Paralysis; Paraplegia; Pregnancy; Spina bifida; Spinal cord; Urinary tract and disorders**

Neurasthenia

Questions and Answers

Why does my doctor object to the term "neurasthenia"?

Probably because laypeople tend to use the word as if it were a specific diagnosis. It is not. There is no disorder or disease that can be called neurasthenia.

What does neurasthenia mean?

"Asthenia" means "weakness" or "debility," and "neur-" can mean "nerves" or "the nervous system." However, people described as neurasthenic are not suffering from an organic nerve disorder. It might be said that the nervous system has a functional weakness, but few doctors would be satisfied with this view. The operation of the brain is too complex to be described in such a crude way.

The symptoms of a person with neurasthenia are very real. Is there a cause for the symptoms?

Certainly. All such effects have a cause. The disorders that produce these symptoms may have various different causes, most of them psychological or social.

Is neurasthenia a purely psychological condition?

In most cases, yes. However, a complex set of symptoms of this kind can be caused by one of several different disorders, some of which are organic in origin.

Would it be wrong for a doctor simply to dismiss a case as being neurasthenia?

Yes. It is a mistake to assume, without sufficient evidence, that a person is suffering from a purely psychological disorder. Doctors are increasingly aware that organic disease can simulate what used to be called neurotic disorders.

An obsolete term, "neurasthenia" does not describe a specific medical condition but rather describes a collection of symptoms that could indicate a variety of physical or—more commonly—psychological disorders.

Because the term "neurasthenia" does not correspond to a specific medical condition, its meaning has altered over the years. When it was introduced toward the end of the 19th century, it meant a state of debility produced by vague causes such as stresses upon the functioning of the mind. In the early 1920s, Freud identified neurasthenia as one of the three pure forms of actual neurosis. The other two were anxiety-neurosis and hypochondria.

Later the term was widened to include conditions such as the obsessional neuroses. In the 1960s one author wrote: "Neurasthenia is observed with such frequency in housewives who are bored and feel neglected by their husbands that it has often been called 'housewives' neurosis.'"

Today, the term is used by doctors only as a euphemism. However, it may be defined as a state of fatigue, weakness, and irritability, sometimes with symptoms that are seemingly related to a particular organ or body system. Other manifestations include anxiety, insomnia, multiple aches and pains, headache, dizziness, and intolerance of noise.

Doctors describe such symptoms as being nonspecific. In general, however, neurasthenia is so often accompanied by unhappiness, alienation, and disaffection that it is thought likely, in most cases, to arise from psychological or social causes. For this reason, it is often considered a form of neurotic depressive disorder. In view of the vagueness of the term, it is necessary to consider several known disorders that could give rise to the symptoms of neurasthenia.

Fatigue

It is always abnormal for an individual to suffer from a feeling of extreme tiredness that is unrelated to work of any kind, physical or mental. The tiredness that follows sustained physical

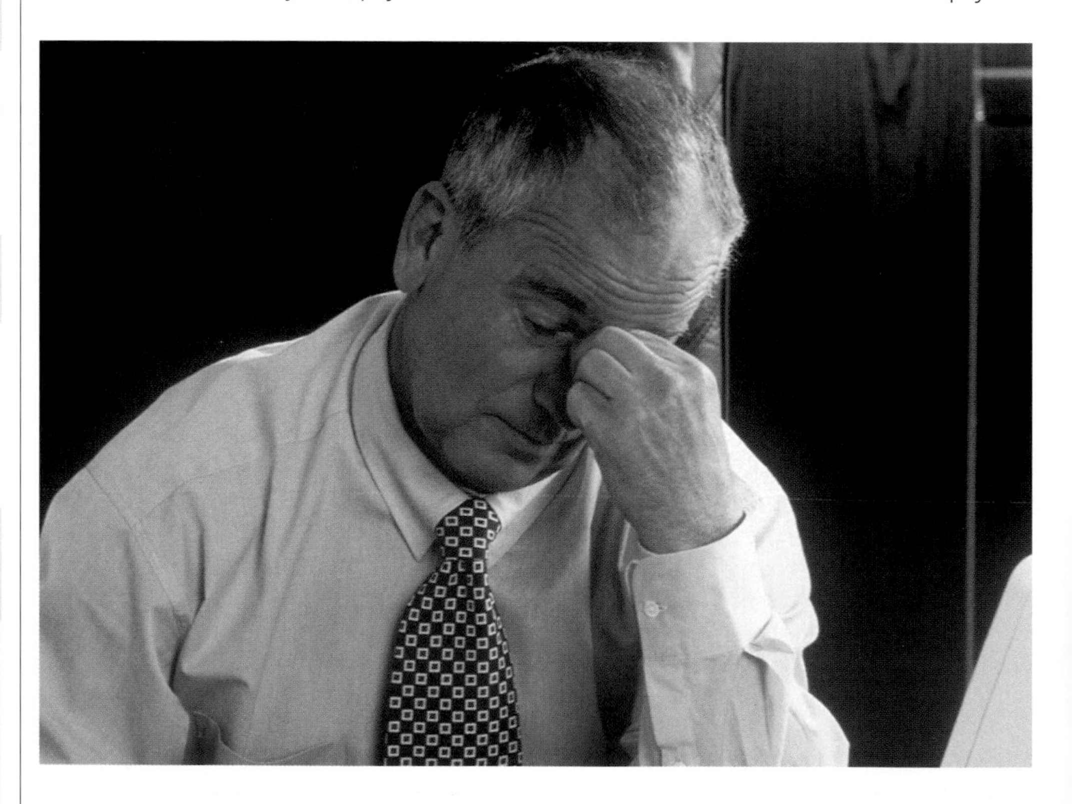

▲ *Chronic fatigue, anxiety, loss of vigor, chest pains, stomach disorders, and shortness of breath are all symptoms that may arise as a reaction to stress and boredom.*

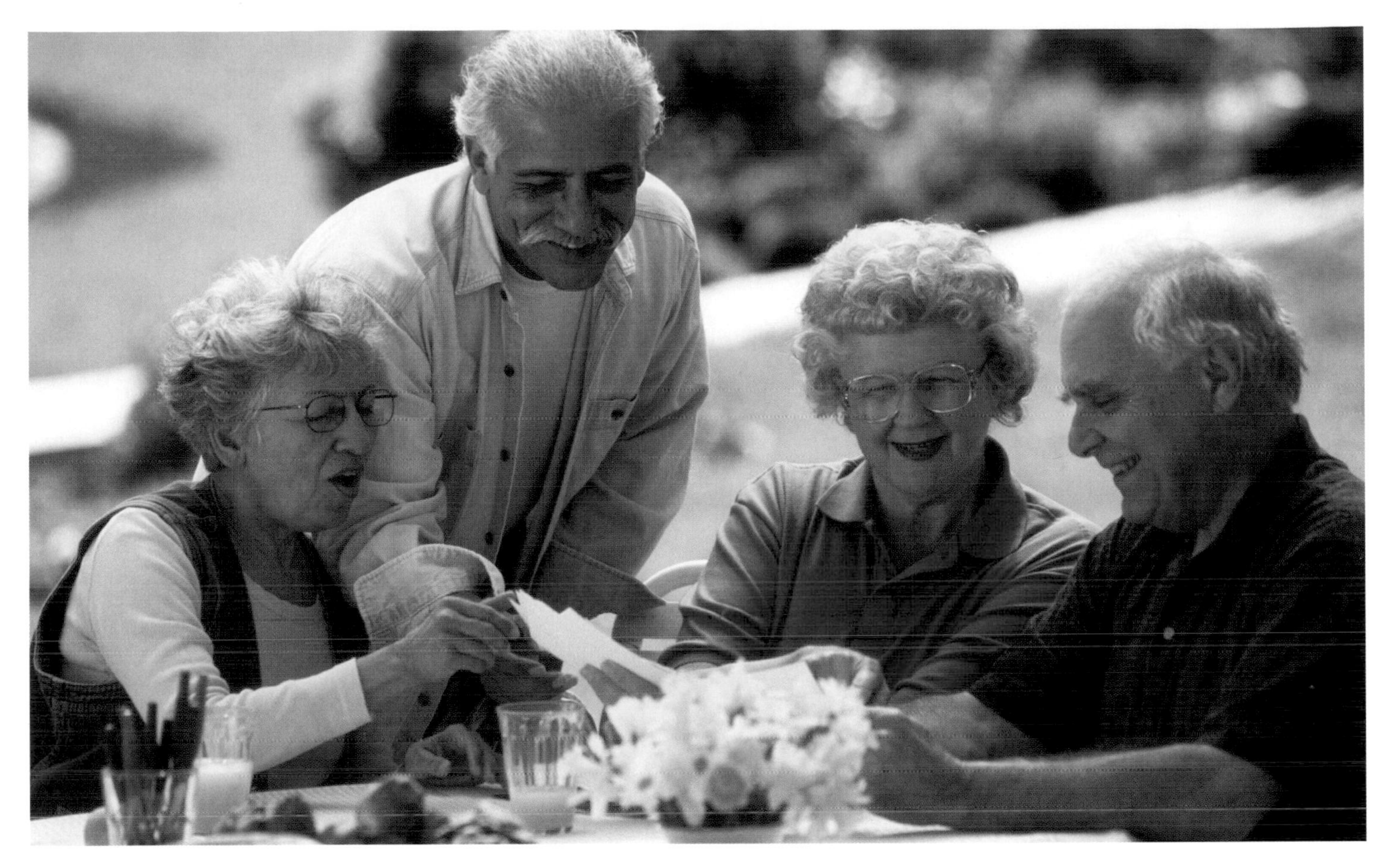

▲ *When the symptoms of neurasthenia have been found to be of purely psychological origin, a change of lifestyle or therapy may encourage a more positive attitude in sufferers.*

exertion or lack of sleep, by contrast, is normal and disappears with rest. Similarly, sustained intellectual work can produce a sense of fatigue. This, too, is normal, and simple rest will bring relief.

However, most cases of nonphysical fatigue actually have nothing to do with the overuse of mental faculties. Such cases are far more often caused by being severely bored, by concentrating on a single task for too long, or by feeling anxious, frustrated, fearful, or disinclined to perform a particular piece of work or chore (see Fatigue).

Chronic fatigue syndrome

The term "chronic fatigue syndrome" is one of the many synonyms for a neurasthenic disorder or—as many experts argue—a range of disorders that includes post-viral fatigue syndrome, epidemic neuro-myasthenia, Otago mystery disease, Icelandic disease, institutional mass hysteria, or benign myalgic encephalomyelitis (ME).

Whether these disorders are identical or a range of overlapping conditions and whether or not they are of organic origin are issues of some controversy among doctors. However, there is a common entity, affecting mainly women, that is characterized by severe fatigue and emotional disturbance and is made worse by exercise. In such cases a single act of exertion may cause fatigue for weeks. The phenomenon is now becoming common in children, too. In different cases, this type of fatigue is associated with many other symptoms, psychological and physical, thereby adding to the controversy.

Dysthymia

A common cause of neurasthenia, dysthymia is a form of depression without psychotic manifestations (see Depression). The term "dysthymia" means ill humored, and dysthymic people are morose and introverted with low self-esteem, fatigue, poor concentration, and poor motivation. In some cases, there is a family history of mood disorders. In others, the problem stems from environmental factors or from difficulty in adapting to adolescence and adulthood.

The so-called seasonal affective disorder syndrome (SADS), in which neurasthenia is said to be brought on by winter, is believed by some people to be a genuine medical entity but is dismissed by others.

Dysthymia is treated with antidepressant drugs and behavior therapy aimed at replacing the suffer's helpless response to life with a more positive attitude. Cognitive therapy may also be used.

Known physical causes

Physical causes of neurasthenia include a range of organic brain diseases, head injury, persistent infections, glandular disorders, nutritional disorders, drugs for high blood pressure, cancer, anticancer drugs, large-dose steroid drugs, and long-term alcohol and drug abuse. Few of these conditions are, however, likely to be missed as a cause of neurasthenia because most involve obvious additional symptoms. Because of the possibility of such organic causes, it is important for doctors not to assume that neurasthenic symptoms are of psychological or social origin. Full medical investigation is required in all new cases.

See also: **Anxiety; Chronic fatigue syndrome; Neuroses; Seasonal affective disorder**

Neurology and neurosurgery

Questions and Answers

I have to go to the hospital for a neurological examination, and a friend told me that neurological wards are like the wards of a mental hospital. Is that true?

No. Very few people admitted to a neurological ward have any degree of mental abnormality: they are there because, like you, they have a neurological symptom that needs investigation. Neurological wards tend to be more relaxed than general wards, where there is a rapid succession of very ill people.

I have to have a brain operation, and my hair will be shaved off. Will it grow back and cover the scars?

Yes; in fact, most people who have had this operation report that their hair grows back better than before and that, in time, all scars are hidden. When the hair loss is caused by drugs, the condition can be permanent, but this is rare in brain operations.

Do metal plates that are put into people's skulls ever have to be replaced, and do they corrode?

No. Most skull replacements are made of either hardened plastic or noncorroding metal alloys such as titanium, chosen for their lightness. Once in place, skull replacements are usually permanent, although they may need adjustment if the surrounding skull grows over them. For this reason their insertion is often delayed several months.

Is there any surgery for depression?

Psychosurgery is not legal in the United States. Electroconvulsive therapy may be used on patients with acute depression who are resistant to drug therapy. A convulsion is induced by passing an electric current through the brain. The patient has no memory of the shock on awakening.

Neurology is concerned with diseases of the brain, the spinal cord, and the peripheral nerves of the body. Neurosurgery deals with the same diseases when they need to be treated by surgery.

In earlier years, neurology and psychiatry were often practiced by the same specialists. Today, however, neurologists are concerned mainly with disorders that are clearly the result of some physical malfunction of the nervous system; the same disorders become the province of neurosurgery when they need surgical treatment.

Neurology units

Neurologists and neurosurgeons usually share the same unit because their work overlaps so much. Units are generally arranged on a regional basis, but in some places there may be a number of units associated with a major teaching hospital as well as with an exclusively neurological hospital. These centers act as units for the referral of patients and as centers for research and training.

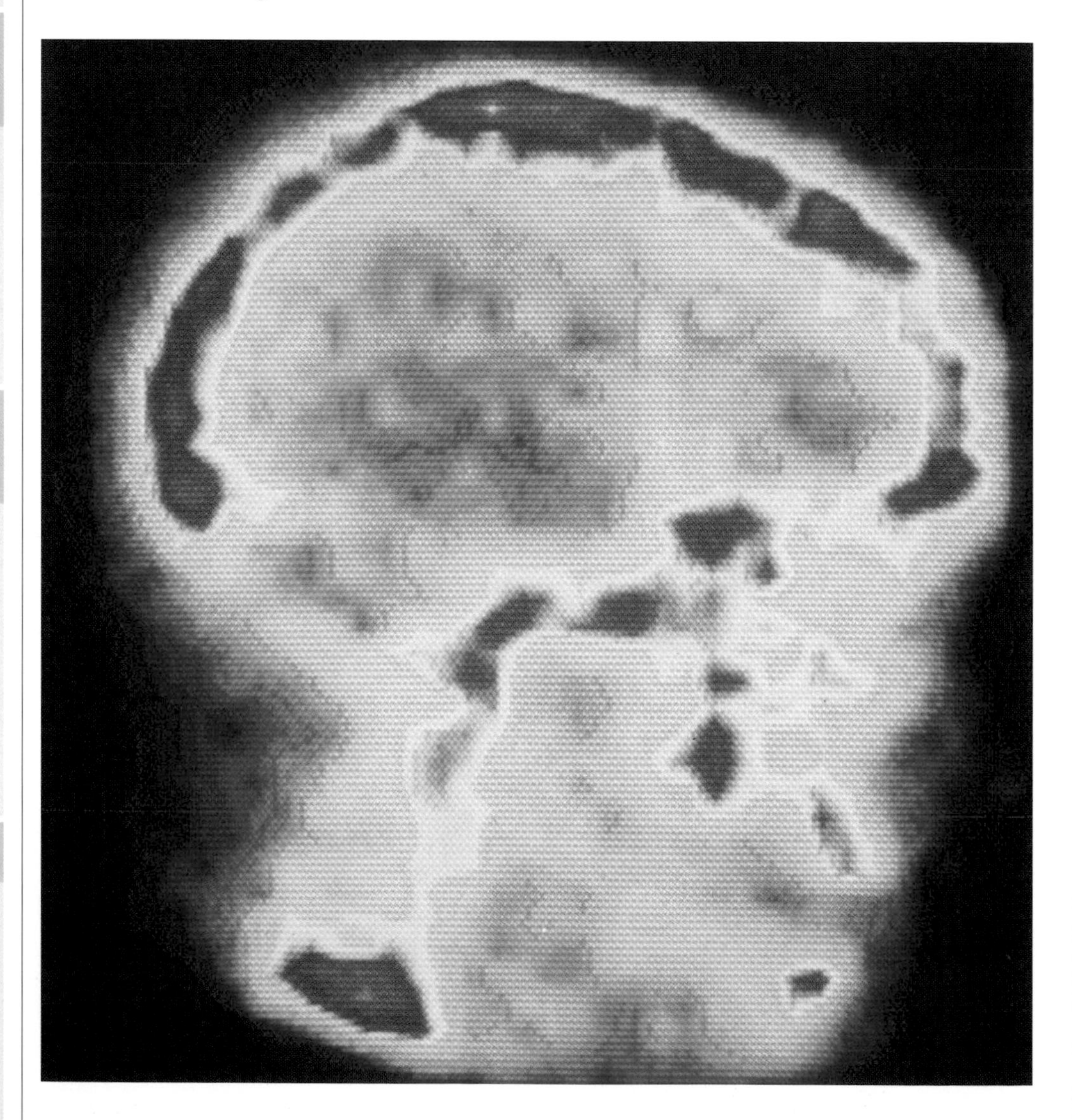

▲ *This brain scan records radioactivity distribution in the brain after injection with an isotope. Disease is indicated if circulation of the radiochemical is affected or interrupted.*

Special features of neurology

When the examination begins, the neurologist has a short list of the conditions that may be at the root of the symptoms. After the examination, the neurologist may feel that certain tests are necessary in order to be more certain of the diagnosis before treatment is started. For example, if someone complains of weakness down the left-hand side of the body, the neurologist will know, from the anatomy of the nervous system, that the actual disorder is situated on the opposite, right side of the brain. Further clues, such as speech disturbance, will make it possible to plot the site of brain lesions, often extremely accurately.

SKULL REPLACEMENT SURGERY

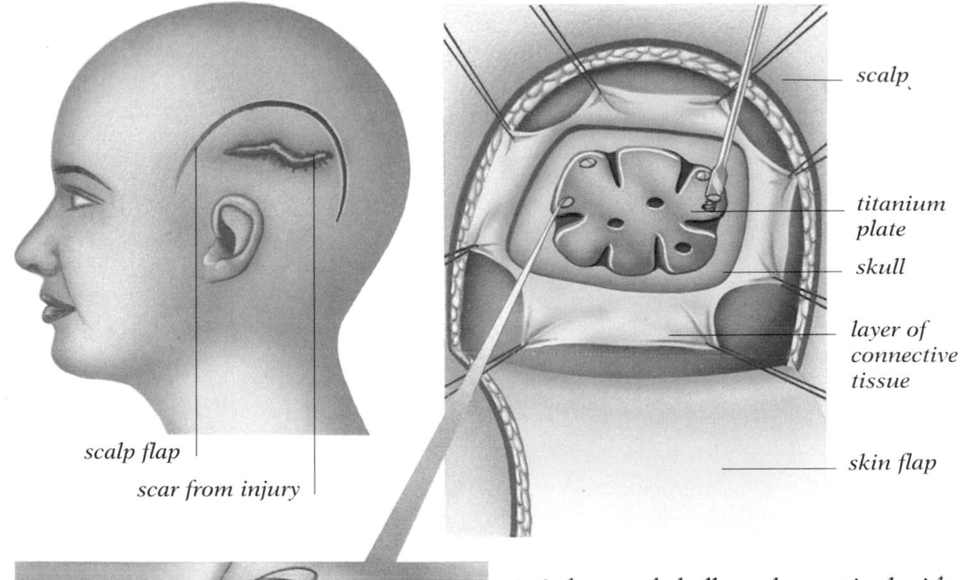

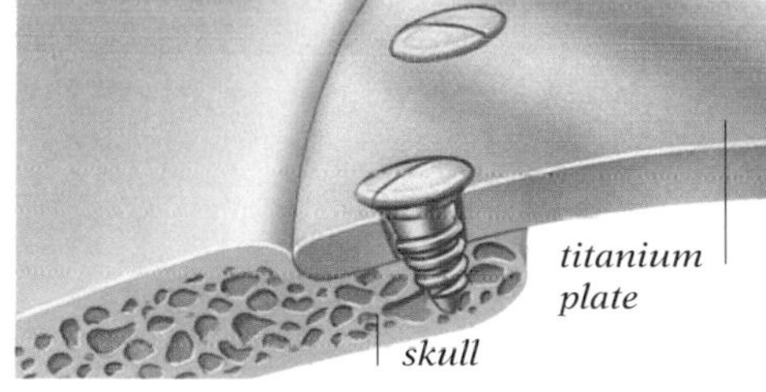

▲ *A damaged skull can be repaired with a plate (cranioplasty). Tissues are allowed to heal; then the head is shaved and the bone exposed. A plate made of plastic or a light alloy is screwed in to lie flat with the skull. The scalp is sewn back and new hair grows to cover the scar.*

Techniques of diagnosis

Neurologists use a range of tests, some of which assess the structure of various parts of the nervous system while others assess function. In the first group are the various X-ray and scanning techniques; in the second are tests of the electrical activity of the nervous system.

X rays: Ordinary X rays of the skull and spine are frequently performed in the initial assessment of many complaints, since the bones of the head and back may show signs of what is causing the trouble. It is often necessary to use X-ray dye to show up arteries, veins, or the space around the spinal cord in order to make a diagnosis: this procedure is called angiography.

When dye is introduced into the space around the spinal cord, by a lumbar puncture, the procedure is called myelography. This method is used to assess disorders of the spinal cord, especially when it is thought that there may be pressure on the nerves coming out of the spinal cord, as there is in sciatica, for example (see Sciatica).

Brain scans: Basically there are two main types of brain scan in use. Computerized tomography (CT) scans use a computer to assemble the information obtained by passing a series of X rays through the head to produce cross-sectional images or slices called tomograms. They create a detailed map or image of the inside of the brain.

An MRI scan produces pictures of the brain by picking up minute disturbances in the way its component atoms behave when they are subjected to radio waves from a magnet. No ionizing radiation is used, and no harm can come to the patient.

A further type is positron emission tomography (PET). A PET scan measures the uptake by the brain of molecules labeled with a radioactive substance, providing information on the functioning of the brain as well as structure.

Finally, isotope scans pick up the minute amount of radiation given off by a radioactive chemical injection and translate it into pictures that indicate the amount of blood circulating in the various compartments of the brain. Whole-body isotope scans are widely used to detect secondary cancer when a primary tumor is known to be present or is suspected (see Tumors).

Tests of nervous system function

These tests are designed to detect faults in the electrical working of different parts of the nervous system. For example, the

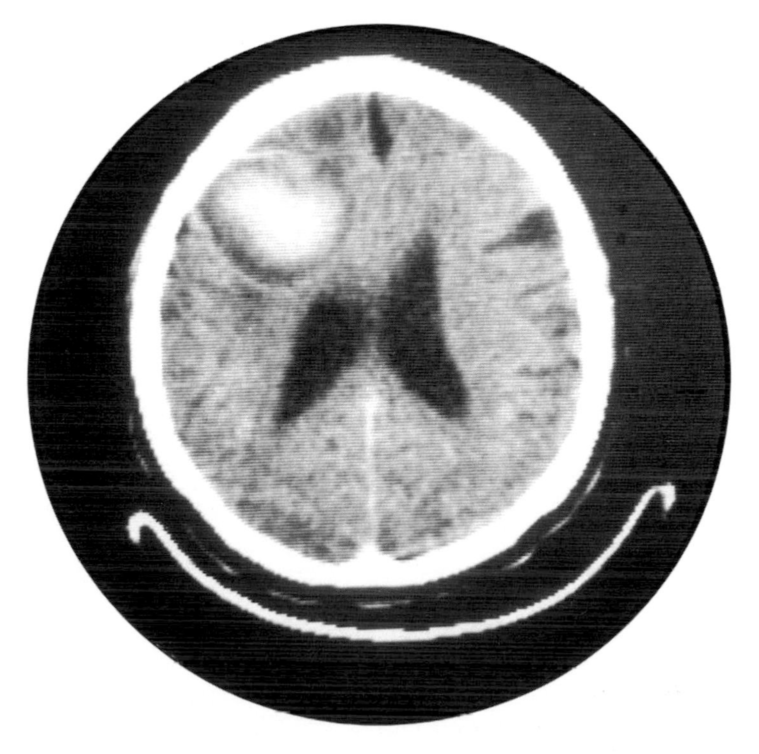

◄ *Computerized tomography (CT) is a form of brain scan. An X-ray tube exposes "slices" of the head, and a computer builds a picture or map of the interior of the brain.*

Questions and Answers

I need to have an angiogram. Will the dye that is injected cause me any harm?

Before you have your arterial X ray (angiogram), your doctor will ask you whether you are allergic to iodine, since the dye used is usually an iodine compound. Most people do notice a sensation of warmth in their bodies after the injection, but this soon passes.

Is it true that brain surgery can be performed under local anesthetic?

The brain itself can be probed and cut without its owner's feeling any pain. It is sometimes necessary for the patient to be conscious during a brain operation so that after the brain has been exposed, different parts can be gently stimulated electrically and by the sensations or movements produced, surgeons can identify the part they need to look at. Usually this procedure is carried out for severe epilepsy. However, most brain surgery is done under a general anesthetic.

My brother has been told he has a brain tumor and needs surgery. Will it cure him?

This very much depends on the type of tumor, how extensive it is, and where it lies in the brain. Many slow-growing tumors can be removed completely and only rarely recur. However, if even a benign tumor is in an awkward spot in the brain—say, near the speech centers—the surgeon may be reluctant to remove the lump completely if this would cause such extensive damage that the patient would become more disabled than if nothing had been done. Instead, the surgeon may opt for a limited operation, knowing that it may have to be repeated in the future.

Does a neurologist have to examine a patient to say brain death has occurred?

Brain death protocols require an EEG, but two doctors can declare someone brain-dead.

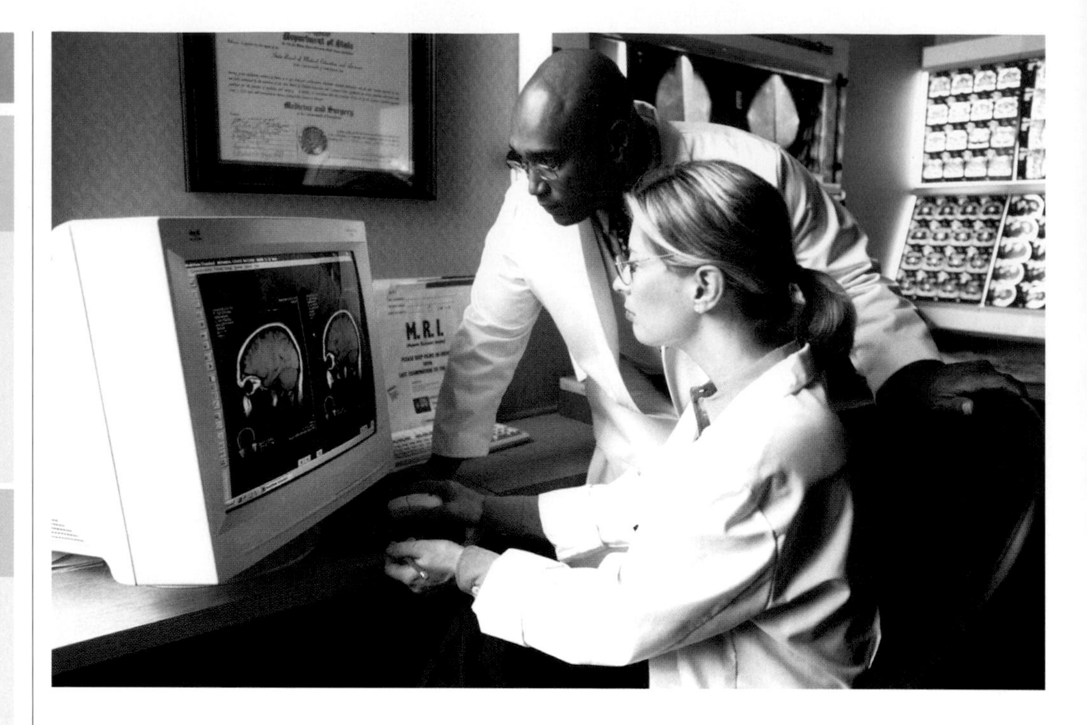

▲ *Doctors examine the results on a computer of a brain scan taken using magnetic resonance imaging (MRI).*

electroencephalogram is used to assess a patient who may be having a seizure at the time of the test. It is also possible to record EEGs over periods of 24 hours, thus picking up signs of seizures that may otherwise be overlooked (see Electroencephalogram).

In nerve conduction studies, the electrical functioning of the peripheral nerves is tested by stimulating them with a small electric current and measuring the speed with which this is conducted down the nerves. Both the EEG and nerve conduction studies are entirely harmless and painless.

Electromyography (EMG) tests the condition of the muscles by passing very fine needles into them and recording their activity. This causes only slight discomfort and gives useful information about inflammation or any other disorder in the muscles or their nerves (see Inflammation).

Blood tests can give much useful information about a person's general health, and a wide variety of blood tests are performed in the neurological unit.

Neurosurgery

Neurosurgery deals with disorders, including injuries to the nervous system, which require some kind of surgery for their treatment. The range is wide, taking in various congenital abnormalities such as spina bifida (in children), head injuries caused by war or traffic accidents, and the removal of tumors.

Neurosurgeons first train in the techniques of general surgery, then undergo a long specialized training. The most important advance in surgery in general and neurosurgery over the last few years has been the development of the technique of microsurgery.

Surgery of the nervous system uses special techniques, such as entering the brain by means of a bone flap in the skull, which can then be replaced after the operation. When parts of the skull itself have to be removed or have been severely damaged, a replacement can be made out of plastic or a light alloy such as titanium. Because of the costliness of hospital care, many people with neurological problems are given scans, EEGs, and other tests as outpatients. For those with disabilities, speech therapy, physical therapy, and occupational therapy can be provided in the home, backed up by general nursing help from a nurse practitioner. A patient's own physician will generally supervise these arrangements with the help and advice of neurological colleagues.

See also: Brain; Diagnostic imaging; Epilepsy; Head and head injuries; Lumbar puncture; Microsurgery; Nervous system; PET scanning; Scans; Spina bifida; X rays

Neuroses

Questions and Answers

I have always thought of myself as neurotic, and my previous doctor agreed. My new doctor says there is no such thing as a neurotic person. What am I to believe?

Experts no longer call nonpsychotic psychological disorders neuroses, because they now have more useful, descriptive terms. However, changing the names of disorders doesn't change their nature.

My aunt has a severe compulsive neurosis and is convinced that she is going insane. Is there a real risk that this will happen?

No. This kind of problem can cause severe disability because of the way it makes people behave, but it does not progress to a psychosis. There are effective treatments for this condition.

I suffer from a major phobic anxiety problem. I have been seeing a Freudian psychoanalyst for two years, and although he says that I am doing very well, I am not sure that there is any improvement. Should I continue?

There is no evidence that classical Freudian psychoanalysis can cure phobias. The current trend has moved away from this kind of treatment for any form of anxiety, since other treatments are more effective. Whether or not you continue depends on whether you are deriving any other benefit from the treatment. You must decide for yourself.

My psychiatrist says I have Briquet's syndrome. This sounds alarming. What is it?

Briquet's syndrome is one of several terms that have been used to describe what is now called a somatoform disorder. Another term for the condition is hysteria.

Psychiatrists in the United States seldom use the term "neurosis" anymore, but in popular language the word is still widely used to describe many psychological disorders of varying types.

The Scottish physician William Cullen introduced the term "neurosis" in 1769. By the end of the 19th century the term had been refined and limited to psychological disorders that were not psychotic or caused by organic disease (see Psychoses). Sigmund Freud made a further distinction between actual neuroses and psychoneuroses, categorizing anxiety neurosis and neurasthenia as actual neuroses, and anxiety hysteria (phobic anxiety), obsessive-compulsive neurosis, and pure hysteria as psychoneuroses.

In the late 1980s the term "neuroses" was almost abandoned in the United States, being replaced by several diagnostic classes such as anxiety disorders, mood disorders, somatoform disorders, and dissociative disorders. One difficulty with the new classification, however, is that it leaves no general term that covers the whole of this important group.

Anxiety disorders

Anxiety is a normal part of life, and it causes various familiar symptoms such as fast heart rate, dry mouth, diarrhea, sweating, wide pupils, restlessness, tingling in the fingers, "butterflies in the stomach," undue frequency of urination, shakiness, and fainting. Such everyday anxiety is called reactive anxiety, and it usually serves to alert people to danger.

Anxiety in the absence of a rational external cause is abnormal, and anxiety disorders include generalized anxiety disorder, panic disorder, agoraphobia, simple and social phobias, obsessive-compulsive disorder, and post-traumatic stress syndrome.

People who experience constant excessive or unrealistic anxiety over the normal circumstances of life are said to suffer from generalized anxiety disorder. This is differentiated

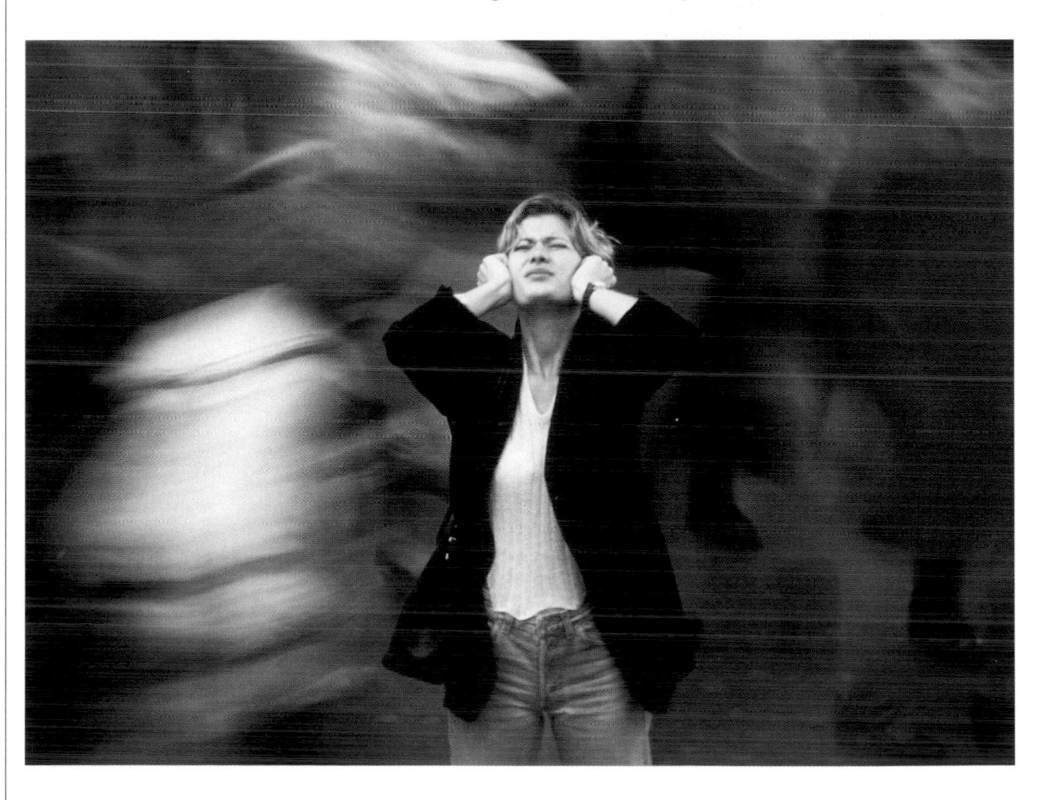

▲ *Agoraphobia is a specific type of anxiety disorder in which the affected person suffers from an exaggerated fear of being alone or being trapped in public places.*

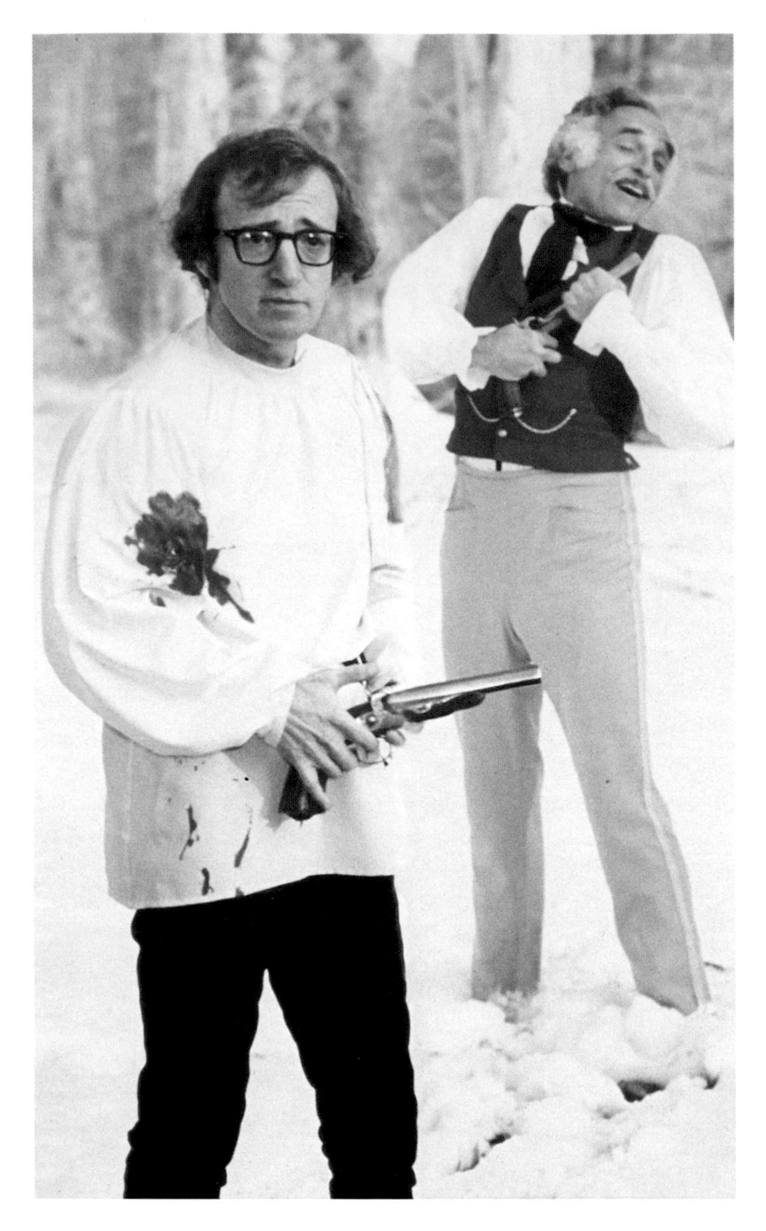

▲ *Woody Allen, who starred in* Love and Death, *has built his career on the caricature of an amusing neurotic. However, a neurotic's anxieties should always be taken seriously.*

from panic disorder, which is characterized by spontaneous episodes of intense anxiety that commonly occur about twice a week and usually last for less than an hour. Panic disorder is more common in women than in men and usually follows a traumatic episode. It is also closely associated with agoraphobia—a fear of venturing alone into public places or being trapped in a public place.

Phobias are abnormal and irrational fears that cause people to avoid normally harmless situations. Simple phobias are irrational fears of harmless objects; social phobias include fears of activities such as eating, speaking, or performing in public.

In a person suffering from an obsessive-compulsive disorder, the anxiety is associated with a repeated, uncontrollable urge to perform an unnecessary action, such as getting up at night, over and over, to check whether a door is locked. The affected person may keep changing a route to work out of a conviction that his or her presence might distract other drivers and cause an accident. The disorder may also involve a recurrent, usually unpleasant, thought that cannot be dismissed, such as a conviction of contamination that leads to obsessive hand-washing.

Post-traumatic stress disorder is a condition caused by a major traumatic event such as serious injury, assault, rape, or involvement in a disaster in which there has been much loss of life. The condition known during and after World War I as "shell shock" was post-traumatic syndrome. The disorder involves uncontrollable and persistent recollection of the details of the event, accompanied by frequent nightmares and a feeling of guilt.

Mood disorders

Extreme mood disorders, severe depression, and bipolar disorder fall into the class of the psychoses. However, there are two less serious mood disorders that could be considered neuroses. Dysthymia is a depressed mood with low self-esteem, feelings of hopelessness, constant fatigue, poor appetite or a tendency to overeat, and insomnia or a tendency to sleep too much. In children and adolescents it may involve irritability. Cyclothymia is similar to bipolar disorder but does not involve any true psychotic elements and is not caused by overuse of alcohol or recreational drugs.

Somatoform disorders

These disorders cause physical symptoms and signs in the affected person, which may sometimes be severe. However, the symptoms are not the result of organic disease but are brought on by purely psychological factors (see Hysteria).

Dissociative disorders

Disorders in this group are brought about by intolerable life circumstances. They include psychogenic amnesia, in which there is apparent loss of memory for selective past events; fugue, in which the affected person wanders off from his or her normal environment to start a new life elsewhere; and multiple personality disorder, in which two or more distinct personalities occur.

Treatment

Drugs that abolish or reduce the physical manifestations of fear can greatly relieve anxiety, and beta-blocking drugs that prevent adrenaline from acting are commonly used. Antidepressant drugs have been found to be helpful in treating panic disorder.

Anxieties, phobias, and compulsions can also respond to behavior therapy: a form of treatment in which the affected person is deliberately and repeatedly exposed to the stimuli that bring on the symptoms. These exposures are accompanied by skilled counseling and by training in relaxation and sometimes meditation (see Behavior Therapy), and the sufferer is gradually desensitized by the process. In some cases the whole family may have to be involved in the treatment. Insight-oriented therapy is designed to help the victim understand the origins of the anxiety. By such means, many of these distressing disorders can be brought under control in a far shorter period of time than was possible with earlier forms of treatment.

See also: **Anxiety; Bipolar disorder; Multiple personality; Neurasthenia; Obsessive-compulsive disorder; Phobias; Post-traumatic stress disorder; Therapy**

Nicotine

Questions and Answers

If nicotine is a stimulant, why do people need a cigarette to calm their nerves?

Nicotine produces an initial surge of adrenaline that increases heart rate and blood pressure. However, it also relaxes the muscles and causes dizziness, which leads to a feeling of lethargy and relaxation. If the dose is increased—when the smoker continues to smoke the cigarette—the original "up" reaction is countered by a "down" in bodily functions. When smokers want a cigarette to calm their nerves, they usually take long drags, unconsciously making sure they are taking in large doses of the drug to produce these calming, or sedative, effects.

Can I take such a large dose of nicotine that I will kill myself?

Not from smoking. You would need to smoke almost two packs of cigarettes, not just at a time, but in one huge inhalation. However, in spite of the almost immediate vomiting reflex, children can harm themselves by eating cigars or cigarettes. If you smoke, keep your cigarettes in a safe place so that small children cannot get hold of them.

If I stop smoking, will my body recover from the effects of nicotine, or will the damage cause effects later in life?

Most effects will pass. Your pancreas will return to normal, so if you do not already have duodenal ulcers, you may not develop them. Thickened arteries, due to nicotine, may cause problems later, but they will stop getting worse. The coagulation effect that nicotine has on the blood does not stop when nicotine is no longer taken into the body. The effect of nicotine on a fetus can be stopped when the mother quits smoking.

Nicotine is a highly toxic, addictive drug. Smoking can cause serious damage to smokers, to their children, and to a fetus. The stark reality is that smoking should be avoided at all costs.

Nicotine is obtained from the dried leaves of the tobacco plant (*Nicotiana tabacum*). The leaves contain 2 to 8 percent nicotine, which can be extracted as a colorless or pale yellow, oily liquid. Nicotine has an unpleasant, pungent smell and a persistent, sharp burning taste. Nicotine has been used as an insecticide, but because it is so dangerous it has largely been replaced by much safer substances.

Most people come into contact with nicotine through smoking. Inhaling tobacco smoke is a highly efficient means of absorbing nicotine into the body because the lungs are specialized organs for infusing the body's blood supply with inhaled gases; the surface of moist tissue brings oxygen—and nicotine—directly into contact with the blood supply.

Smokers absorb up to 95 percent of the nicotine they inhale. The fact that a smoker's heartbeat and blood pressure increase as early as one minute after the first puff of a cigarette gives some idea of how quickly the drug goes to work on the body. Small quantities of nicotine can also be inhaled by nonsmokers when others near them are smoking.

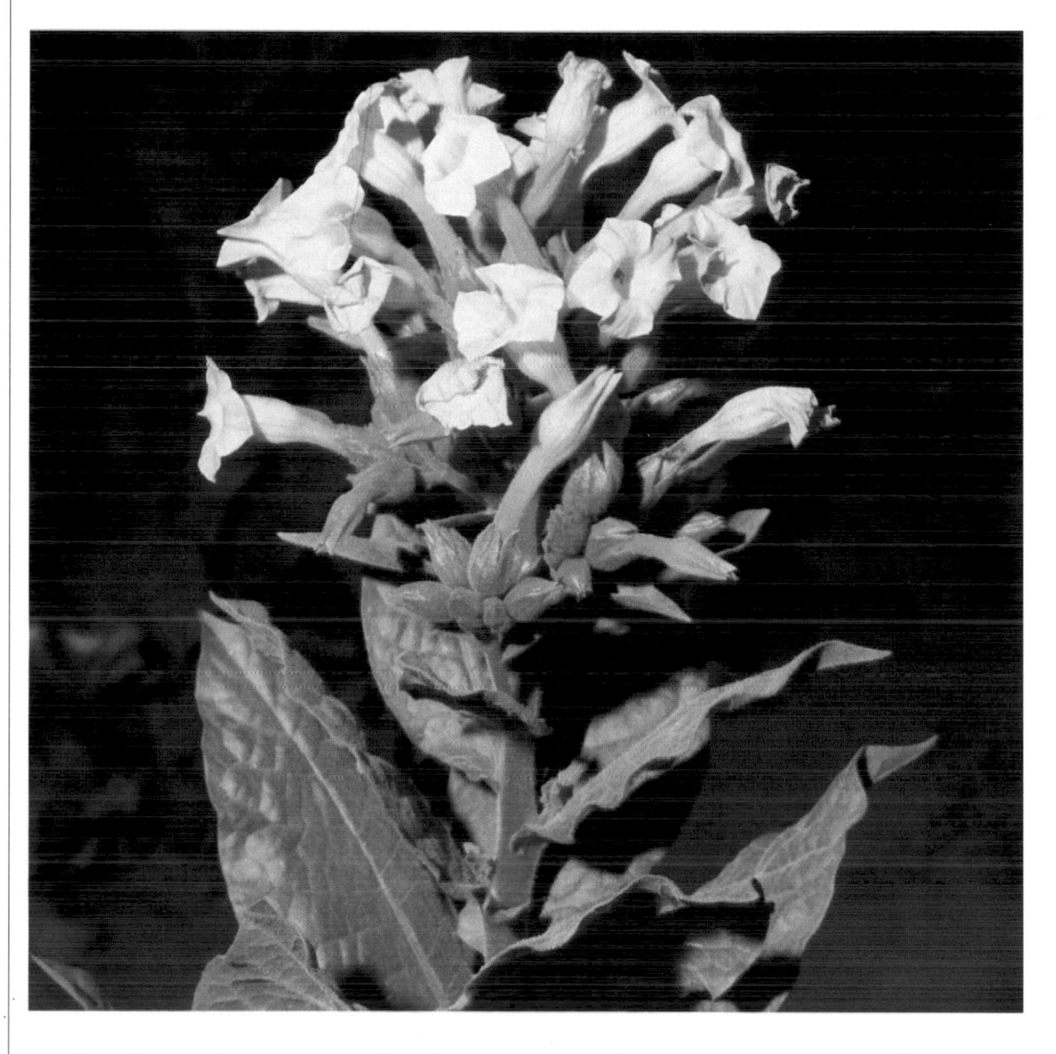

▲ *The tobacco plant originated in the Americas and was brought to Europe by 16th-century explorers.*

Stimulant and sedative

Nicotine has puzzling and contradictory effects on the body; it can both stimulate and sedate. The effect that is produced can depend either on the dose (small doses will stimulate, and large doses will sedate or even paralyze) or on the interval between doses. Sometimes a period of excitation is followed by a depression of bodily functions. At other times nicotine appears to reinforce the mood a person is in when he or she smokes a cigarette. For example, if a smoker is frightened or angry, nicotine will maintain this state of mind (see Moods).

How the body is affected

Nicotine stimulates the nerves that are activated by acetylcholine, a chemical transmitter of nerve impulses. Since these nerves radiate throughout the body, in the brain itself, and in the autonomic nervous system, the effects of nicotine on the body are widespread and diverse. Nicotine acts just like acetylcholine (see Nervous System).

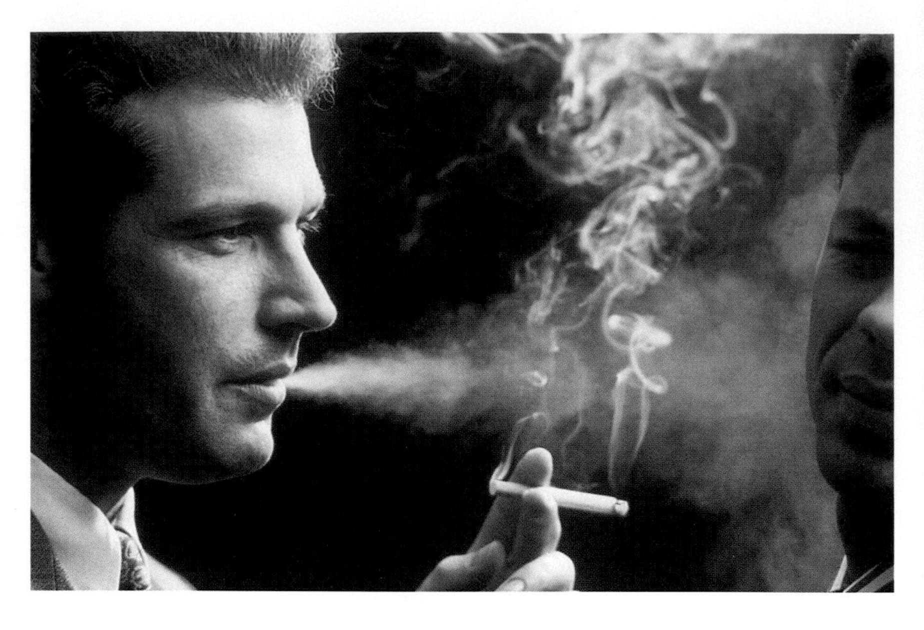

▲ *Cigarette smoke can irritate nonsmokers, and may cause them harm. For this reason, nonsmoking areas and smoking bans are very common.*

HOW NICOTINE AFFECTS THE BODY

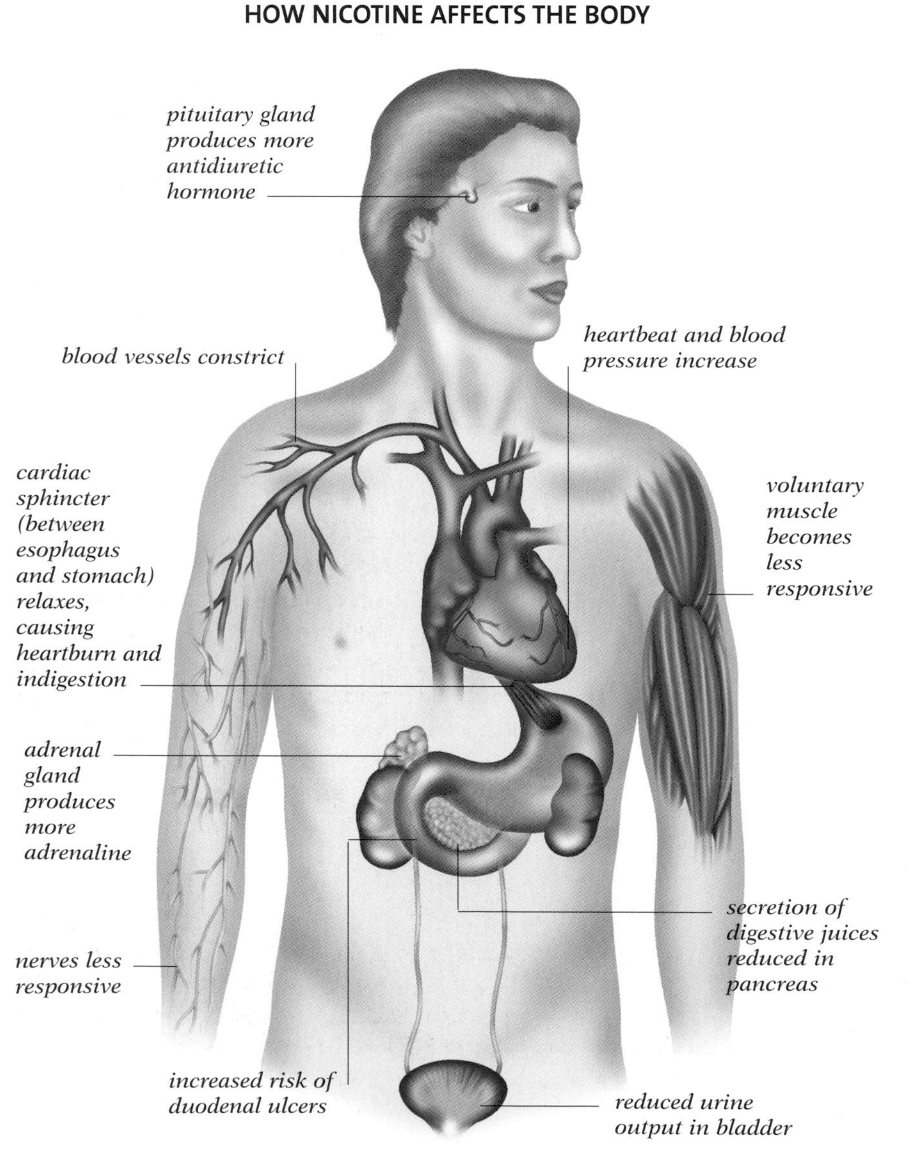

◄ *Some of the effects of nicotine on the nervous system, glands, muscles, and some of the major organs. Nicotine stimulates the adrenal glands to produce more adrenaline and the pituitary gland to produce antidiuretic hormone that reduces urine output. Nerves and muscles are less responsive; heartbeat increases.*

Nicotine stimulates the adrenal gland to produce adrenaline and noradrenaline, causing increases in blood pressure and heartbeat. It also constricts the arteries through which the blood pulses and increases the concentration of fatty acids in the blood. These acids encourage blood platelets (the part of the blood that coagulates) to stick together and to the walls of the blood vessels—the early stage of thrombosis.

Not only does smoking help to cause heart disease; it may have other undesirable effects on the heart. It speeds up the heart and, if the coronary arteries are already narrowed, it may cause the symptom angina as a result of the increased demand by the heart muscle for blood. It can also cause premature heartbeats, which are followed by a compensatory pause. It is possible that these effects might be caused by secondary smoking, which is the passive inhalation by nonsmokers of smoke exhaled by smokers (see Heart Disease).

It is important to understand, however, that although nicotine is the reason why people smoke, it is not the principal reason why smoking is so dangerous. Tobacco smoke tar contains more than 2,000 distinguishable ingredients, and some of these are cancer-causing agents. Some are extremely damaging to the cells lining the air passages to the lungs. They are the principal cause of chronic

► *It is easy to see that the concentration of nicotine in the blood and the heartbeat rate both rise sharply when a cigarette is smoked and both take about an hour to return to normal.*

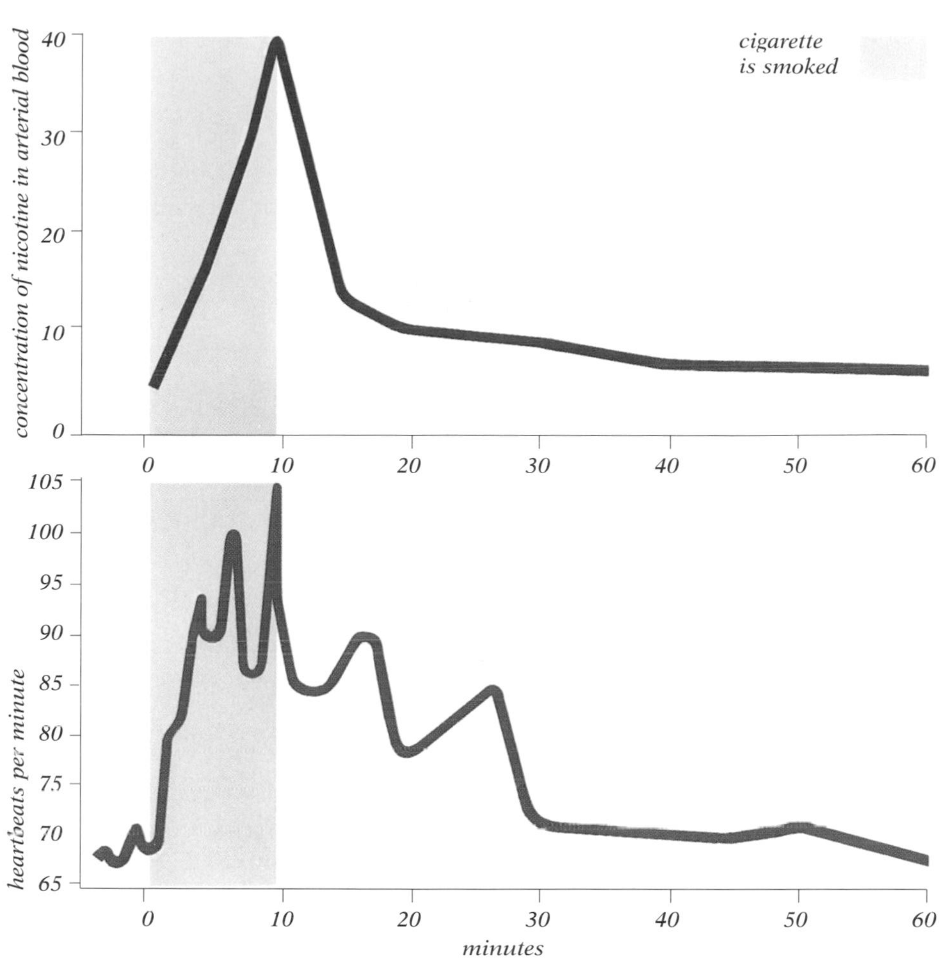

bronchitis, emphysema, and a potentially fatal condition, chronic obstructive pulmonary disease (COPD).

Smokers are not the only ones at risk. In pregnancy the fetus can be affected. Nicotine and other tobacco products have been found in the amniotic fluid of mothers who smoke but are absent in all nonsmokers. These pass through the placenta and may cause congenital malformations.

Animal studies showed that high doses of nicotine caused fetal abnormalities, although the doses were much higher than those that would be inhaled by cigarette smoking. However, nicotine can drastically affect the fetus by causing the mother's brain to release the hormone oxytocin, which causes uterine contractions and constricts the flow of blood to the uterus and placental bed. Babies of smokers can thus be starved of oxygen and have a much higher chance of being born with a lower-than-average birth weight, of being stillborn, or of dying very young.

Nicotine poisoning

In its pure form, nicotine is rapidly absorbed through the skin. A fatal dose brings death from respiratory failure in a matter of minutes. Less severe poisoning results in nausea, stomach pains, diarrhea, dizziness, mental confusion, disturbed hearing and vision, faintness, convulsions, and sweating. Chronic poisoning, a condition found in exceptionally heavy smokers, has in the past been thought to be the cause of local irritation of the respiratory tract as well as digestive and nutritional disturbances, constriction of blood vessels, high blood pressure, and sometimes impairment of sight. The current view, however, is that most of these effects are due to substances other than nicotine. Tobacco amblyopia (blindness) is no longer believed to be an effect of nicotine.

For nicotine to have the toxic effects mentioned, a person would need to take about 0.02 ounce (567 mg) in a single dose. The nicotine from one small cigar, if it was injected intravenously, would kill an adult. When it is smoked, only 10 percent of the drug is actually inhaled. An average medium-tar cigarette yields 1–2 mg of nicotine for absorption, so it would be necessary to smoke 20 to 30 cigarettes very quickly to produce a toxic dose. However, the long period of time it takes to smoke a fatal dose allows the body enough time to deactivate some of the drug. The level of nicotine in the body and the dramatic effects nicotine produces fall as rapidly as they rise. Nicotine in cigarettes cannot be used as a means of suicide—even when children have swallowed large numbers of cigarettes, this rarely leads to death, because the body reacts quickly, and vomiting is the first indication that nicotine poisoning has occurred.

Addiction

The vast majority of researchers now agree that nicotine is addictive and that generally smokers unconsciously establish a nicotine level. For example, when smokers are given high-nicotine cigarettes, it is noticeable that they will involuntarily decrease the number of times they inhale; when they are given low-nicotine cigarettes, they will increase inhalation until the desired amount of nicotine is absorbed.

People who give up smoking show marked withdrawal symptoms. Craving is followed by tension, irritability, restlessness, depression, and difficulty in concentrating. Physically, there is a fall in blood pressure and heart rate, and gastrointestinal changes take place that often lead to constipation and sleep disturbances. Motor functions can also be impaired, leading to poor performance of activities such as driving a car or operating machinery.

Nicotine addiction is a habit that can be broken, and the body will recover from most of the harmful effects. To help overcome the physical symptoms of withdrawal, some people find that over-the-counter nicotine chewing gum or patches can help to reduce the craving (see Withdrawal Symptoms). The problem can be discussed with a doctor; he or she should be able to advise on how to obtain these aids and how to use them to their best advantage.

See also: **Arteries and artery disease; Heartburn; Lung and lung diseases; Pancreas and disorders; Poisoning; Pregnancy; Smoking; Thrombosis; Vomiting**

Night blindness

Night blindness, in which the eye cannot adjust quickly from bright to dim light, poses a problem chiefly for people who drive at night. This rare condition usually results from poor nutrition and is easily treated in most cases.

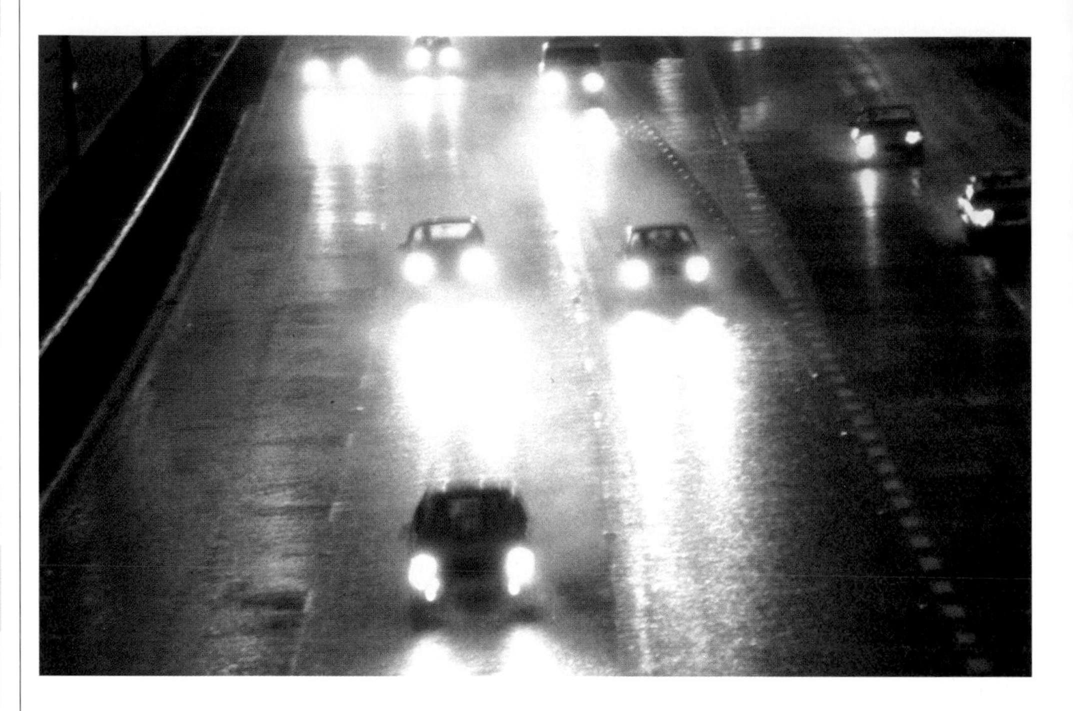

▲ *Anyone affected by night blindness should seek treatment before driving after dark.*

The term "night blindness" is misleading, since the condition does not involve a total loss of sight at night. A person affected by the disorder will, however, experience greater loss of vision when lighting is restricted than is usual for most other people.

The most common cause of night blindness is a deficiency of vitamin A in a person's diet. Vitamin A is vital in the transition from day to night vision.

In the retina—the light-sensitive area at the back of the eye—there are two types of sight nerve endings: cones and rods. The cones are densely clustered around the center of the retina and are stimulated only by bright light. Their function is to perceive color and fine detail. The rods—found mainly on the outside of this area—are almost unable to operate in daylight. They respond to very low levels of light intensity, thus enabling objects to be seen in poor light.

Rods contain a light-sensitive pigment called rhodopsin, or visual purple, which needs to be activated to achieve night vision. Vitamin A is needed for this activation—hence a lack of it results in a decreased visual adaptability to dim lighting. A genetic deficiency of rhodopsin is another relatively rare but important cause of night blindness (see Blindness and Braille).

Symptoms and treatment

In most people the transition to "rod vision" takes up to 30 minutes. People with night blindness not only see less far and in less detail but also take much longer to adapt to night vision.

This reduced adaptability is particularly important in relation to night driving. A driver with night blindness sees the headlights of an approaching vehicle as well as anybody else. However, when it has passed he or she will take longer to adjust to the renewed darkness, and for a while will be able to see only a short distance ahead.

Most cases of night blindness are treated with vitamins A and D. Improvement is quite rapid and is usually permanent.

See also: **Eyes and eyesight; Vitamin A**

Questions and Answers

Do people with night blindness have normal vision in the day?

Yes. People with night blindness have nothing wrong with their vision as such and can see perfectly well in daylight.

Is it true that night blindness has something to do with glaucoma?

No. Glaucoma is a condition in which the pressure of the fluid inside the eye rises so that the retina may become damaged. One form of glaucoma can cause the sufferer to see colored haloes around lights—this is perhaps how the confusion has arisen.

If I take extra vitamin A, will I see better at night?

Not unless you already have some degree of night blindness due to vitamin A deficiency. People who work at night sometimes eat foods rich in vitamin A in the belief that it will improve their night vision, but there is no evidence that this will happen unless they are deficient in the vitamin.

I find it difficult to distinguish objects in the dark. What can I do?

If you have night blindness due to vitamin deficiency, the quickest cure would be to take halibut liver oil capsules. This oil is one of the best sources of vitamin A.

Other than a poor diet, what else can cause vitamin A deficiency?

A high-protein diet may cause a deficiency because the body uses up the vitamin much faster when converting protein into body tissue and energy. Vitamin A stores are also used up during a high fever, or by taking certain drugs. Some intestinal diseases can interfere with vitamin A absorption.

Noise

A dripping tap, the roar of traffic, or midnight music from the apartment next door are all examples of noise, a form of pollution that is at best an irritation and at worst a serious danger to health.

Noise can be defined as any unwanted sound. It may include continuous city traffic, an inconsiderate neighbor's late-night party, or damaging infrasound—noise below the level that people are able to hear—from aircraft. In extreme cases, the irritation caused by unendurable noise can lead to violence, damage to the body, and even mental illness.

Noise sends unwanted energy impulses along the hearer's auditory nerves. These impulses can give rise to feelings of anger; for example, people who are unable to get to sleep because of noisy neighbors can become infuriated to the point of using actual violence.

Studies suggest that some people are more sensitive to noise than others; it is thought that a more outgoing person is able to tolerate a greater degree of noise. Nevertheless, governments in developed nations are aware that noise is a form of pollution from which everyone needs protection at some point.

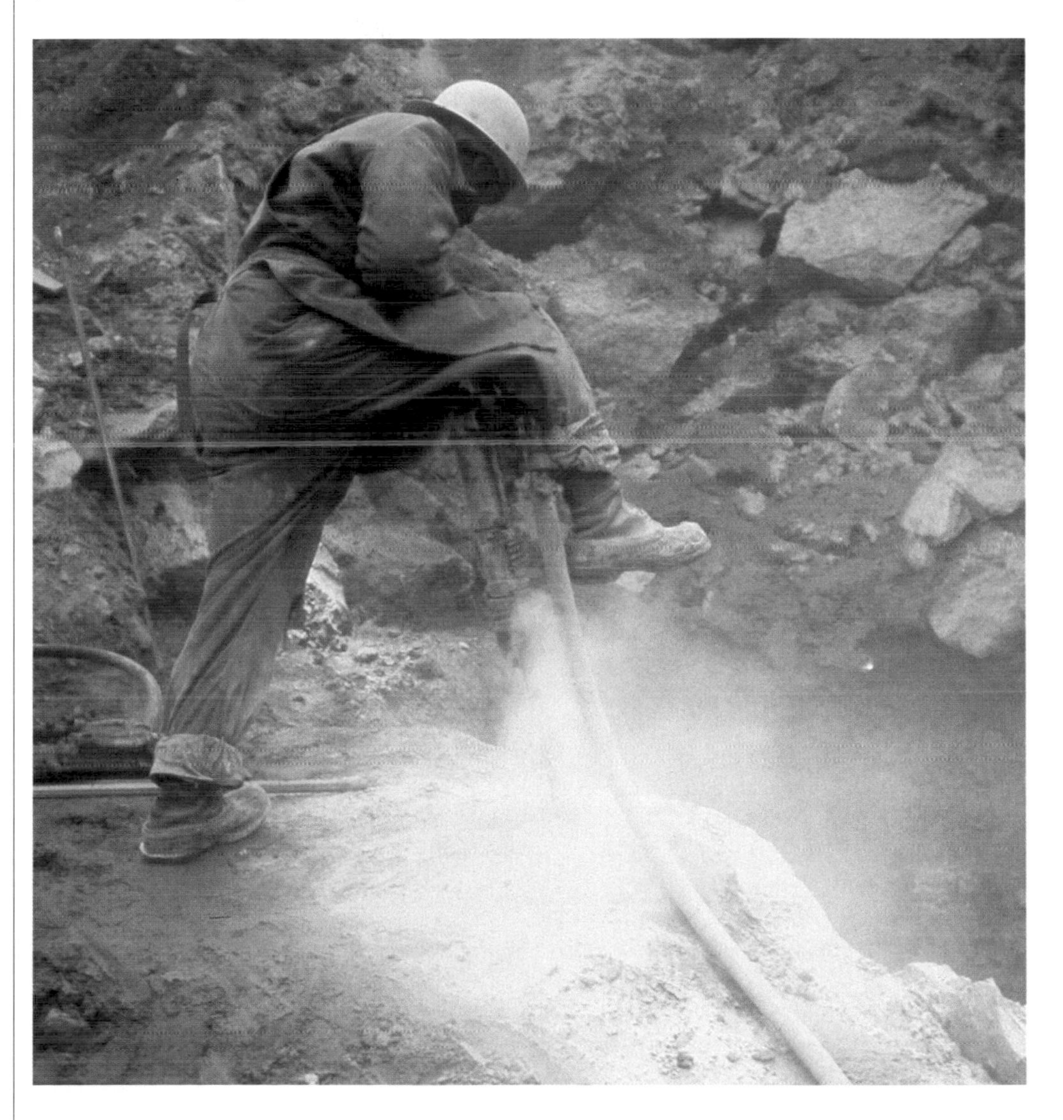

▲ *The noise from a pneumatic drill is annoying to passers-by and is dangerous for operators unless they wear some form of protection for their ears.*

Questions and Answers

My teenage daughter loves to go to nightclubs. Could her hearing be damaged by loud music?

Some nightclubs have amplified music pounding at well over the danger level. Try to persuade your daughter to take a few nights off between clubs to give her hearing time to recover. Also, she should not get too close to any band that is playing or to the amplification system, where the noise is loudest. Some musicians and DJs are themselves in danger of going deaf as a result of many years' exposure to loud music.

I can't sleep at my sister's house because of the chiming of her grandfather clock, yet she says she never hears it. Is this unusual?

No, not at all. One person's annoying noise can be another's lullaby. We all become used to familiar noises in our environment and almost cease to hear them. City dwellers who visit the country may find it difficult to sleep in the relative silence and are kept awake by the occasional moo of a cow, whereas at home they slumber happily against a background of loud traffic noise. Because people vary so much in the sort of noise they can tolerate, it is very difficult to gather data on the subject.

My son works in a factory where employees are given ear protection against the noise of machinery, but my son will not wear his; he says they are uncomfortable. How can I persuade him to wear them?

Try explaining to him in vivid terms what damage to hearing is like. For example, it might involve not being able to hear the top notes in favorite pieces of music; not hearing a sports commentary on television clearly; and not being able to converse with friends in a noisy environment.

Questions and Answers

I have to be at work by 6:00 A.M., so I have to get to bed early; however, my next-door neighbor plays his stereo until very late and often has all-night parties. I am not antisocial, but how do I get some uninterrupted rest?

This is a difficult problem because people feel entitled to their own way of life. Try inviting your neighbor in and calmly explaining the problem. If possible, let him hear just how much noise is audible from his house when he is playing music. Make your tone reasonable, not complaining: if he is a considerate person, he will appreciate your problem.

If the neighbor ignores your request, you will have to call the police. They will probably issue a warning and stop the noise for the time being, but it may not be a permanent solution.

I find that I can tolerate loud traffic noise and all the other noise hazards of living in a city, but a small, continuous noise—such as an unidentified rattle in the car or a dripping faucet—drives me frantic. Is this odd?

No. Humans are adaptable, and many city dwellers are accustomed to noisy surroundings. It is when we expect an environment to be free of unwanted sound and find that it is not that we react with irritation. It is wise to try to deal with unwanted sound as soon as possible, because hearing it constantly can lead to tension.

I've been told that sound we can't hear is just as dangerous as audible noise. Is this true?

No, it isn't. In general, audible noise is a far more serious danger. However, people exposed to infrasound—sound so low that they cannot actually hear it—often suffer from headaches, fatigue, and visual disturbances. Also, if the intensity of the nonaudible sound were increased sufficiently, it could cause such damage to the internal organs that death would follow.

The effects of audible noise

Research into noise has found that it can produce various effects on the human body, including inflammation of the lining of the stomach and the brain, and constriction of the precapillaries (tiny blood vessels). In a laboratory experiment, volunteers were subjected to "white noise"—noise that is a mixture of different frequencies of 90 decibels (dB). ("Frequency" refers to the number of vibrations of a sound wave per second. Decibels are units of comparison; in the case of noise they compare loudness with an accepted standard.) The experiment found that there was a change in the volunteers' diastolic pressure—the background pressure of the blood measured when the heart is relaxed between beats.

Experiments on volunteers in Italy showed that exactly three seconds after a noise of 87 dB started, arterioles (small blood vessels) contracted, cutting the blood in them by half. After the noise had ceased, the arterioles took a full five minutes before they returned to normal.

Noise affects the heart directly through stimulation of the nervous system and indirectly by changing the dynamics of the vascular (circulatory) system. It is thought—although research on this is not yet conclusive—that noise may contribute to heart attacks and possibly strokes.

Tests on the impact of noise on the eye showed that the blood vessels on the retina dilate and so affect the functioning of the eye. It was found that workers in a noisy environment had to readjust their depth of focus continually, and that this could possibly be the cause of headaches.

Infrasonic noise

The above are the effects of noise at levels that are audible. There are also the effects of infrasonic noise, which is loosely defined as noise below the threshold of hearing, or nonaudible noise. Infrasound works on the body through the internal organs, setting up a kind of friction (rubbing) between them. It can provoke an irritation so intense that for hours afterward any low-

NOISE LEVELS

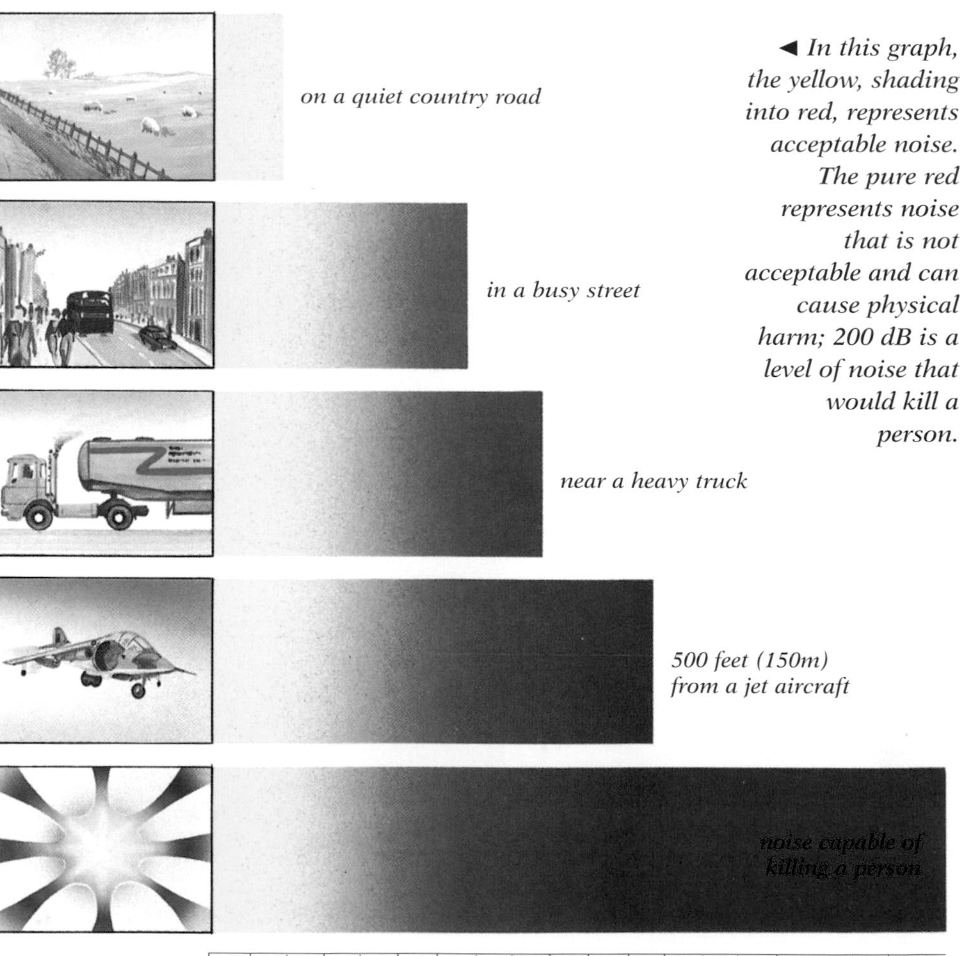

◄ *In this graph, the yellow, shading into red, represents acceptable noise. The pure red represents noise that is not acceptable and can cause physical harm; 200 dB is a level of noise that would kill a person.*

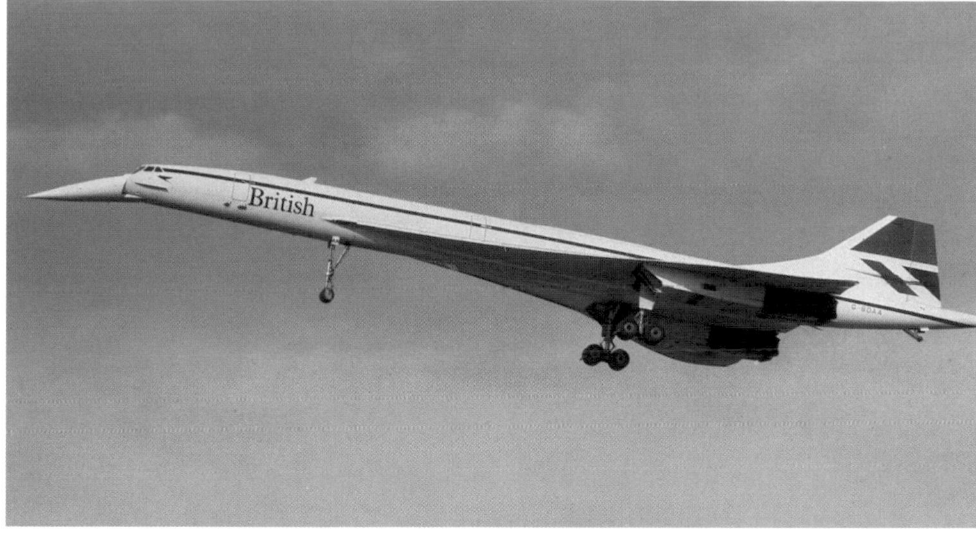

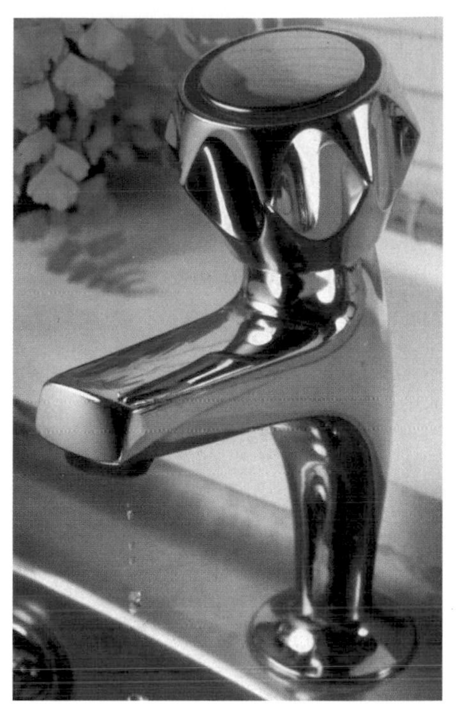

▲ *Sonic booms from supersonic aircraft are often startling; however, in some circumstances they can also cause actual damage to livestock and property.*

► *A dripping faucet may disturb the sleep of someone who can tolerate other noises.*

pitched sound seems to echo through the body. Tests of infrasonic noise on volunteers cause reactions such as headaches, choking, coughing, visual blurring, and fatigue. If a person is subjected to infrasonic noise at a very low level, he or she is unable to do any mental work, even simple arithmetic. As the intensity of the noise is increased, the person develops dizziness, nervous fatigue, and the symptoms of seasickness. At very high intensities, a person's internal organs would vibrate and the final result would be a quick, but painful, death.

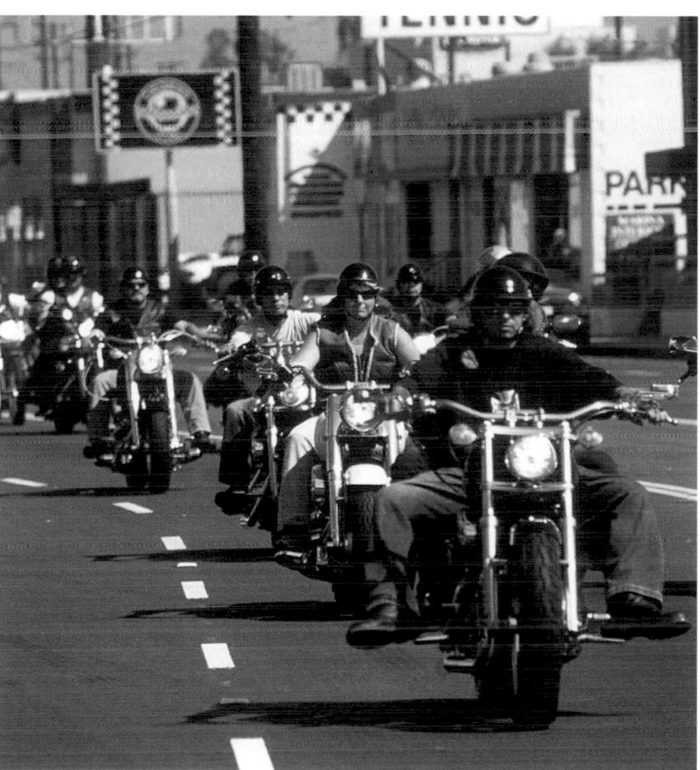

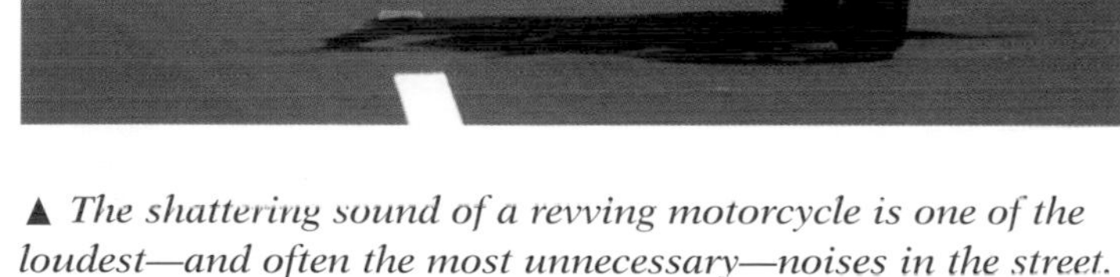

▲ *The shattering sound of a revving motorcycle is one of the loudest—and often the most unnecessary—noises in the street.*

Industrial hazards

Damage to hearing due to working in a noisy environment has been recognized for a long time, but it is difficult to quantify. Many employees have come to accept noise as just an unavoidable working condition. In many such cases, hearing impairment has been put down to age. However, it is now widely accepted that prolonged exposure to noise during the working day can result in a greater or lesser degree of hearing loss. This is particularly true of people who work with noisy machinery.

High levels of acoustic power—over about 90 dB—are known to cause actual destructive changes to the hair cells of the hearing mechanism in the cochlea. An explosion close to the ear can totally destroy the hearing function by literally shaking the hearing mechanism to pieces. For example, military personnel have been deafened by unprotected exposure to the sound of nearby gunfire, and children can be deafened by a slap on the ear.

A pattern of gradual hearing loss has emerged from studies of people in various occupations. Initially, it has been found, there is temporary dullness of hearing after a day's exposure to noise at work, and there may also be some noise in the ears (tinnitus). These are the first signs that some damage is being done to a person's hearing. The tinnitus can take various forms—it may be a rushing or hissing sound, or it may be more musical; it can also persist for minutes or even hours after severe exposure to noise. However, since both dullness of hearing and tinnitus tend to disappear after a few hours away from noise, such symptoms are likely to be ignored by the worker. In addition, symptoms tend to diminish as he or she gets used to the noisy environment. The next stage is reached when the individual notices that his or her hearing has become impaired—however, by this point the damage is irreversible.

Protective equipment and legislation against unduly high levels of noise have been introduced in most developed countries.

However, there is a problem in that much machinery still needs to be modified or redesigned if acceptable noise levels are to become the norm. This entails more research into the problem, since there are probably too little data available at present to convince industry of the necessity to make what will inevitably be costly changes.

Experiments with noise levels in offices have shown that with noise reduction comes an increase in efficiency. When noise levels in one office were reduced by 20 percent, it was found that the keyboardists' output was considerably greater than that of others working at the original high level of noise.

Traffic problems

As towns and cities increase in size, so too does the traffic traveling through them. Private transportation—automobiles and motorcycles—can be noisy, but by far the greatest proportion of noise comes from commercial diesel-engine vehicles such as trucks. The major source of high-frequency noise on the roads is airborne engine noise resulting from the combustion process and the design characteristics of engine structures. The main source of low-frequency noise is engine exhaust and engine inlet noise.

Highways have brought not only convenience but also a high level of traffic noise into previously quiet areas, disturbing many people's lives. It has been estimated that 8 dB can be considered a typical level of noise of this type. Therefore, many small towns and country areas now come into the loud-noise category, with the resultant disturbance to people's sleep and privacy.

Aircraft noise

Aircraft noise is second only to traffic noise as a source of annoyance. As more people are on the move worldwide, air travel is increasing constantly. Supersonic jets have added to the noise problem.

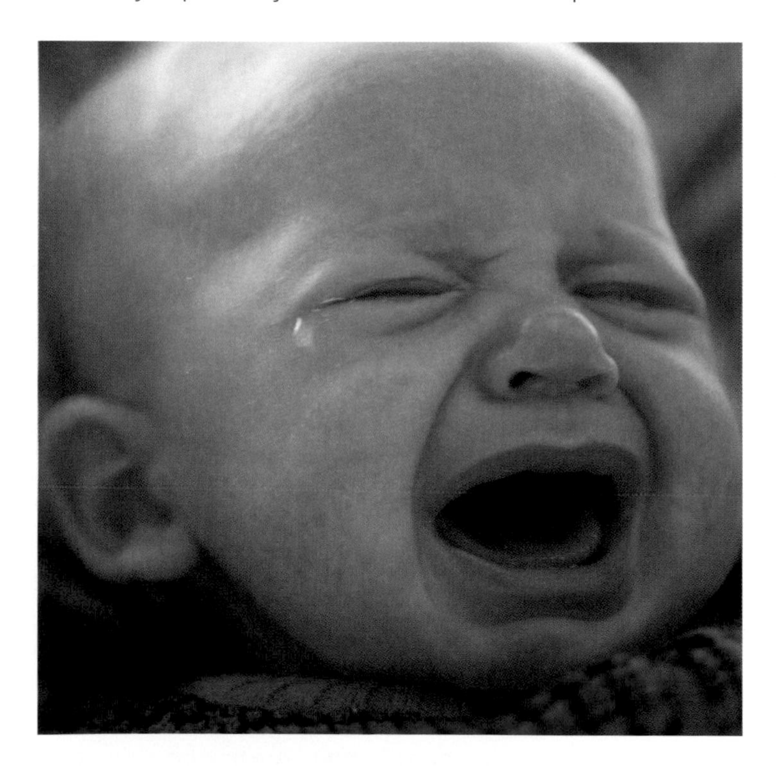

▲ *A baby's cry is particularly stressful to endure. However, it seems to be nature's way of ensuring that the child's needs will be met by parents or caregivers as quickly as possible.*

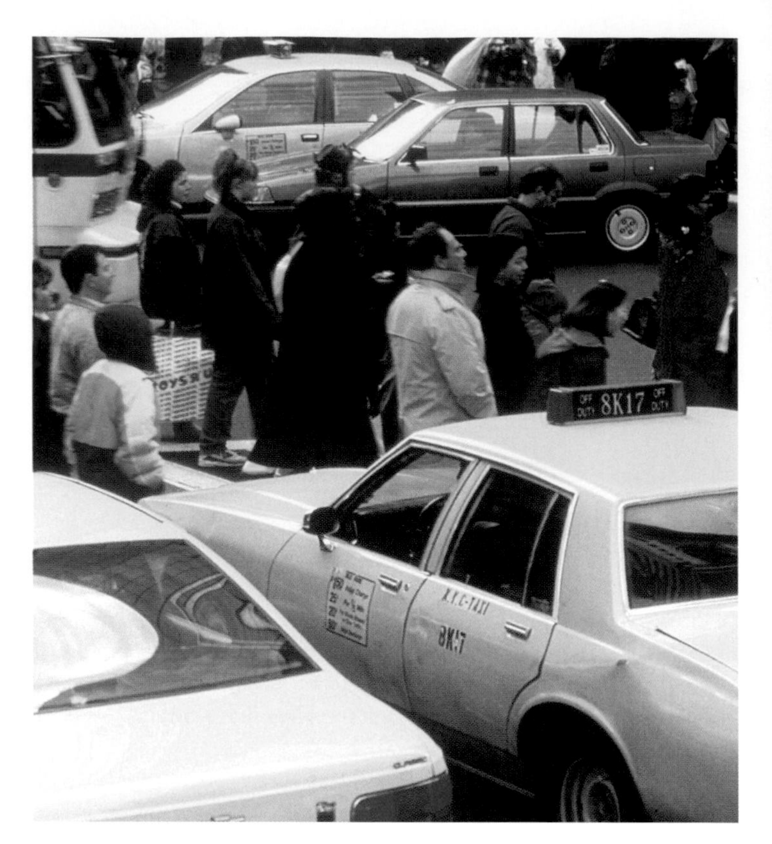

▲ *The ever-increasing volume of automobiles on urban roads has added to the noise pollution suffered by city inhabitants.*

Many airports are situated in built-up areas; as a result, the inhabitants of those areas are subjected to constant aircraft noise. According to a survey carried out near Heathrow Airport on the outskirts of London, eight times as many people living in the area were admitted to mental hospitals as living in places not affected so badly by noise.

While it may prove impractical to reduce present levels of air traffic or noise from aircraft, more can be done in planning for future control. Wherever new airports are planned, people are putting pressure on the authorities to locate them away from densely populated areas. In addition, new planes are being designed to be much quieter than present models.

Currently, people who live near airports have to put up with the noise and its disturbance to their sleep and lives more generally. House insulation is not a full solution. They also have to live with the underlying fear of the possibility of plane crashes in their area.

Outlook

As more people become aware of the hazards of noise and more research is carried out that confirms the dangers, greater pressure can be put on governments and other authorities to reduce noise levels in society. Noise pollution tends to be rather a vague subject with which to contend, since there is no average reaction to any one type of noise. However, people are much more likely to protest against pollution of all kinds and damage to their environment, and this should lead to future improvements.

See also: **Deafness: Headache; Hearing; Occupational hazards; Pollution; Tinnitus**

Noninsulin-dependent diabetes

Questions and Answers

My cousin developed diabetes at the age of 12 and has had to take insulin shots ever since. She has had eye complications with internal bleeding. I have now been diagnosed with type II diabetes, but I have been assured that similar complications are unlikely in my case. Is this true?

Very likely, but complications can occur in this kind of diabetes. The essential thing is to keep blood sugar levels within normal limits. If this is done, complications should not occur.

I am very overweight and have developed diabetes. My doctor has not prescribed insulin but tells me that the condition can be cured if I lose weight. She says that the disease is caused by my obesity. My three sisters are also very heavy but none of them has diabetes. How is this possible?

The kind of diabetes you have is called noninsulin-dependent diabetes, and most cases are caused by obesity. Different people produce different amounts of insulin; your sisters produce enough for their needs, but you can't, so you must lose weight.

I'm worried by all this talk about the complications of diabetes. What are they, exactly?

Complications develop usually over a period of years, so they are more common in older people who have been diabetic from youth. But they can also affect people who become diabetic later in life. They include eye damage that can lead to blindness, kidney damage, and damage to arteries that can lead to heart attacks, strokes, and gangrene. They can be avoided if diabetes is properly controlled.

Not all diabetics need insulin injections, but for those not taking insulin it is essential to ensure that the body's own insulin production is adequate. Noninsulin-dependent diabetes (NIDD) is not a trivial condition and it can have serious complications.

Diabetes is a condition in which blood glucose is too high and insulin, which helps glucose from food get into the cells, is either absent or inadequate in quantity. Insulin-dependent diabetes or type I diabetes is a common type of diabetes that is usually first diagnosed in young people. The insulin-producing cells of the pancreas no longer make insulin, because they have been destroyed by an autoimmune disease process, in which the body's own immune system attacks the insulin-producing cells.

Noninsulin-dependent diabetes is a type of diabetes that usually affects older people. Insulin is still produced by the pancreas but in quantities insufficient for the body's overall needs. It is also known as type II diabetes, or maturity-onset diabetes. The latter term is less often used today, because it is now recognized that noninsulin-dependent diabetes can also

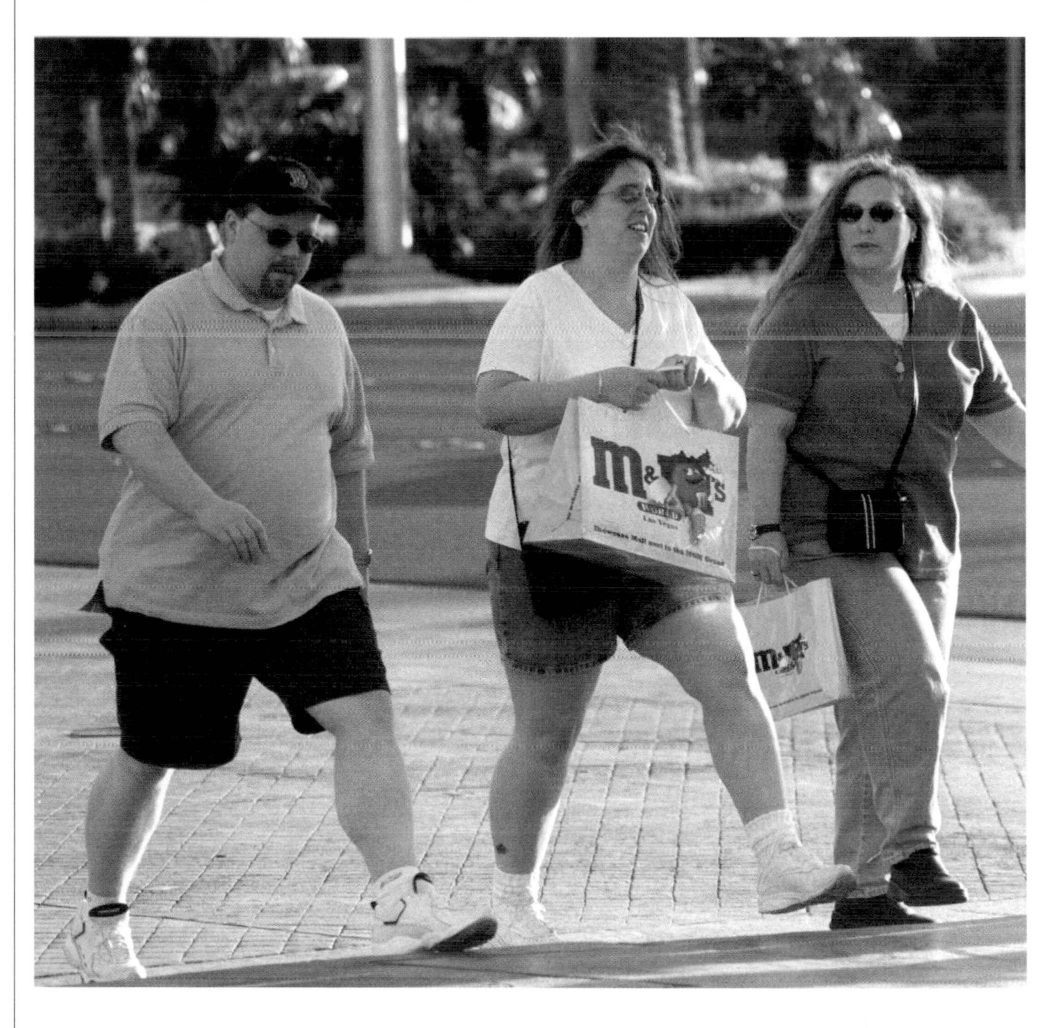

▲ *Overweight people are more likely to develop noninsulin-dependent diabetes. Because it develops slowly, the condition may be undetected for years.*

affect young people, even those as young as 15. Noninsulin-dependent diabetes, however, usually starts between the ages of 50 and 65. It may occur in people older than 65, and it may also have a genetic factor and run in families. This type of diabetes usually starts with insulin resistance, a condition in which the cells cannot use insulin properly. At first, more insulin is made to compensate, but eventually the pancreas loses the ability to secrete insulin.

Diabetes can be best understood by a simple account of the action of insulin. The outer membranes of many body cells, including muscle, fat, liver, and brain cells, are penetrated by shaped sites called insulin receptors. Part of the receptor is on the exterior of the cell and part is in the interior of the cell. The outer parts are shaped to fit insulin molecules exactly. When an insulin molecule locks onto a receptor site, a sequence of reactions occurs within the cell; these include production of proteins and DNA and the movement of glucose transporter units to the outer membrane, where they can pick up glucose and carry it into the cell.

Glucose is the principal energy-giving fuel, which is used by all the cells of the body. Insulin locking also promotes the passage into the cell of amino acids, which are the building bricks of proteins.

None of these reactions can happen unless insulin locks onto the insulin receptors. If there is no insulin, or if the supply is inadequate, the effect on cells is very serious; and because glucose cannot get into the cells, it accumulates in the tissue spaces and in the blood, and then is excreted in the urine.

Causes of noninsulin-dependent diabetes

A principal, but not the sole, cause of NIDD is obesity. About 80 percent of people with NIDD are obese. For reasons that are not fully understood, obesity is associated with a state known as insulin resistance. It may simply be that the number of insulin receptor sites is inadequate, or it may be that the mechanisms triggered in the cell by insulin locking are adversely affected.

In people with NIDD, a rise in the levels of glucose in the blood does not result in a normal healthy increase in the production of insulin. A simplified explanation is that, while the limited amount of insulin the pancreas can produce may be enough to keep a thin person healthy, there will not be enough insulin if that person should become obese. There is also evidence that there is a genetic element in the causation of NIDD, and about one in three people with NIDD has a relative who is also affected with the disorder. It is known that people with severe insulin resistance often have mutations (errors) in the genes that code for the insulin receptors. Another factor in the cause of NIDD is that a wealthier society tends to take in more food, leading to a rise in obesity, and hence a rise in the condition (see Obesity).

Symptoms

The symptoms are similar in the two types of diabetes. The basic symptoms are an excessive output of urine, persistent and severe thirst, loss of weight, and lassitude. Weight loss may be substantial even though the patient is still obese. This results mainly from muscle wasting because of a failure of protein production.

Because the urine contains large amounts of sugar, dried splashes of urine appear white and crystalline. Fungus infections such as thrush are encouraged by the sugar and are common in the genital region, especially in women. Thrush can cause severe itching in the area. Men will occasionally develop an inflammatory swelling of the glans of the penis (balanitis). Other symptoms of NIDD include muscle cramps, tingling in the fingers, constipation, and sometimes a craving for sweet foods. Older people may suffer blurring of vision and changes in the focus of the eyes.

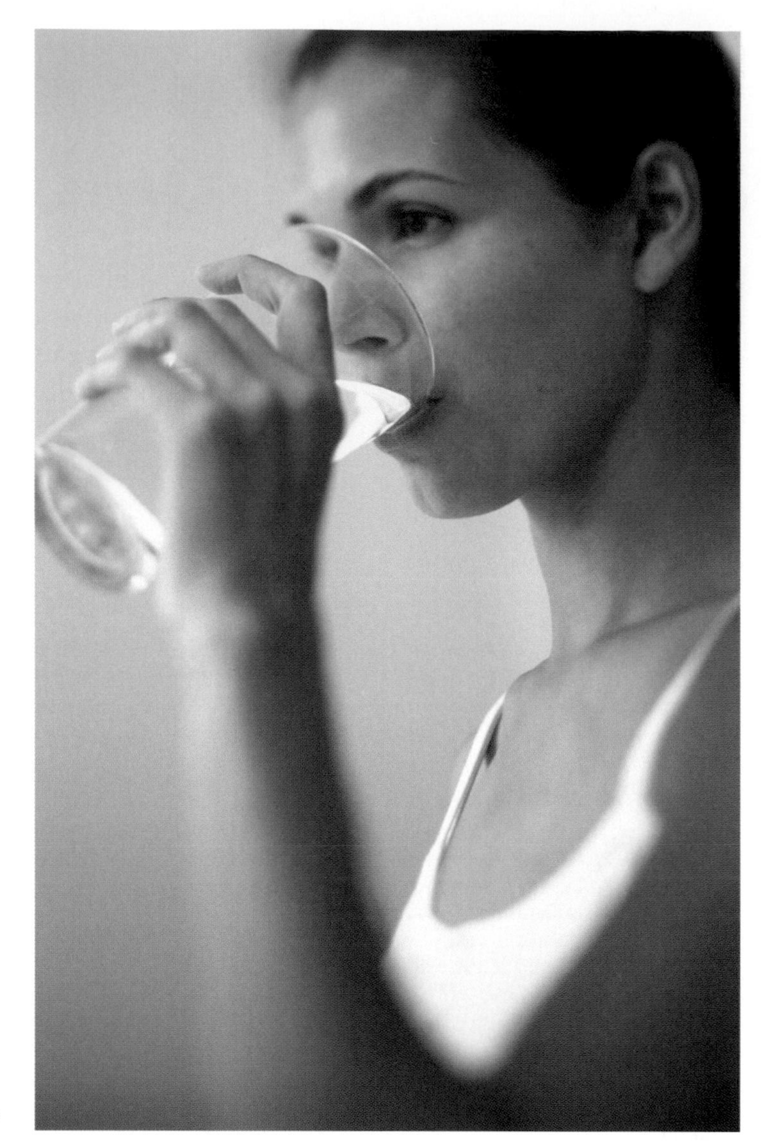

▲ *One of the symptoms of noninsulin-dependent diabetes is thirst and a dry mouth. Because of drinking extra fluids, someone with the condition also urinates excessively.*

Treatment

The object of treatment is to keep blood sugar levels within normal limits so that complications do not occur. Exercise, in conjunction with a healthy diet to maintain an appropriate weight, plays an important part in controlling blood sugar levels. In many cases NIDD can be completely controlled by diet alone. What is eaten is just as important as how much is eaten. The aim is to control the blood sugar without drugs, but if necessary, production of insulin can be boosted by sulfonylurea drugs such as tolbutamide, chlorpropamide, or other drugs. If these drugs fail, insulin injections will then become necessary.

See also: **Glucose; Insulin**

Nonsteroidal anti-inflammatory drugs

Questions and Answers

My son is a biochemist and has been talking about "COX." This appears to be related to the nonsteroidal anti-inflammatory drug (NSAID) ibuprofen. What is the connection?

"COX" is an abbreviation for cyclo-oxygenase. Like nearly all words ending in "-ase," it names an enzyme. The fatty acid arachidonic acid is a long straight chain, and COX converts it into a ring compound called a prostaglandin that causes pain and inflammation. Ibuprofen is one of the NSAID drugs that block this conversion.

My daughter, who is only 11 years old, has started to have periods and is taking a lot of Motrin. Is this safe?

No. NSAIDs should never be given to a child under 12, because, following a virus infection in children, they can cause a serious condition called Reye's syndrome. This condition is characterized by brain inflammation and liver damage and can be fatal. It is more commonly caused by aspirin than other NSAIDs, but none of the NSAIDs are recommended for children.

Can NSAIDs cause severe bleeding?

Yes. NSAIDs interfere with blood clotting and prolong bleeding. This can be useful in preventing heart attacks (which are caused by blood clotting in the coronary arteries of the heart). However, it can sometimes be dangerous. People with a tendency to stroke might be saved from a cerebral thrombosis (clot) but might be at greater risk from a more serious cerebral hemorrhage.

Citizens of the United States consume more nonsteroidal anti-inflammatory drugs than any other class of medication, taking more than 30 billion tablets of NSAIDs every year.

The term "nonsteroidal anti-inflammatory drug (NSAID)" is misleading because such drugs are most commonly taken for their painkilling action. The name came about because, prior to the development of this large range of medications, the only class of drugs effective in combating inflammation was steroid drugs (corticosteroids). One member of the NSAID group, aspirin (acetylsalicylic acid), has been known for many years, but its full range of actions has only recently been discovered.

How do NSAIDs work?

When tissue cells are damaged or inflamed, an enzyme present in cells called cyclo-oxygenase acts on the fatty acid arachidonic acid in the cell wall to convert it into a powerful, short-lived substance called a prostaglandin. Prostaglandins are involved in an inflammatory process and cause many of the symptoms of inflammation. By directly stimulating sensory nerve endings they also cause the experience of pain (see Nervous System). NSAIDs block the action of cyclo-oxygenase and so are effective in controlling inflammation and its symptoms. An NSAID will have no effect on the pain caused, for instance, by a prick with a needle because this directly stimulates the pain nerve endings. Neither will an NSAID relieve the pain caused by an injection of a prostaglandin (see Pain).

As treatment for painful inflammatory conditions such as rheumatoid arthritis, osteoarthritis, rheumatic disorders, headaches, menstrual pain, postoperative pain, and secondary bone cancer, NSAIDs are, in general, effective and safe (see Headache; Postoperative Care). They have largely replaced many more dangerous painkillers. In addition to controlling pain and inflammation, NSAIDs also act to lower temperature in fevers

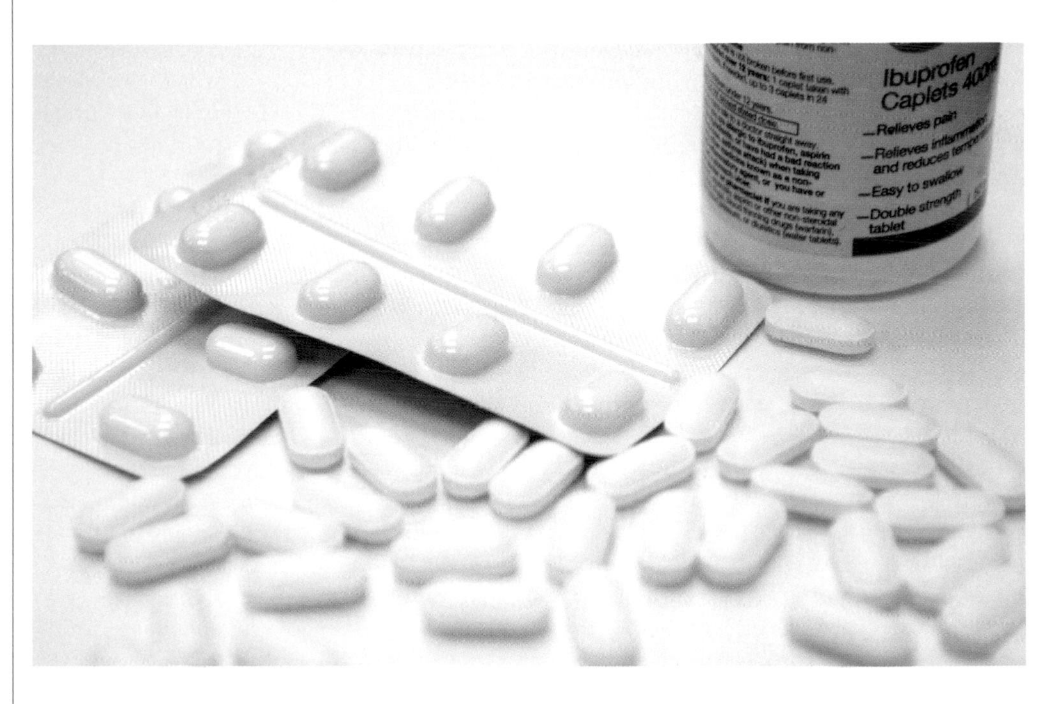

▲ *Ibuprofen, also known under brand names Advil, Motrin, and Nuprin, is popular in the treatment of arthritis, backache, gout, headache, menstrual pain, and muscle aches.*

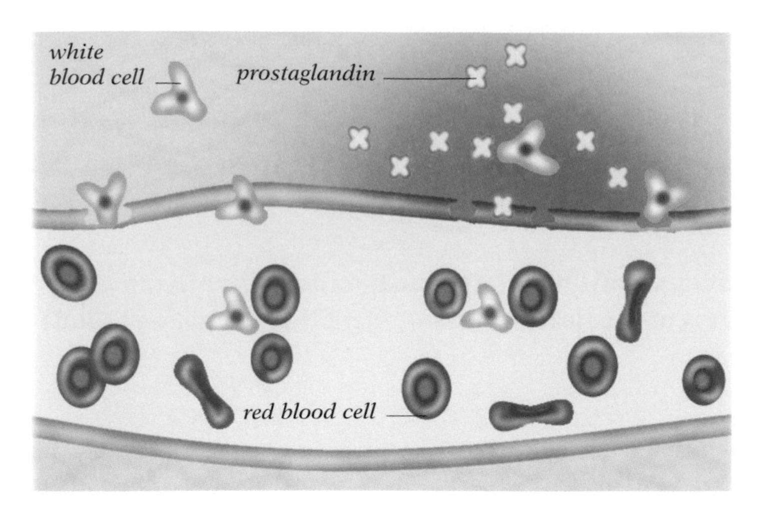

▲ *Prostaglandins cause the blood vessels to widen and leak fluid. White cells move into the tissue, which becomes red and swollen.*

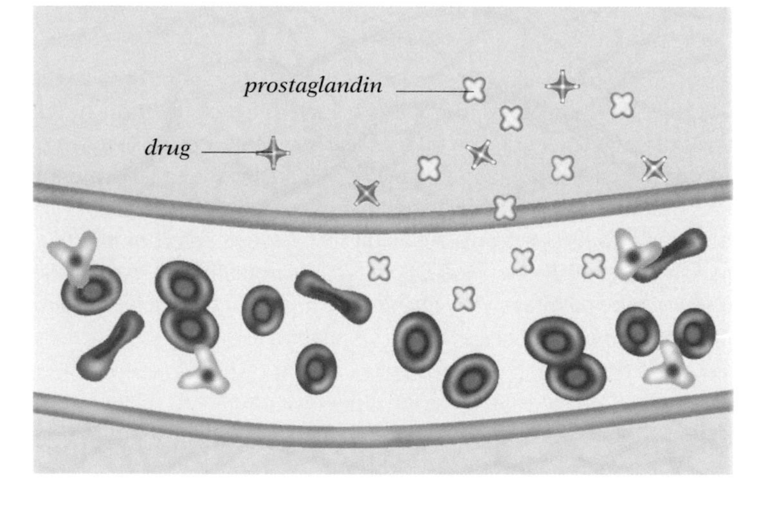

▲ *NSAIDs limit the release of prostaglandins. The blood vessels return to normal, and swelling and redness decrease.*

Different NSAIDs have slightly different properties, and if one fails to produce pain relief in the full recommended dosage, another should be tried. They should not be used in combination.

Identifying NSAIDs

NSAIDs are a very large drug class, and each member of the class has at least two names—the generic name and the common name or trade name. The trade name is usually more familiar. For each generic name there are several, sometimes many, trade names.

Side effects

Any drug that interferes with a fundamental body process such as the synthesis of prostaglandins is likely to have side effects, and NSAIDs are no exception. They have an effect on blood clotting which can be useful to prevent thrombosis in arteries but which, in some cases, can be dangerous. On the positive side, a small daily dose of a drug such as aspirin can substantially reduce the risk of heart attack. But in eye injuries, for instance, in which there has been some leakage of blood into the eye fluid, NSAIDs should not be given. To give them is to risk severe and sight-threatening bleeding within the eye. A single aspirin tablet can double the bleeding time for as long as a week.

Common NSAIDs

COMMON NAME	GENERIC NAME
Ansaid	Flurbiprofen
Butazolidin	Phenylbutazone
Clinoril	Sulindac
Dolobid	Diflunisal
Feldene	Piroxicam
Indocin	Indomethacin
Lodine	Etodolac
Meclomen	Meclofenamate
Motrin	Ibuprofen
Nalfon	Fenoprofen
Naprosyn	Naproxen
Orudis	Ketoprofen
Ponstel	Mefenamic acid
Relafen	Nabumetone
Rimadyl	Carprofen
Tolectin	Tolmetin
Toradol	Ketorolac
Voltaren	Diclofenac

The most common and best-known side effect of the NSAIDs is abdominal pain, often with nausea and diarrhea. These symptoms are mainly due to gastric irritation resulting from the withdrawal of the protective effect of prostaglandins on the stomach lining. In some cases this effect may be so severe that it causes gastric ulcers and even perforation. Patients with a history of indigestion or ulcers should therefore avoid NSAIDs.

Prostaglandins are important in helping the uterus to contract in childbirth, so using NSAIDs during labor is likely to prolong the process of giving birth. Other possible side effects of NSAIDs include allergic rashes, sleep disturbances, headache, and dizziness. Occasionally, they can interfere with the production of white blood cells in the immune system. Aspirin allergy is uncommon but may occur in people with other allergies. It can cause alarming and often dangerous reactions, including severe difficulty in breathing.

NSAID interactions

It is often necessary for people, especially old people, to take several different medications. However, NSAIDs have many interactions with other drugs. When taken with steroids and anticoagulant drugs, NSAIDs may increase the risk of bleeding from the stomach or bowel. They can cause kidney damage when taken with some diuretic drugs or with ACE inhibitors, and they can reduce the rate at which some other drugs are eliminated from the body in the urine, thereby increasing the effects of these drugs, sometimes dangerously (see Kidneys and Kidney Diseases). Drugs that interact in this way include oral hypoglycaemic drugs for type II diabetes; heart drugs such as digitalis; cimetidine, for stomach acidity; cyclosporin; butyrophenone antipsychotic drugs; the antidepressant lithium; the anticancer drug methotrexate; and quinolone antibiotics.

See also: **Arthritis; Aspirin and analgesics; Inflammation; Painkillers; Pain management; Prostaglandins; Ulcers**

Nose

Questions and Answers

I have had a congested nose for weeks. What could be the cause?

There could be hundreds of causes. The three most common irritants are dust, alcohol, and tobacco. These are followed by cosmetics (especially face powders, talc, and perfume), smoke, and gases. You should consult your doctor, who may refer you to a specialist.

What causes a runny nose when I have a cold?

The inside of the nose is constantly washed with mucus and swept with cilia (the "brush border" on the lining cells). A cold increases watery mucus production in an attempt to get rid of the infection, and a runny nose results.

My son has begun to pick his nose. When should I start being severe with him?

Nose-picking is unhygienic and antisocial, and you should put your foot down now. Train him to carry a hankie or tissue and to always use it when he sneezes or wants to get rid of excess mucus.

My neighbor says that a nosebleed is a sign of pressure on the brain. My son has had several nosebleeds in quick succession. Is this serious?

Nosebleeds are common in children, perhaps because they are so active and thus are likely to have many minor injuries. Some children are more prone to nosebleeds than others. A frequent cause is that blood vessels just inside one or both nostrils have burst, after becoming weakened and enlarged through rubbing and picking, or because of previous nosebleeds. Pressure on the brain is not a cause. However, recurrent bleeding can be a symptom of disease, so you should consult your doctor.

In addition to being a distinctive facial feature, the nose is a highly sensitive organ. It detects odor, then sends nerve impulses to the brain. Together with the eyes, ears, and throat, the nose can influence a person's health.

The nose is an important organ that has three main functions. First, it is the natural pathway by which air enters the body through breathing. The air is warmed, moistened, and filtered there before entering the lungs. Second, the nose acts as a protective device—if irritants such as dust enter, they are expelled by sneezing and do not have a chance to pass into the lungs, where they may cause damage (see Sneezing). Third, the nose is the organ of smell. The nose also acts as a form of resonator, helping to give each person's voice its individual characteristic tone.

Structure

The external part of the nose consists partly of bone and partly of cartilage. The two nasal bones, one on each side, project downward and also form the bridge between the eyes. Below

SIDE VIEW OF THE NOSE

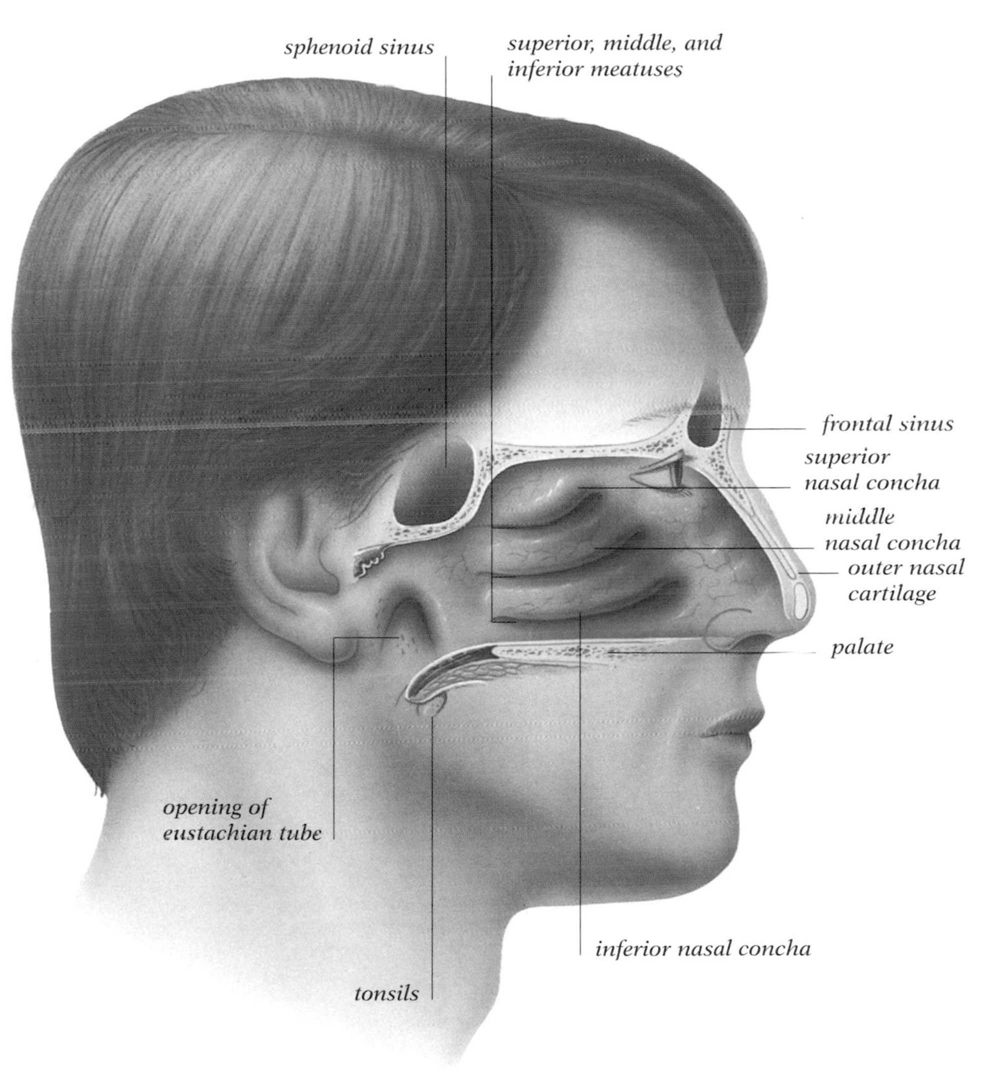

▲ *This cross section of the face shows the important parts of the nose and how it is linked to other areas of the face.*

Treating nosebleeds

A nosebleed occurs when a small blood vessel inside the nose is ruptured by a blow, by picking the nose, or by a bout of sneezing. It can happen for no apparent reason, especially to teenage girls who have just started to menstruate. People who have hay fever or a nasal infection may get nosebleeds. Although the blood loss looks great, it is not, in fact, copious, and it is rarely very serious. It will generally clear up in five to 15 minutes—in other words, in the time it usually takes blood to clot. Very heavy bleeding may follow damage to an artery at the back of the nose. In this case the nose has to be packed in a special way by a doctor. Nosebleeds that occur within a week of a tonsil or adenoid operation are particularly serious and should be treated immediately, as are nosebleeds that follow a blow to the head, which could indicate a fractured skull. Tell your doctor if the bleeding was caused by a blow. Otherwise:

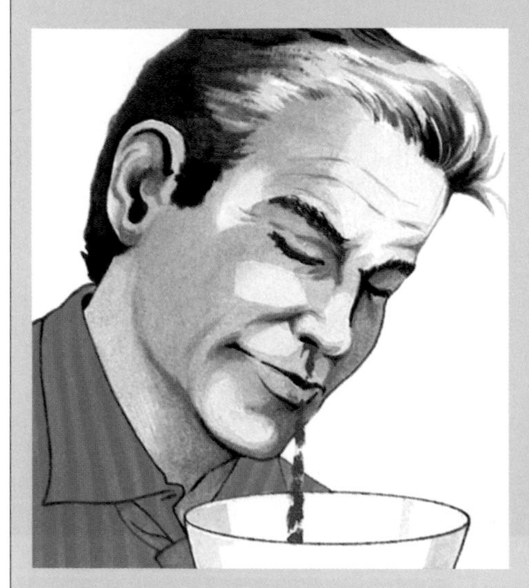

- Sit the patient down, loosen his or her clothes around the neck, and incline the head slightly forward so that the blood drips into a bowl or any other receptacle that will catch the flow of blood.
- Try to prevent the patient from swallowing too much blood.

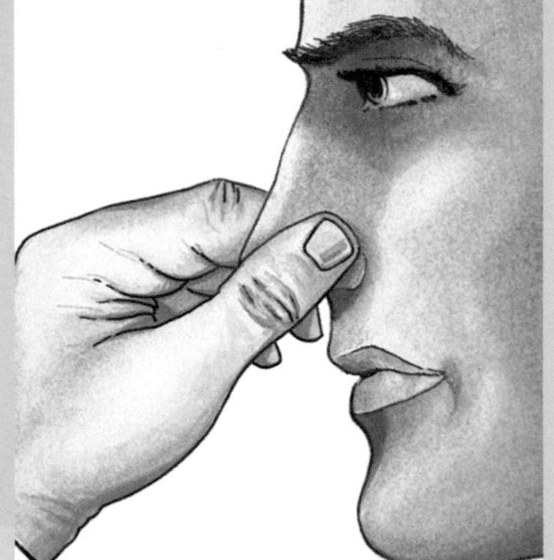

- Get the patient to breathe gently through the mouth and lightly pinch the nostrils closed for approximately five minutes.
- Apply ice wrapped in cloth to the nose.

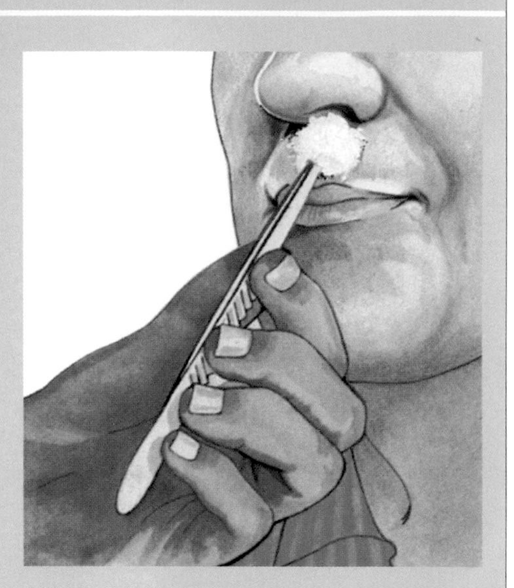

- If the bleeding is severe, put a small packing of sterile cotton gauze into each nostril. Make sure the packing is tight, and press the nostrils together for 10 minutes.
- If the bleeding persists for 20 minutes, call your doctor or take the patient to the hospital.
- When bleeding stops, make sure the patient leaves the nose alone.
- Remove packing 12 to 24 hours later.

throat. It leads from the nose to the middle ear; that explains why an earache sometimes occurs with a sore throat.

Colds and hay fever

The common cold is caused by a virus. It leads to acute inflammation of the nose, and excessive production of watery mucus, which causes nasal congestion.

Hay fever, or allergic rhinitis, is an allergic form of head cold, which is generally more unpleasant and longer-lasting than a cold caused by a virus. However, the hay fever disappears if the patient is able to pinpoint the cause and then avoid it in the future. Dust, animal dander, and irritating smells are also common triggers of nasal inflammation.

With colds, prevention is often better than treatment. It is best to avoid being around people with colds whenever possible. People who have colds themselves should stay at home until they feel better. Acetaminophen and commercial cold medicines are soothing and relieve the discomfort and inflammation (see Painkillers). A nasal spray will relieve the pain, and inhalation of menthol is also beneficial. Douching the nose is particularly helpful if dry crusts have formed inside it.

Repeated colds, or colds that linger, may be caused by a polyp, a deviated septum, or sinus trouble, all of which can be corrected by minor surgery.

Injuries and malformation

A broken nose is one of the most common sports injuries and requires immediate medical attention (see Sports Injury). Almost invariably a broken nose will be out of shape. If it is allowed to heal without being reset by a surgeon, it will, in most cases, lead to other problems such as chronic runny nose or sinusitis. Resetting the break usually requires at least one night's stay in the hospital.

The cavities on either side of the septum are rarely of equal size, because the septum usually leans to one side. If the septum actually touches the conchae, irritation may arise and perhaps lead to a runny nose. This type of problem can be corrected by an operation.

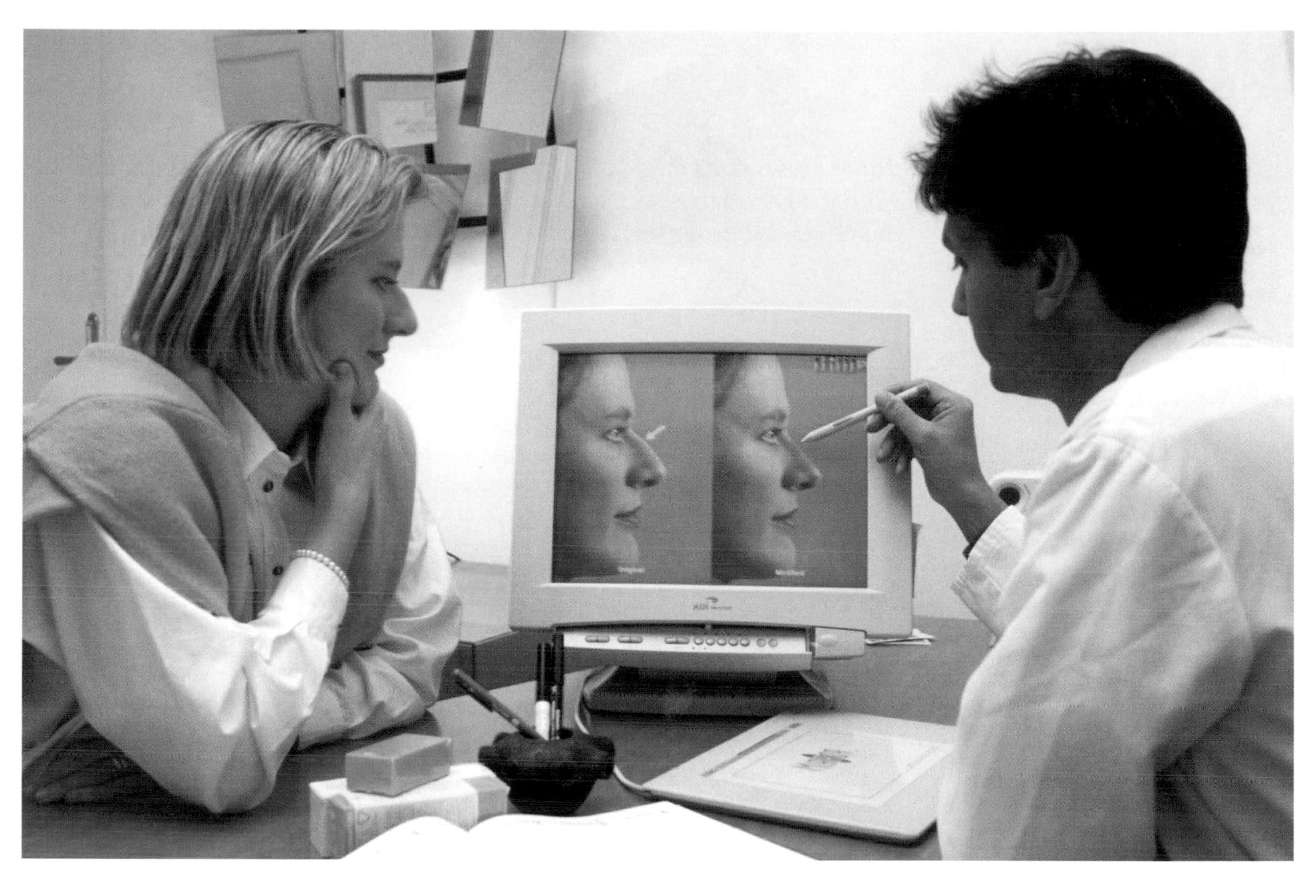

▲ *A nose job may resolve a deep psychological need in a person.*

Adenoids

Adenoids are two glandular swellings at the back of the nasal passage, which are made up of lymph tissue. If the adenoids become infected, they block the nose, so that the sufferer is forced to breathe through the mouth. Chronic mouth-breathing in children is often caused by adenoids.

Adenoidal children snore when they are asleep, and they are prone to bronchitis. The point of the nose becomes pinched, and the nostrils narrow, because so little air is passing through them. As mouth-breathing requires less effort than nose-breathing, the rib muscles of affected children will develop poorly. They may become round-shouldered and may stoop or be pigeon-chested. They may also be slightly deaf. Removal of the adenoids is a simple surgical procedure and will bring tremendous relief.

Polyps

Although harmless, polyps are a nuisance and interfere with breathing. These soft growths of a jellylike texture, which are usually on a short stalk, are generally found in the middle concha. They rarely occur singly, and when one polyp is removed other polyps nearby may enlarge. Because of this, it may take several trips to the physician or ear, nose, and throat doctor to treat polyps. However, it is worth persevering with treatment. Some people worry that polyps are cancerous. This is not the case. They are benign tumors that respond well to surgery.

Foreign bodies

Small children have been known to push objects such as peanuts, buttons, lumps of foam from stuffed toys, wax crayons, peas, small stones, and other similar objects up their noses. The objects may cause no symptoms at first but will eventually result in swelling, discharge, headaches, and facial pain.

Children who have pushed something up the nostril should be made to sneeze while the opposite nostril is blocked. If this does not work, they should be taken to a doctor.

Sinusitis

Bacterial infection is most common in the sinuses behind the eyebrows and those at the side of the nose. The condition usually develops as a complication of a viral infection, such as a cold.

The symptoms of sinusitis include headaches, a discharge into the nose or throat, weakness, toothaches, and facial pain. Acute attacks may be precipitated by colds, hay fever, and damp weather. Acute sinusitis needs prompt treatment to avoid the risk that the infection will spread backward and cause meningitis to develop (see Meningitis).

Sinusitis usually responds to menthol inhalation, but more severe cases may require the use of antibiotic treatment or an operation to wash out the sinuses (see Antibiotics).

See also: **Adenoids; Common cold; Cosmetic surgery; Hay fever; Mucus; Pigeon chest; Polyps; Rhinitis; Sinusitis; Smell**

Numbness

Questions and Answers

I have a large scar on my knee that feels numb. Is this because the nerve has been damaged, or is it because the blood supply is poor or has been cut off?

It doesn't really have anything to do with either of these things. Numbness in the area around the scar would be caused by nerves' being cut in the accident; numbness in the scar itself is a different matter. A scar is made up of new tissue that grows out from either side of the cut to fill the gap and restore the continuity of the protective skin surface. Some, but not many, blood vessels will have grown out into the scar to supply the new tissue. It is because of this that scars look pale and do not turn red when you take a hot bath. The lack of nerves in the scar is what accounts for its numbness.

I sometimes wake up in the morning with complete numbness in part of my arm. I have difficulty in moving it and if I touch it, it has a dead feeling. Why is this?

The numbness has occurred because during the night the position of your body has caused pressure on a nerve or the artery to that part of the body to be squeezed and the blood supply cut off. Once the pressure has been removed, or you move your arm continuously, the feeling should return. If the numbness is accompanied by other symptoms, see your doctor.

Some months ago I cut my finger deeply. The cut has healed but the top of my finger is still numb. Will the feeling in it ever come back?

Probably not. The sensory nerve to the area must have been severed, and it seems that the cut nerve ends have not rejoined. Some feeling can return, but it should have returned by now.

Numbness is not a disease, but it is a symptom that something is interfering with the nerves that normally carry sensations to the brain. The causes of numbness can range from a response to cold temperatures to a serious disease.

Numbness of one kind or another is something everyone has experienced. The cause is usually obvious—banging a finger or working with bare hands in cold weather—and the condition does not last long. However, numbness can be an indication of disease and may have unpleasant consequences if it is not taken seriously and dealt with promptly. Any numbness that lasts for a week or more should therefore be reported to the doctor for further investigation.

In the medical sense, numbness means a loss of sensation, and it usually refers to interference with the sense of touch. If the loss of feeling is complete the condition is called anesthesia; if the loss is only partial, as in the familiar sensation of pins and needles, it is called paresthesia.

Causes

Basically, numbness is due to some problem in the function of the sensory nerves. These pass messages to the brain about what is happening in and around a part of the body (see Brain). If the sensory nerve is damaged or interfered with in some way, the message cannot reach the brain and loss of feeling, or numbness, will result.

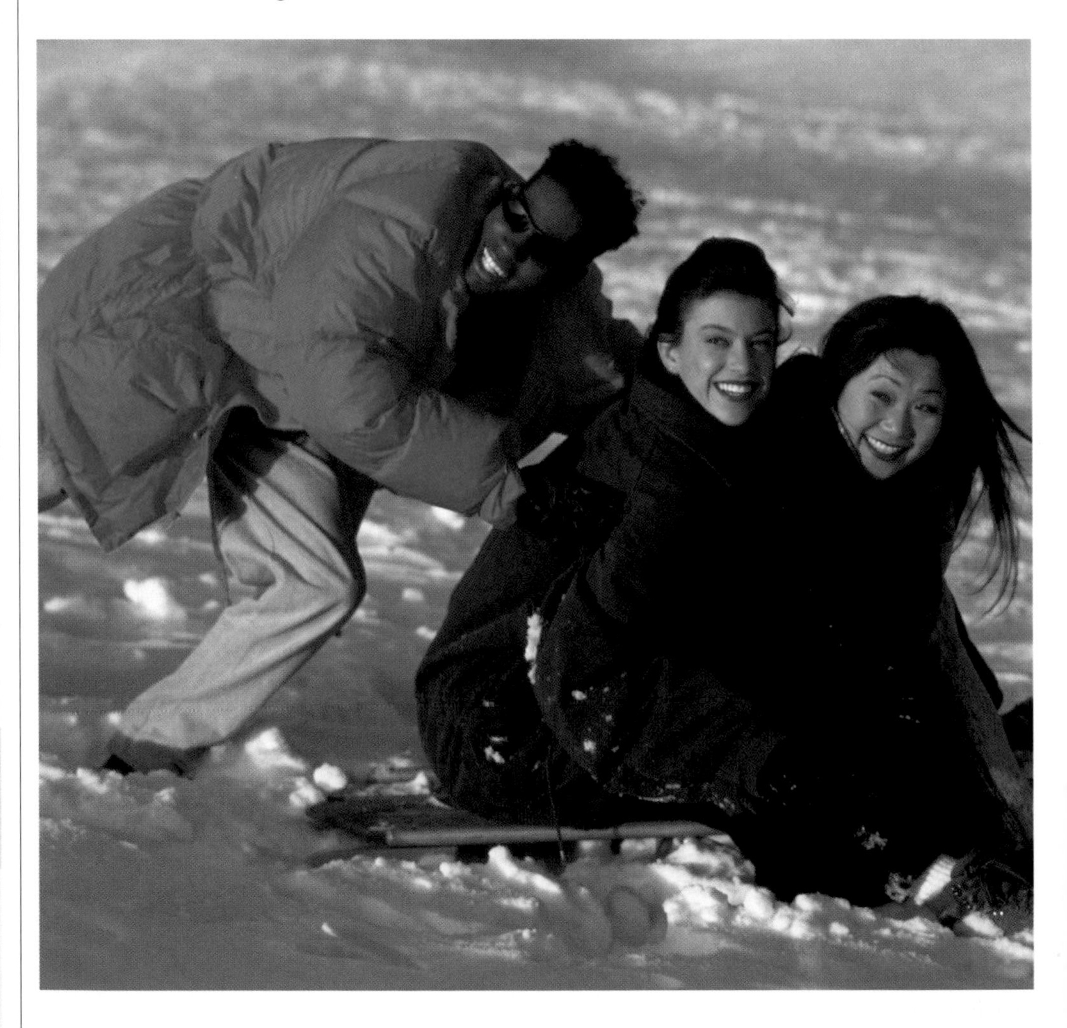

▲ *Hands become numb in the cold because the arteries contract, reducing circulation, and the sensory nerves cease to function.*

How numbness occurs

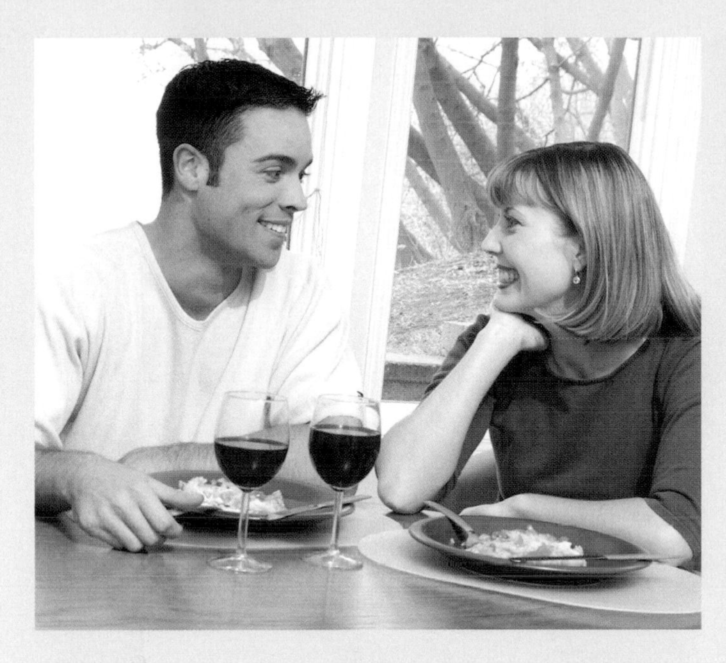

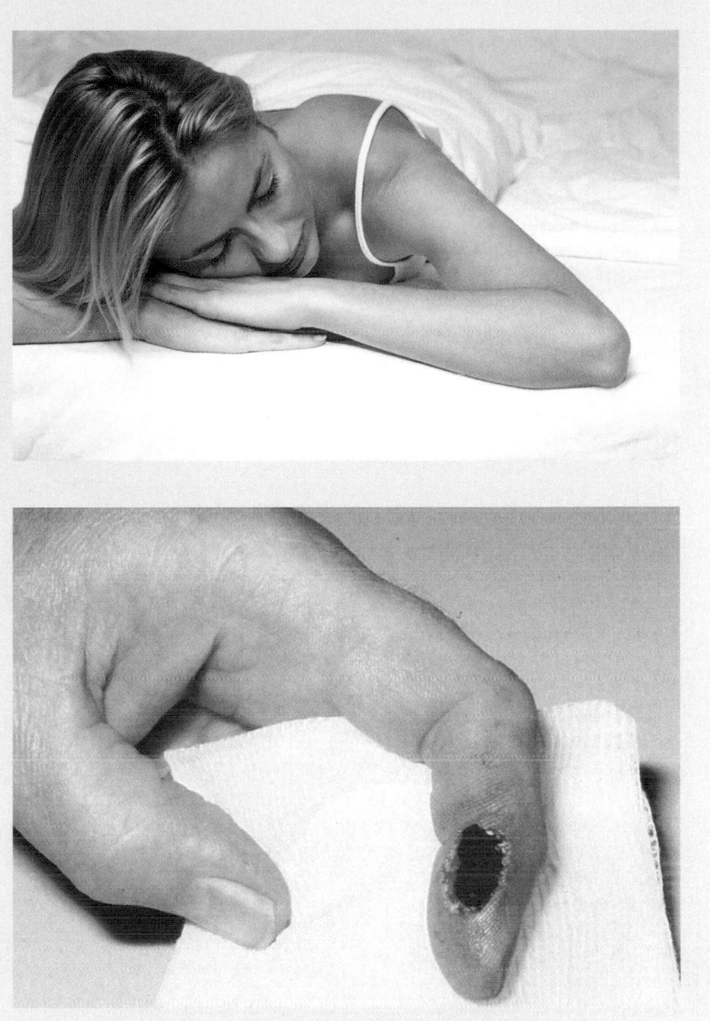

Numbness, or a loss of sensation, arises because there is some problem with the working of the sensory nerves. For example, if you have slept on your arm through the night (above right), either pressure on the nerve or the cutting off of blood circulation will result in numbness in the limb. This is only temporary. Drinking to excess will inhibit the normal working of the nerves (above). This will lead to neuritis, a nerve inflammation, which can often be successfully treated by stopping drinking. Finally, numbness can occur when the nerves are cut, as happens when some portion of the body, like a finger, is wounded (right). Here the resulting loss of sensation may be temporary or permanent, depending on the damage done to the nerves.

Damage to the sensory nerves is usually accompanied by a loss of function in the motor nerves that serve the same part of the body. When the brain receives a message from the sensory nerves, it activates the motor nerves to carry messages to the muscles, so that a specific movement can be made (see Muscles).

Loss or interruption of function in the motor nerves will result in the total inability to move the part concerned (paralysis) or weakness and loss of power if the effect is not total. Numbness and paralysis frequently occur together, since in many parts of the body the sensory and motor nerves run close to each other and are likely to be affected by similar types of damage.

Common disorders

Numbness can result from several disorders of the sensory nerves. One of the most obvious is that the nerve is cut. A deep cut or gash in the skin, for example, will sever the nerves that are present in the area, causing a feeling of deadness.

Sustained pressure on a sensory nerve can also cause numbness and is usually preceded by "pins and needles." A common example of this is often found with a slipped disk. One of the cushioning disks between the vertebrae becomes displaced in such a way as to press on a major nerve trunk as it leaves the spinal column. The patient feels the pain along the course of the nerve and also has a patch of numbness in the ankle region.

The normal working of a nerve can be interrupted by neuritis, which is inflammation of a nerve. Disorders in which neuritis may occur include diabetes, malnutrition, alcoholism, other chemical poisonings, and certain virus infections.

The nerve can also cease to function if the supply of blood is cut off. This can be demonstrated by winding a piece of string or a rubber band tightly around the base of a finger. In a few minutes the finger will become very numb. This happens because the pressure of the string or rubber band around the finger is great enough to squeeze the walls of the blood vessels together, thereby cutting off the blood supply.

Treatment and outlook

Treatment for numbness depends on whether the damage to the nerve is permanent or temporary. When nerves are cut they will sometimes join again as the wound heals, and feeling will return. Often the loss of sensation is permanent because the nerves do not manage to reconnect.

Questions and Answers

Why is it that after I go to the dentist and have a local anesthetic, my lip feels enormous, although it looks normal?

As you say, your lip is not really swollen. After a period of total numbness, when the local anesthetic begins to wear off, sensation returns gradually rather than suddenly. There is a phase of only partial feeling, which involves the same sensation that occurs when the skin and its nerves are stretched by an area of swelling. This is why your lip will feel much larger than usual.

I have been getting numbness in my fingers for weeks. Can I take anything to remove the sensation?

There is no specific medicine that can be taken for numbness. It is not a disease but a symptom that something is wrong with the working of the nerves in your fingers. Most of the diseases that cause numbness are not serious—but a few are, so it is important to tell your doctor about any feeling of numbness that lasts for more than a few days.

When the disorder that is causing the numbness has been treated, the feeling will probably return to your fingers.

I seem to get numbness in my hands and feet every winter, at temperatures that don't affect other people. Is there anything seriously wrong with me, and what should I do about it?

It sounds as though the circulation in your hands and feet is not as good as it should be. When any part of the body is exposed to severe cold, the arteries contract automatically to cut heat loss to a minimum. If for some reason your arteries are already narrow, this additional narrowing will cause insufficient blood to get to your hands and feet. If the numbness follows changes of color from red to white to blue, the problem is probably the Raynaud phenomenon, and you should see your doctor as soon as possible.

HOW A FINGER IS ANESTHETIZED

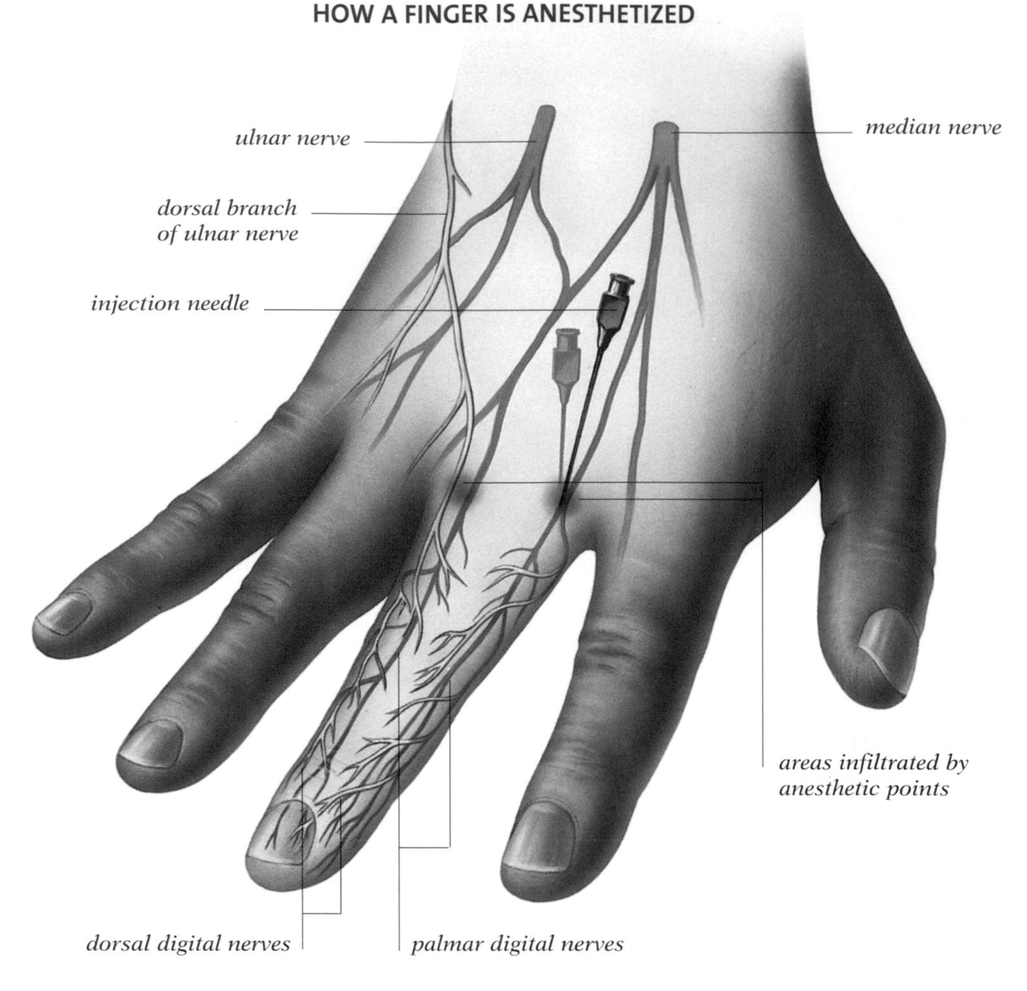

▲ *When a cut finger is to be stitched, all four of its nerves must be numbed first by local anesthetic. A needle is inserted on either side of the finger and gently manipulated so that it reaches the two nerves at different depths on both sides.*

There are two reasons for this. First, the nerve filaments to the skin are extremely fine and are likely to be displaced as well as cut in the course of the accident. If this happens, it is unlikely that they will be able to link up again. Second, nerve tissue has the least capacity for repair of all the body's tissues. When large nerves are severed—for example, in very deep gashes in the arms or legs—attempts are usually made to sew the cut ends together.

Numbness that is due to pressure on a nerve usually disappears completely, with a full return of feeling once the source of pressure has been removed. However, if the pressure has been very heavy and has continued for a long time, it is possible that some of the nerve fibers will have died and therefore the numbness will be permanent.

Treatment for numbness resulting from neuritis consists of dealing with the condition that caused it. The feeling usually returns fully because these conditions only interfere with the normal working of the nerves rather than destroying them. Similarly, when pressure on the nerve is the cause, once the pressure is removed and the blood supply is restored, the nerve begins to function.

Local anesthetics

Numbness is sometimes created artificially so that surgery can be performed painlessly. This is called local anesthesia as opposed to general anesthesia, which makes the patient unconscious. The local anesthetic agents that are most commonly used are synthetic opiates such as novocaine. They can be administered by injection or in the form of a spray, an ointment, or even a lozenge.

See also: Alcoholism; Anesthetics; Circulatory system; Diabetes; Local anesthetics; Nervous system; Paralysis; Pins and needles; Slipped disk; Touch

Nutrition

Questions and Answers

I would like to become a vegetarian. Would my nutritional requirements be properly met without eating animal protein?

Animal proteins are convenient sources of essential amino acids in a normal diet. However, a vegetarian diet composed of a mixture of proteins from cereals, grains, nuts, and dairy products will give you a proper balance of all the nutritional elements and vitamins, if you consume enough of these foods.

Is it true that pregnant women have special food requirements?

Yes. A growing fetus in the uterus needs extra calories and proteins as well as additional calcium, iron, and vitamins. If the expectant mother is deprived of these, her body will give priority to the fetus and deficiencies will develop.

Do illnesses have any effect on our nutritional needs?

Yes. Many illnesses, especially infections, increase the body's demands for calories, proteins, and certain nutrients. This accounts for the weight loss that often accompanies some chronic infections, since the appetite is often reduced at the same time. Some tumors may increase the need for certain nutrients by stepping up the turnover of specific chemicals in the body.

An elderly neighbor of ours was treated in the hospital for scurvy. Isn't scurvy rare nowadays?

Vitamin C deficiency, which causes scurvy, still occurs, especially in elderly people who live on their own. The reason is that their nutrition is unbalanced; they are eating too few foods that are rich in vitamin C. Friends and family should help with food shopping.

The body is like a factory that needs maintenance and fuel, which is supplied by the food we eat. Nutrition is the study of different kinds of foods and the ways that the human body utilizes them.

A list of the body's components will give some idea of the complex chemical structures of which humans are made. For the average person they are: protein (17 percent); fat (13.8 percent); carbohydrate (1.5 percent); water (61.6 percent); minerals (6.1 percent). In fact, the cells of the body are factories that use chemical reactions to convert the components supplied to them in the diet into the products necessary for life and growth of the body.

There are about 48 substances that must be supplied ready-made in the diet, including oxygen and water. All the rest can be manufactured, given these basic essentials. In addition, the body needs a constant reserve of energy to function efficiently. For nutrition to be adequate, it is important not only that adequate nutrients are supplied in the diet but also that the body absorbs them properly.

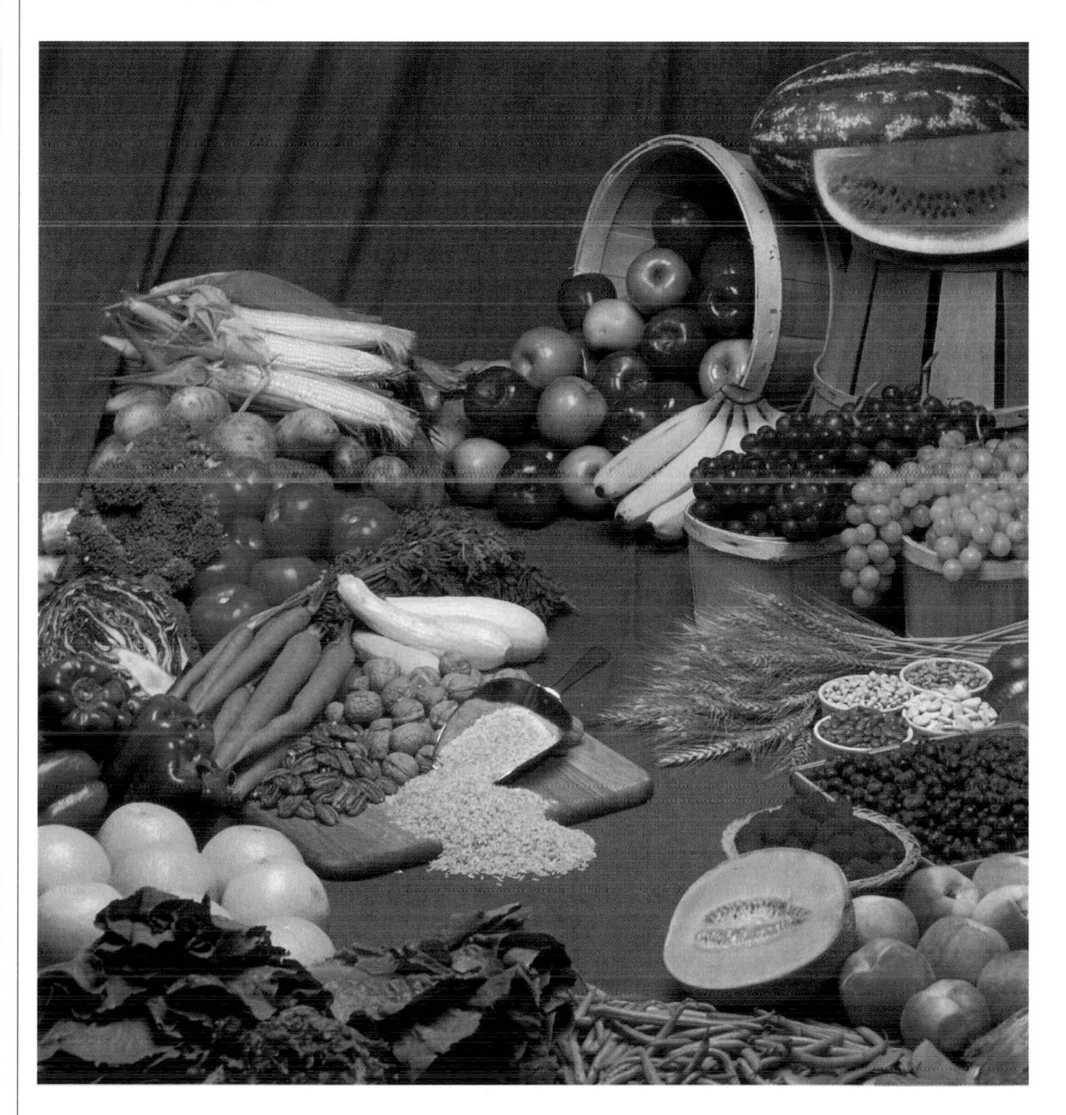

▲ *A healthy vegetarian diet includes vegetables, fruits, nuts, and grains. The Community Nutrition Research Group recommends three to five servings of vegetables, two to four servings of fruit, two to three servings of nuts, and six to 11 servings of grains each day.*

Packed lunches for schoolchildren

A packed lunch can meet children's nutritional needs during the day, but a nourishing meal in the evening to supplement this must be provided. Sandwiches are ideal—bread contains vital nutrients and the fillings can contain a sufficient amount of protein—but lunch ideas need not be restricted to sandwiches alone.

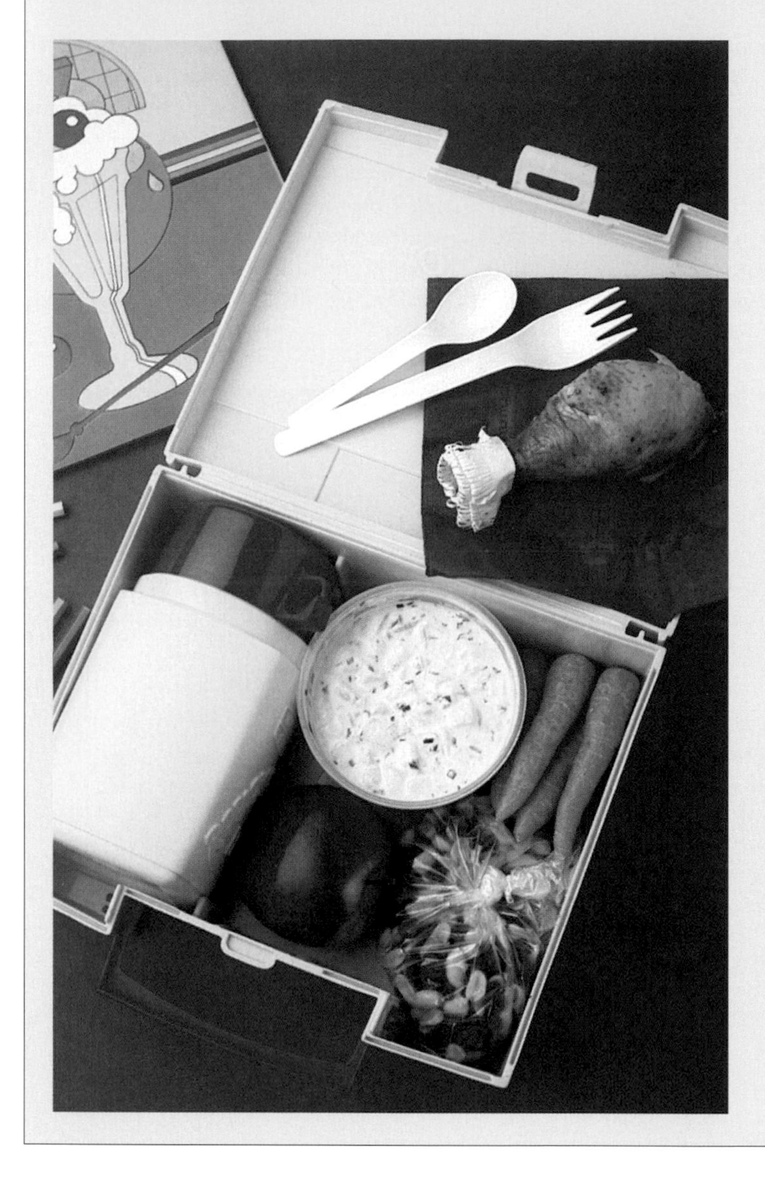

INCLUDE:

- Meat, fish, nuts (containing protein for growth)
- Dairy products (protein and fat for growth and energy)
- Whole wheat bread (carbohydrates, protein, and fiber)
- Fruit and vegetables (vitamins and minerals)

AVOID:

- Candy, jam, cookies, chocolate (all these sweet foods can be replaced with foods that have natural sugars, such as fruit, honey, potatoes, and bread)

A VARIETY OF LUNCHTIME IDEAS:

- Chicken drumsticks
- Cooked meatballs
- Hard-boiled eggs
- Small meat pie
- Slice of quiche
- Tuna salad

FOR COLD DAYS:

- Thermos of hot soup (with chunks of meat and vegetables) plus a fresh buttered roll or bagel

FOR DESSERT:

- Fruit yogurts
- Fruit salad
- Peeled and segmented orange
- Seedless raisins and nuts

PACKING:

- Use plastic boxes or save yogurt, margarine, or cottage cheese containers.
- Wrap carrots or celery in wax paper. Use aluminum foil for sandwiches.
- Remember to pack a fork, a spoon, and some napkins or tissues for wiping hands.

Fuels for the tissues

The body's basic fuels are fats and carbohydrates, and the energy they produce is measured in calories. People take in these fuels from animal and plant products, and the body converts them into assimilated forms for uptake into the cells.

Fats are converted into fatty acids and triglycerides, which are carried in the blood as complex lipoproteins. These are then taken to the adipose (fatty) tissues for storage; or, if they are needed, they can be "burned" chemically to provide energy.

Carbohydrates are mainly converted into sugars, especially glucose. This is the body's principal fuel. It is easy to transport, and the cells can use it conveniently. Glucose can also be made in the liver and other tissues by breaking down protein. Some cells, especially in the brain, require glucose as an energy source. This is stored in the form of glycogen and can be readily converted to glucose when needed. A minimum level of glucose is essential for the brain cells to function (see Glucose).

Proteins are broken into their basic components, amino acids. From amino acids the cells make their own proteins. They are not usually used as fuel, but when other sources of energy are lacking, they can be metabolized for this purpose (see Metabolism). In cases of starvation the muscles waste away as the body burns up their protein components in an effort to maintain the glucose level of the blood at an appropriate level.

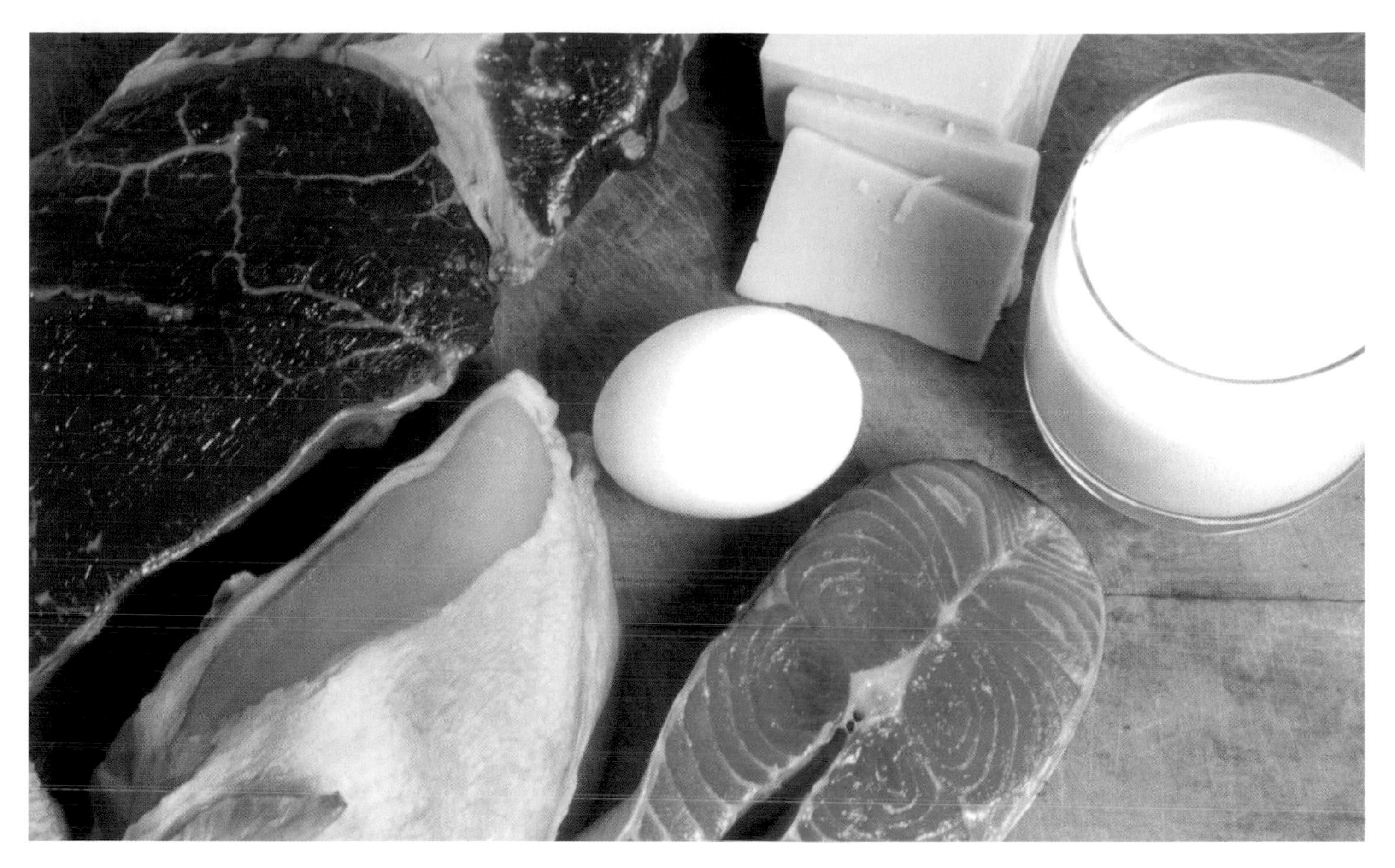

▲ *Meat and fish are a good source of proteins and amino acids. Dairy products such as milk, cheese, and eggs provide vitamin D and calcium, which helps the bones to grow.*

Essential nutrients

The body also requires some chemicals that it cannot make for itself. However, these can usually be stored, so a person may be able to survive for months, or even years, without them before the effect of any deficiency in the diet is felt. Oxygen is necessary at all times, and a lack of water will be felt in a day or two, since this cannot be stored in any quantity. The nutrients that people need include vitamins, essential elements and minerals (including those that are required in only minute amounts), fatty acids, and some amino acids.

Vitamins are essential in small amounts to help the body function. Different vitamins work in different ways. For example, once it is in the body, vitamin D acts like a hormone, coordinating the distribution of calcium and bone growth. Vitamin K helps control the clotting of blood. Vitamins are soluble in either water or fat. This is important, because if the absorption of fat is abnormal, owing to some disease in the intestines, then the fat-soluble vitamins will not be absorbed into the system. The fat-soluble vitamins are A, D, E, and K. Other vitamins are water-soluble.

Some constituents of the diet may interfere with the absorption or use of vitamins. It has been suggested that nicotinic acid, present in cereals, may be chemically bound to some of the other constituents; this binding would make it unavailable for use.

Food preparation may also affect some water-soluble vitamins. Folic acid is often destroyed through prolonged cooking or canning. (Nicotinic acid and folic acid are included in the vitamin B group.)

Mineral elements that are needed for adequate nutrition include carbon and hydrogen, which are so abundant that deficiency is practically impossible.

Sodium and chloride, the constituents of common salt, are essential to human biochemistry. Salt is widely distributed in foods, and deficiencies are found only when the body's requirements are greatly increased through abnormal losses. For example, when people who live in hot climates sweat excessively, the ensuing salt loss may be sufficient to require extra dietary supplements (see Salt).

Calcium is an important constituent of bones and other tissues. The body's calcium usage is carefully regulated by a hormone system that includes vitamin D.

Iron is essential for the manufacture of hemoglobin, the vital oxygen-carrying substance in red blood cells. Some iron is also essential in the makeup of some of the enzyme systems in cells that provide energy to be used by the cells.

Minute quantities of other elements (trace elements) are also needed. Iodine, for example, is essential to the manufacture of thyroid hormone (see Thyroid; Trace Elements).

Fluorine, contained in fluoride, is necessary to prevent tooth decay; and in areas of low fluorine level, this is sometimes added to water supplies (see Fluoride). Other trace elements such as copper, cobalt, and manganese are needed for various enzyme systems.

Amino acids are nitrogen-containing compounds that are the basic building blocks of the much larger protein molecules. The cells can manufacture many amino acids, but nine amino acids must be supplied ready-made in the diet. Different foods have different proportions of these essential substances; a mixture of food proteins must be eaten to ensure an adequate diet.

Linoleic acid and alpha-linoleic acid are fatty acids that are essential for the body to function properly. They are components of cell membranes and are needed for oxygen use and energy production, control of substances flowing in and out of cells, and hormone regulation. Deficiencies of fatty acids are rare.

Principles of good nutrition

It is important to eat the right kinds of food in the right quantities. The maintenance of good health depends on much more than simply getting enough calories and the basic vitamins and minerals.

The first requirement is that a person should not exceed the amounts necessary to maintain an optimum weight. By far the most common form of malnutrition in the United States is caused by excessive overeating, leading to obesity and all its attendant physical and psychological problems. The Centers for Disease Control and Prevention (CDC) report that in 2002, 64.5 percent of American adults aged 20 years and older were overweight and 30.5 percent were obese. Nearly 5 percent were severely obese. A similar increase has occurred in children. Regardless of the type of food that is eaten, obesity occurs when a person's calorie intake consistently exceeds his or her energy expenditure. Obesity is more common in lower-income groups than in high-income groups, and it is twice as common in African-American women as it is in Caucasian women. The difference between African-American and Caucasian men is less marked. Obesity is associated with a reduced life expectancy and a number of serious diseases such as diabetes, atherosclerosis, high blood pressure, and arthritis, in addition to various social disadvantages.

There is no easy answer to obesity nor any miraculous drug that can control food intake. The only effective cure is to establish new eating habits that involve strictly limited amounts of the appropriate foods. Obesity is encouraged by diets that are high in fat. This is because, weight for weight, fats provide nearly three times the calories of carbohydrates or proteins (see Obesity).

The second requirement is to avoid foods that are known to cause diseases. The principal disease of concern is atherosclerosis, which is a disease of arteries that results in a diminished capacity to carry blood. It is the cause of conditions such as heart attacks, strokes, limb gangrene, serious kidney diseases, dementia, and other severe disorders. Atherosclerosis has a number of causes, but among the most important is the excessive intake of saturated fats. Most of these are of dairy origin. It is not the amount of cholesterol in the diet that is of primary concern, but the total intake of saturated fats that a person consumes.

The third requirement is to ensure an adequate intake of dietary elements that prevent diseases. For example, people who eat a diet high in soluble, but nonabsorbable, fiber—such as that found in oats and wheat germ—have a much lower incidence of intestinal diseases such as colitis, diverticulitis, and colon and rectal cancer. Colorectal cancers are one of the three most common causes of deaths from cancer. Fiber also has the advantage that it can bind some of the cholesterol entering the intestine from the liver as a constituent of bile into an insoluble form. Cholesterol that is bound in this way is lost from the body in the feces.

Antioxidants

Another class of dietary elements that can prevent disease are the antioxidant vitamins and the flavonoids. Vitamins A, C, and E are antioxidant vitamins; to be effective as antioxidants, they must be taken in much larger quantities than are necessary to prevent a vitamin deficiency. Less than about 0.05 ounce (1 g) of vitamin C and less than 0.01 ounce (0.3 g) of vitamin E taken daily are unlikely to be of much value as antioxidants. Flavonoids are compounds that are found in many fruits and vegetables and in red wine.

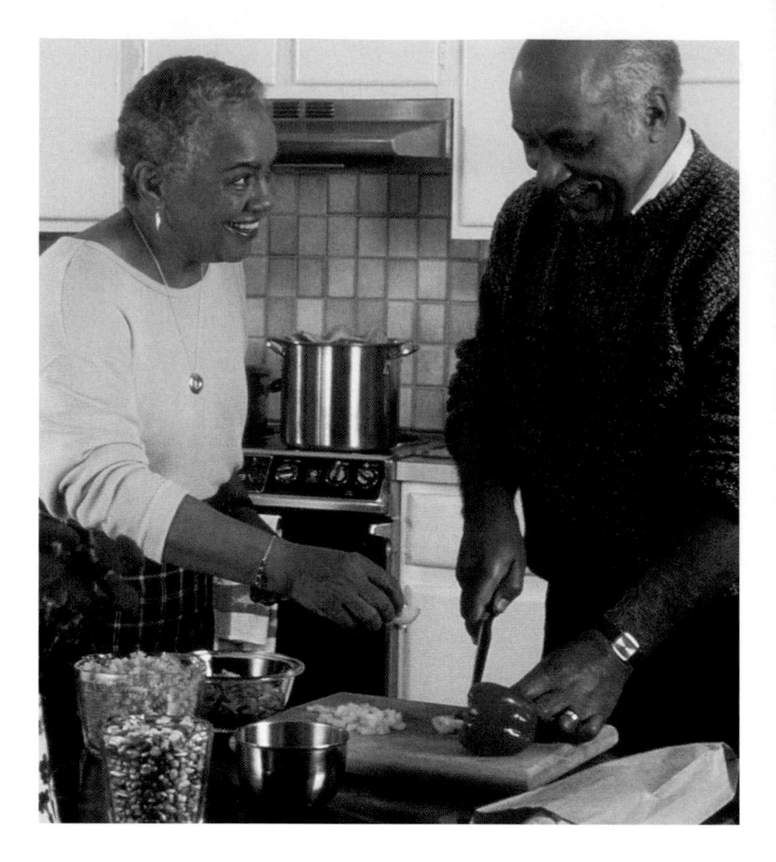

▲ *The key to proper nutrition is an adequate daily intake of protein, carbohydrates, fats, vitamins, and minerals, which should be maintained throughout a person's life.*

Antioxidants are important because many disease processes that damage the body do so by the production of powerful chemical elements called free radicals. These can start destructive chain reactions in the cells and tissues. Antioxidants mop up free radicals before they can cause harm.

The use of antioxidants may decrease the incidence of heart disease and cancer, and it may also remove lipids and cholesterol from the blood vessels, but this is not proved. Excessive intake of vitamins, especially fat-soluble A and D vitamins, is always dangerous because the excess is not excreted as it would be with water- soluble vitamins (see Antioxidants).

A good balance

A healthy balanced diet is one that is high in fruit and leafy green vegetables, to provide slow-release carbohydrates, fiber, and flavonoids. It should be low in fats of all kinds, especially dairy fats and their products, and moderate in protein, such as that found in cheese and red meat, because too much protein is associated with fat; and the diet may be supplemented by antioxidant vitamins.

See also: **Arteries and artery disease; Calcium; Diet; Fats; Iron; Malnutrition; Minerals; Pregnancy; Protein; Vitamins**

Obesity

Questions and Answers

My friend eats the same amount as I do, is about the same height as I am, but is of average weight, whereas I am fat. Why is this?

The way in which people's bodies use food varies widely. People who use their food fuel economically become obese more easily than those who use it extravagantly, because they burn off less energy for the same amount of work. You may also find that you are getting less exercise than your friend, so that you are expending less energy. Finally, you may have acquired an excess of fat as a child, so that even if you eat the same as your friend, you are still not losing your excess stored fat.

My son is seven and is very fat. Will he lose weight as he gets older, or will he be an obese adult?

Unless your son loses weight now, he is likely to be overweight as an adult. Some fat children do lose weight in adolescence, but you can't count on this. Assume that your son is likely to remain fat and help him change his eating habits to prevent this.

Is it true that gland trouble can cause obesity?

People are rarely overweight because of an underactive thyroid gland or overactive adrenal glands, and in these cases there are other symptoms.

Is it true that obese people feel the cold less than thinner people?

Fat tissue is an efficient insulator—in fact this is one of its functions. People who have more fat should not feel the cold as much, since they have insulation under their skin. The exception is people who are overweight as a result of thyroid hormone deficiency: they feel the cold far more than others.

People are called "obese" if more than one-third of their body weight is fat. Obesity can happen to anyone, and not only is the excess weight unattractive, but, more important, it is a serious health hazard.

According to some estimates, in countries like the United States up to half the population carry too much fat and many are obese. Obesity can be prevented by calorie management, although once obesity occurs, it is often difficult for people to achieve their ideal weight.

Causes

Obesity is caused by eating too much, that is, more food than the body uses, so that the surplus is stored as fat. When overeating occurs for many years and the surplus fat is not burned up, weight will be gained. For example, if a person eats one slice of bread more than he or she needs every day, after 10 years the stored food will weigh about 40 pounds (about 18 kg), and the person will weigh 40 pounds more than his or her ideal weight.

To a certain extent, obesity runs in families. The cause may be genetic inheritance—some people are more likely to become obese than others, given the same food intake and energy expended—but often obesity occurs from learning bad eating habits from the family.

Emotional factors can play an important part in causing obesity. When people are depressed, they often turn to food for comfort—and over time, weight gain is the result. Their large size may then be a cause of depression, and they will eat more and get even fatter—making obesity a self-perpetuating condition.

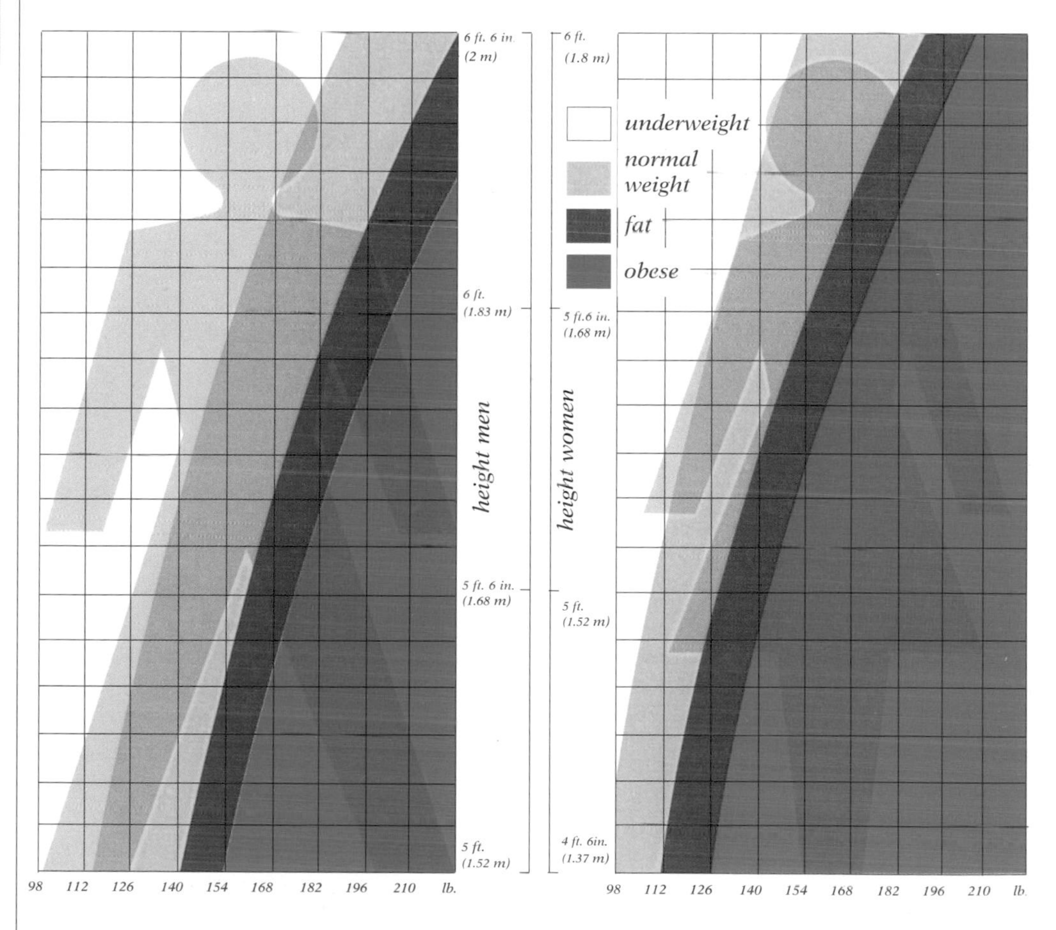

▲ *A simple way of seeing whether you are obese is to check whether your weight is within the recommended range for your sex and height, as shown in the tables above.*

Questions and Answers

I recently stopped smoking and have put on 20 lb. (9 kg). Is this more dangerous to me than if I had continued to smoke?

No. Many people who give up smoking put on weight, usually because they replace addictive smoking with a greater appetite for eating. However, studies have shown that the increase in weight under these circumstances is less dangerous than continued smoking, although clearly it is better to give up smoking without becoming obese.

I am a woman in her forties with three grown children. I don't really overeat, and I seem to be as active as I always was, but I'm obese. How could this have happened?

It happened gradually. If you have been eating only a small amount above your daily calorie requirement, then it will take many years for this excess to accumulate into obesity.

Another possible factor is that women usually acquire weight in pregnancy and may not lose it afterward; therefore, several pregnancies could have left you with a considerable excess, which you will not lose unless you eat less than you require.

Finally, women use up lots of energy caring for young children. If your food intake stays the same, you will put on weight when your children leave home and you have less to do—and as you age and your metabolism slows.

I know that my teenage daughter binges on huge quantities of food at least twice a week, yet she is not obese. Why is this?

Your daughter may be burning up all the calories that she consumes, in which case she should eat smaller amounts of food at regular intervals. Alternatively, she could be suffering from bulimia—binge eating followed by self-induced vomiting. If she seems preoccupied with her weight and you suspect she has bulimia, take her to see your doctor, who may recommend psychotherapy.

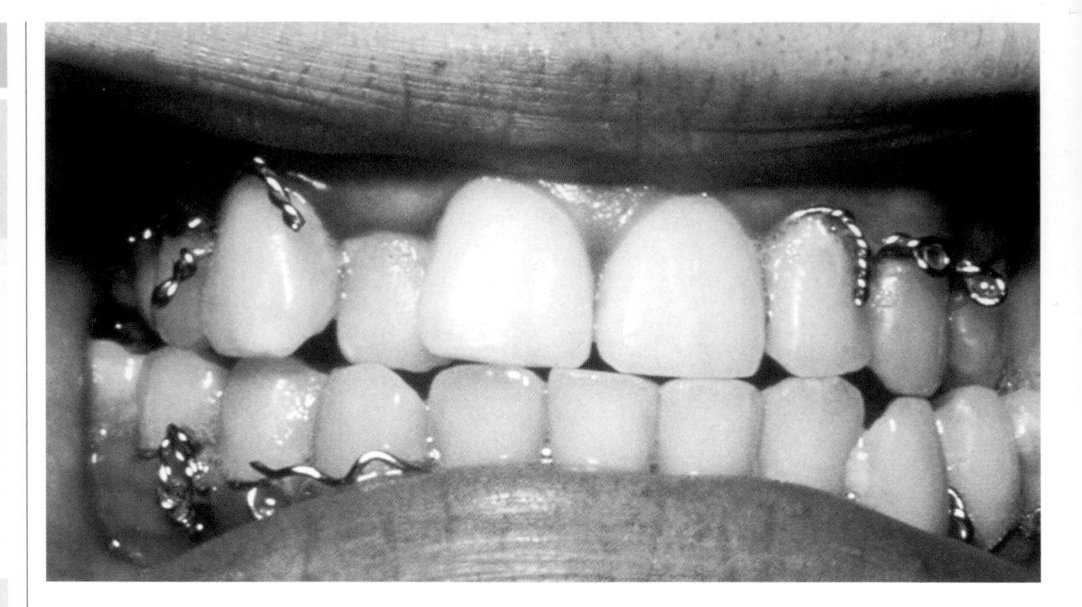

▲ *Wiring together a person's teeth is an extreme measure that can be taken to cure obesity. It is used only as a last resort when all other methods have failed.*

Medical findings

In rare cases a medical problem causes obesity. An underactive thyroid gland or overactive adrenal glands can result in weight gain, as can rare medical causes such as congenital syndromes involving hormonal abnormalities, and birth defects that affect appetite regulation.

Research has also identified a group of proteins called leptins that are involved in the regulation of metabolism and appetite (see Metabolism). Deficiencies of leptins or of their receptors lead to obesity and sometimes cause diabetes in mice. The role of leptins in human obesity is still under investigation.

Development of obesity

When a person consumes more food than the body needs, the liver converts the surplus into fatty acids. These fatty acids are carried in the bloodstream to the fatty (adipose) tissues located around the body, where they are converted into storage fats and kept inside the cells.

When fat is laid down in excess, it appears where the body tissue is most abundant—initially this is usually in the buttocks and the abdomen, followed by the thighs and arms. People may develop fat deposits in slightly different places and at different rates, but most people follow this pattern.

Health risks

Most people dislike being overweight because they feel that it makes them unattractive, but there are also some serious medical dangers that are associated with obesity. Being slightly above the ideal recommended weight for an individual's height, build, and age—by 5 percent or so—is probably not a great risk to health. However, if a person's weight is much over this amount, he or she will be prone to many other complications in addition to the emotional and social problems that obesity can cause.

One problem is that the extra weight an obese person carries is distributed mainly in the central parts of the body, where it puts extra strain on the joints, particularly the knees. This leads to the early development of osteoarthritis (wear and tear of the joints), which is likely to become a painful problem in early middle age (see Osteoarthritis).

In addition to this, obese people who consume large amounts of certain foods and neglect others may suffer from malnourishment due to a lack of protein or essential vitamins and minerals (see Malnutrition).

Obesity can also cause mild diabetes, which in turn may cause serious complications in the small blood vessels of the eyes and kidneys (see Diabetes). Since there is an increase in available fats, especially cholesterol, in the circulation, the obese person also tends to develop gallstones and, to a lesser extent, gout.

Fatty infiltration

More serious problems arise when fatty infiltration impairs the efficiency of the abdominal muscles. This impairment inhibits movement of the diaphragm and makes breathing inefficient, possibly leading to lung disorders and shortness of breath. For similar reasons, obese people have a high incidence of lung complications when they have a general anesthetic before an operation.

Atherosclerosis

Obese people tend to have high levels of fat in their blood, and for this reason they have an increased risk of developing atherosclerosis —thickening and hardening of the arteries that impairs blood circulation (see Arteries and Artery Disease).

As a result, there is likely to be an increased chance of thrombosis of the arteries that supply vital organs such as the brain and heart. This can cause strokes and heart attacks (see Heart Attack; Stroke). If the blood supply to the kidneys is threatened, the blood pressure will rise and kidney failure may result.

Life expectancy

Because of these complications, obese men and women have a reduced chance of living to a healthy old age. Indeed, some insurance companies have calculated that if a man is 25 pounds (11 kg) overweight, his life expectancy will be reduced by one-fourth.

Dieting

The main treatment for obesity is gradual dieting. That is, the gradual overeating that has caused the condition must be reversed so that less food is eaten than is required for the energy expended by the person in his or her daily activities (see Dieting). In addition, the output of energy should be increased through exercise and movement (see Exercise).

Ineffective shortcuts

Dieting is never easy, since it requires extreme willpower to change the eating habits that have been acquired over a lifetime, and for this reason, many obese people try various shortcuts—none of which are an effective alternative to sensible dieting.

The first of these is the crash diet. It is possible for a person to lose a large amount of weight very quickly, but studies have shown that crash dieters almost always gain back the weight and return to their previous size within a year or two of dieting.

Another method is to take amphetaminelike pills. These help reduce a person's appetite, but at the expense of dangerous side effects to the heart and brain. Such pills are also addictive.

Other, much safer, drugs have been developed, including non-absorbable bulking agents, statin drugs such as orlistat that block the action of digestive fat-splitting enzymes, and serotonin reuptake inhibitor anorectic agents such as sibutramine. Although these modern antiobesity drugs can help to control appetite, however, most of them are at least mildly addictive, none actually "burn up" fat, and weight is rapidly regained once the pills are stopped.

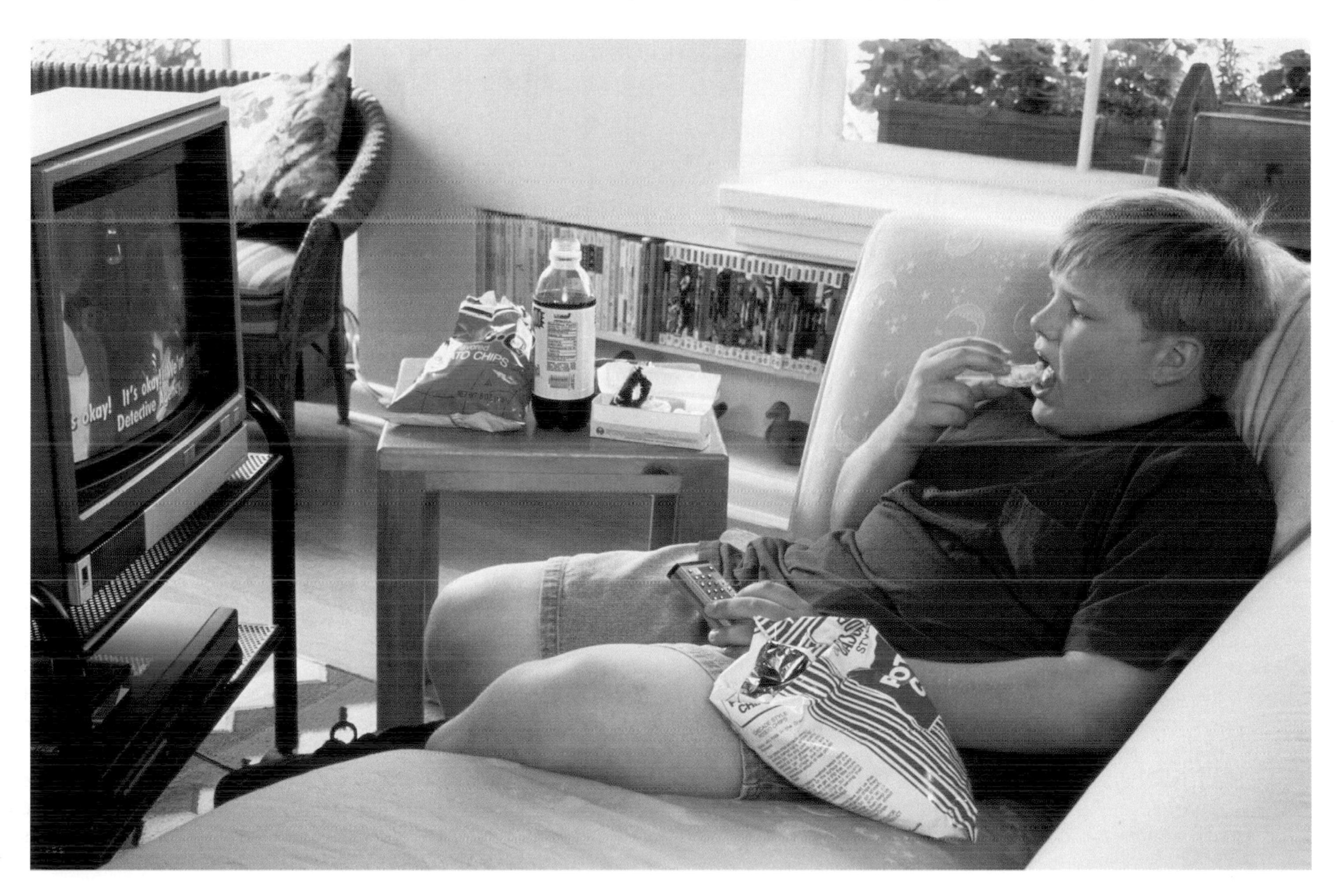

▼ *In recent decades, a dramatic increase in cases of type II diabetes in U.S. children seems to be closely linked to obesity.*

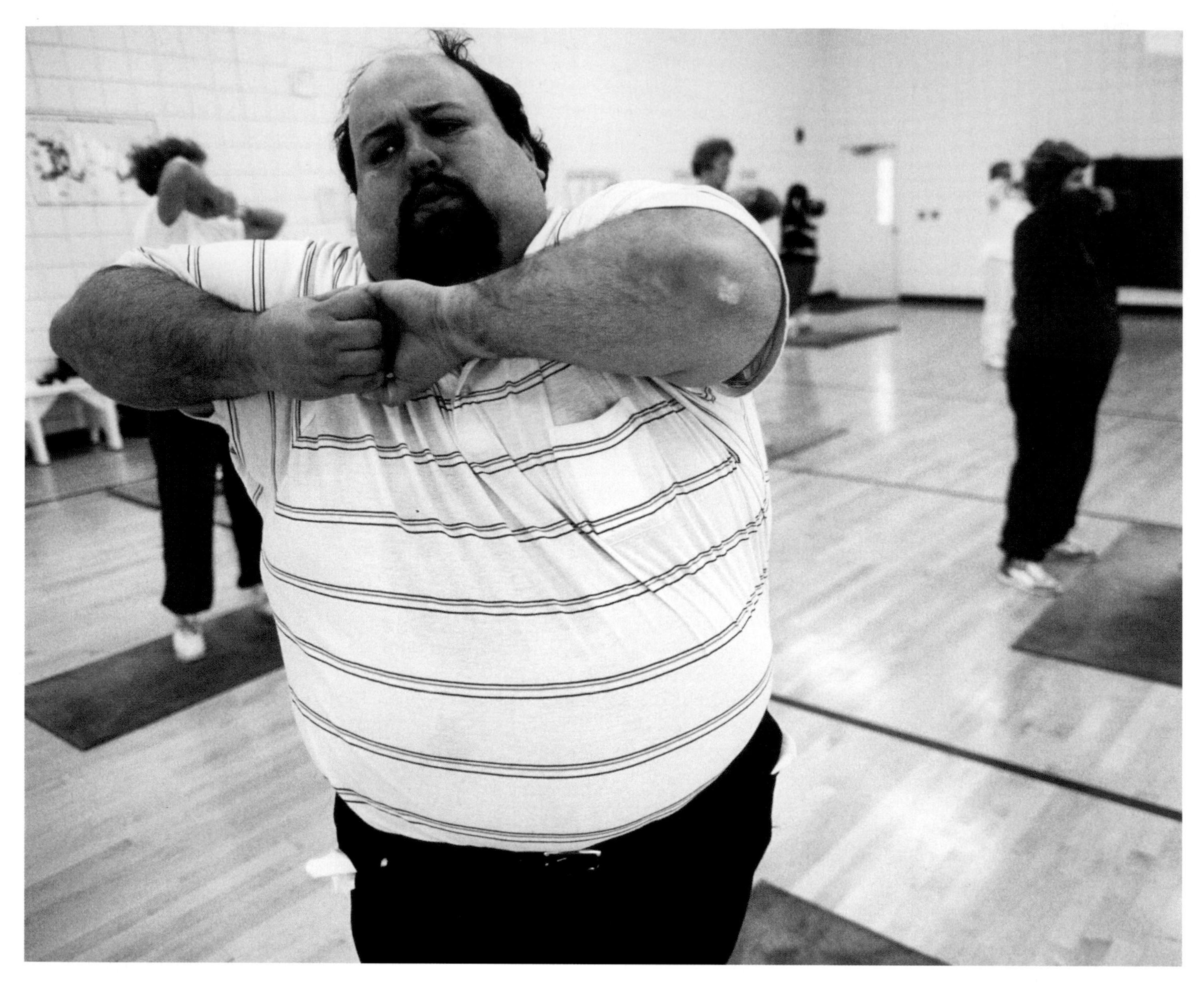

▲ *To achieve long-term weight loss, obese people must consistently eat less and expend more energy through exercise.*

Extreme measures

When obesity becomes life-threatening, people may resort to jaw-wiring, which is the temporary wiring together of the jaws to prevent the person from taking in solid food—resulting in a great loss of weight. However, the weight is usually rapidly regained when the wires are removed.

Various operations have also been tried to help very obese people lose weight when everything else has failed. Sometimes the stomach walls are stapled together to reduce the volume of the stomach so that the person feels full more quickly and stops eating sooner. However, the stomach may still be stretched by overeating, and if the staples break, major surgery may be required. Another method involves removing or reversing segments of the small intestine, or bypassing it, so that less food is absorbed. However, these procedures can cause serious malnutritional problems, and patients risk complications such as leakage of the intestinal fluid, internal bleeding, blockages, infection, and even death.

Lifestyle changes

Obese people who genuinely want to lose weight and to remain slim must completely alter their previous lifestyles and eating patterns. In particular, they must change any bad habits, such as eating only junk food. They may also find it helpful to seek medical advice as to the most suitable diet for weight reduction and for fostering and maintaining sensible and healthy eating habits.

Diet clubs and organizations such as Weight Watchers may help obese people to lose weight and learn about nutrition, which is important, because they need to develop and maintain healthy eating habits after they reach their ideal weight. The clubs also offer the encouragement and support of other members who have a similar problem.

In addition to reorganizing their eating habits, obese people need to increase the amount of exercise that they get—particularly if they lead a mainly sedentary life.

See also: **Anorexia and bulimia; Birth defects; Breathing; Cholesterol; Depression; Fats; Gallbladder and stones; Glands; Gout; Heredity; Kidneys and kidney diseases**

Obsessive-compulsive disorder

Questions and Answers

What's the difference between an obsession and a compulsion?

An obsession is a thought or feeling that keeps recurring over long periods of time. It's an idea which you can't get out of your mind however much you may try, but which has little real relevance to your present life. A compulsion is a constant or repeated conviction that you have to do something, often something that you have already done and, rationally, have no need to do over again. Some compulsions, such as repeatedly checking that you have locked a door or washed your hands, are especially common.

Are obsessions and compulsions always a sign of mental disease?

No; they are both very common, and almost everyone experiences one or both of them, at least to a mild degree, from time to time. Many entirely normal people have long-term mild to moderate obsessions or compulsions.

Are there different kinds of obsessions?

Yes. Most obsessions are just obsessional thoughts, but a person may have obsessional arguments with himself; may experience obsessional images that are often shocking, obscene or antireligious; or may have obsessional doubts. The doubts often concern actions that a person feels responsible for, such as unwittingly causing an accident, accidentally starting a fire, leaving property unsecured, and so on. Obsessional doubts commonly lead to compulsive actions.

Are women more often affected by obsessive-compulsive disorder than men?

No. The sex incidence is equal.

This distressing psychological disorder can, when severe, be seriously disabling. Developments in understanding of the condition have provided effective and drug-free treatment that will be of great benefit to most affected people.

Many people with this condition seriously fear that they may be developing a psychosis and that they will become seriously mentally ill (see Psychoses). It is important for them to be aware that this is not so. It is not common for obsessive-compulsive disorder to progress to a psychosis. In the United States, obsessive-compulsive disorder affects about 500 people in every 100,000 of the population. About 75 percent of all affected people have both obsessive symptoms and compulsive symptoms. The remainder have either obsessions or compulsions alone. The disorder commonly starts at a time of great emotional stress, and it has a slight tendency to run in families. In about one case in 20 a blood relative also has the disorder.

Causes

Very little is known about the causes of obsessive-compulsive disorder. Psychoanalytic theories of causation, claiming that the disorder is a defensive regression to the pre-oedipal anal-sadistic phase, now carry little weight with most experts. It has been claimed that a high proportion of people with this disorder had a difficult or prolonged birth and may have suffered some subtle brain damage. Affected people have a higher incidence of slight but nonsignificant abnormalities in their electroencephalogram (EEG) than those in the general population. Some people with certain forms of epilepsy also have obsessive-compulsive symptoms. However, none of these findings should be taken as conclusive evidence that this is a simple neurological disorder.

Symptoms

Obsessional thoughts tend to follow a well-recognized pattern and commonly relate to one or more of six themes. One of the most prominent is a preoccupation with dirt, contamination, and

▼ *Repetitive hand washing can be a symptom of obsessive-compulsive disorder.*

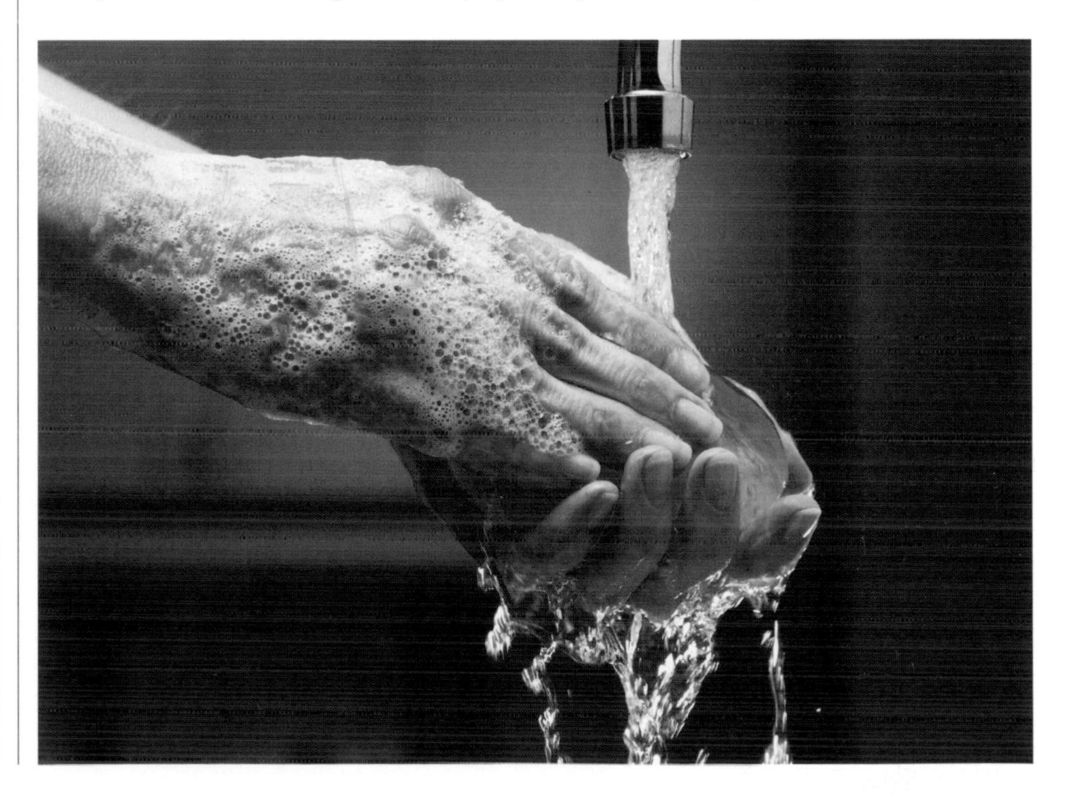

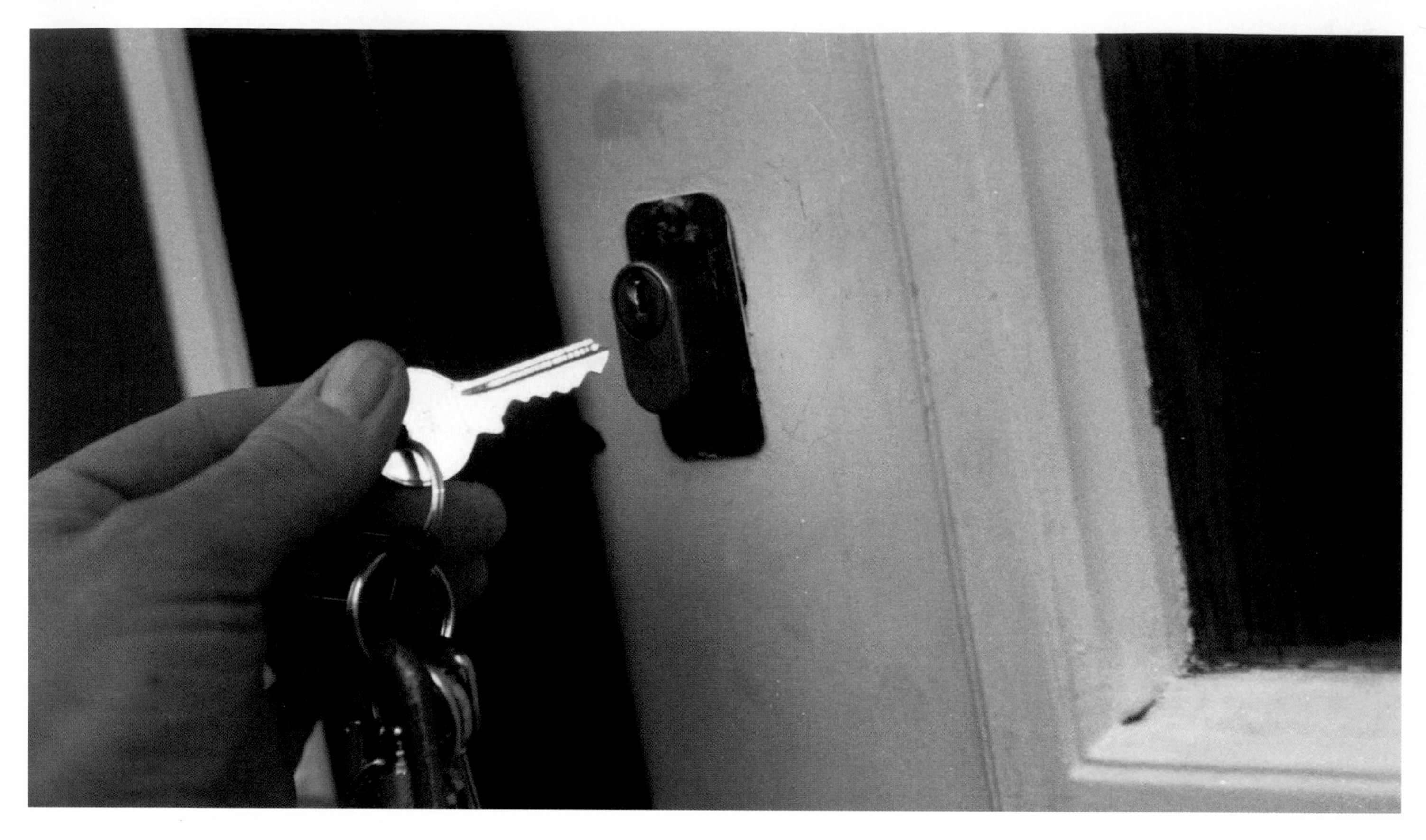

▲ *One type of obsessive-compulsive disorder involves checking and rechecking that a door is locked.*

disease. This obsession usually leads to repetitive compulsive cleaning, washing the hands to the point of severe dermatitis, and other related rituals. The second theme is an obsessive belief that the affected person is suffering from a particular disease, usually cancer. This type of obsession overlaps with hypochondria.

A third theme is obsessive orderliness—the need to have a place for everything and to put everything in its place in a particular way. Any deviation from the recognized standard pattern causes severe mental discomfort and a compulsion to restore the status quo. Sometimes obsessive orderliness involves the fear that others may be harmed unless a particular pattern of behavior is meticulously followed. This may amount to a severe and disabling compulsion. The fourth theme is an obsession that the sufferer may act aggressively, physically or verbally, toward another person. Such obsessions, however, seldom lead to actual aggression.

The fifth and sixth of the common themes relate to religion and sex. Religious obsessions involve doubts and thoughts believed to be blasphemous. Obsessive patterns of behavior in religious observance may also be involved, with the belief that any deviation from a set ritual may have dire spiritual consequences. Sexual obsessions usually take the form of recurrent imaginings of sexual activity that the person concerned finds obscene and disgusting but is unable to banish from the mind (see Sex).

People with obsessive-compulsive disorder should be aware that however strong one of their more serious impulses may be, they are most unlikely to act on it. Therefore, people with a compulsion to perform an act they would normally find abhorrent, or to commit a crime, are most unlikely to give way to the impulse.

Outlook

About 70 percent of all those newly affected by obsessive-compulsive disorder improve substantially within a year. The others suffer prolonged but often intermittent symptoms, with periods of total or partial recovery lasting for months or years. The most severe and persistent cases are those in people whose personality has always been obsessive, and the outlook is worst for those with the most severe symptoms who have particularly stressful lives.

Treatment

Patients should be aware that rituals and magical thinking are their worst enemy and actually perpetuate the obsessive-compulsive disorder. Both should be strongly resisted. Magical thinking is the belief that by thinking of something an event can be made to happen in the real world. An affected person can do much to improve his or her condition by deliberately refraining from engaging in any meaningless ritual, and by rejecting the belief that thoughts can directly influence events. With the agreement of the sufferer, all members of the family should be aware of the harmful effects of persisting in abnormal rituals. Stressful factors should be eliminated as much as possible.

If professional treatment is needed this is most likely to be successful if it takes the form of behavior therapy, supplemented, if necessary, by a serotonin reuptake inhibitor drug such as fluvoxamine (trade name: Luvox) or fluoxetine (trade name: Prozac). Behavior therapy is largely concerned with personal training in the avoidance of ritual behavior.

See also: **Behavior therapy; Complexes and compulsions; Hypochondria; Mental illness; Neuroses; Psychiatry; Stress; Tranquilizers**

Obstetrics

Obstetricians and nurse-midwives are trained in obstetrics; they specialize in the care of women throughout pregnancy and labor, and up until after the birth. Most babies in the United States are delivered by obstetricians.

The term "obstetrics" refers to the branch of medicine that deals with the emotional and physical well-being of a woman during her pregnancy, her labor, and the period of adaptation to the new baby. Equally important, obstetrics is also concerned with the health and welfare of the unborn child and his or her safe passage into the world.

Physicians who specialize in this field are known as obstetricians. A nurse-midwife—who is often the main medical staff member present during births in Europe, but who is involved in only about 4 percent of births in the United States—is a nurse who has trained extensively in obstetrics. He or she is qualified to conduct normal prenatal care and deliveries in cooperation with an obstetrician. Also involved are such professionals as family doctors.

Prenatal care

Obstetricians and nurse-midwives work very closely together, and many areas of their work overlap, especially in the prenatal clinic. It is here that the expectant mother receives regular medical checkups to ensure that she is fit and that the baby is developing normally. The staff members give her information about diet during and after pregnancy and advice on any vitamin

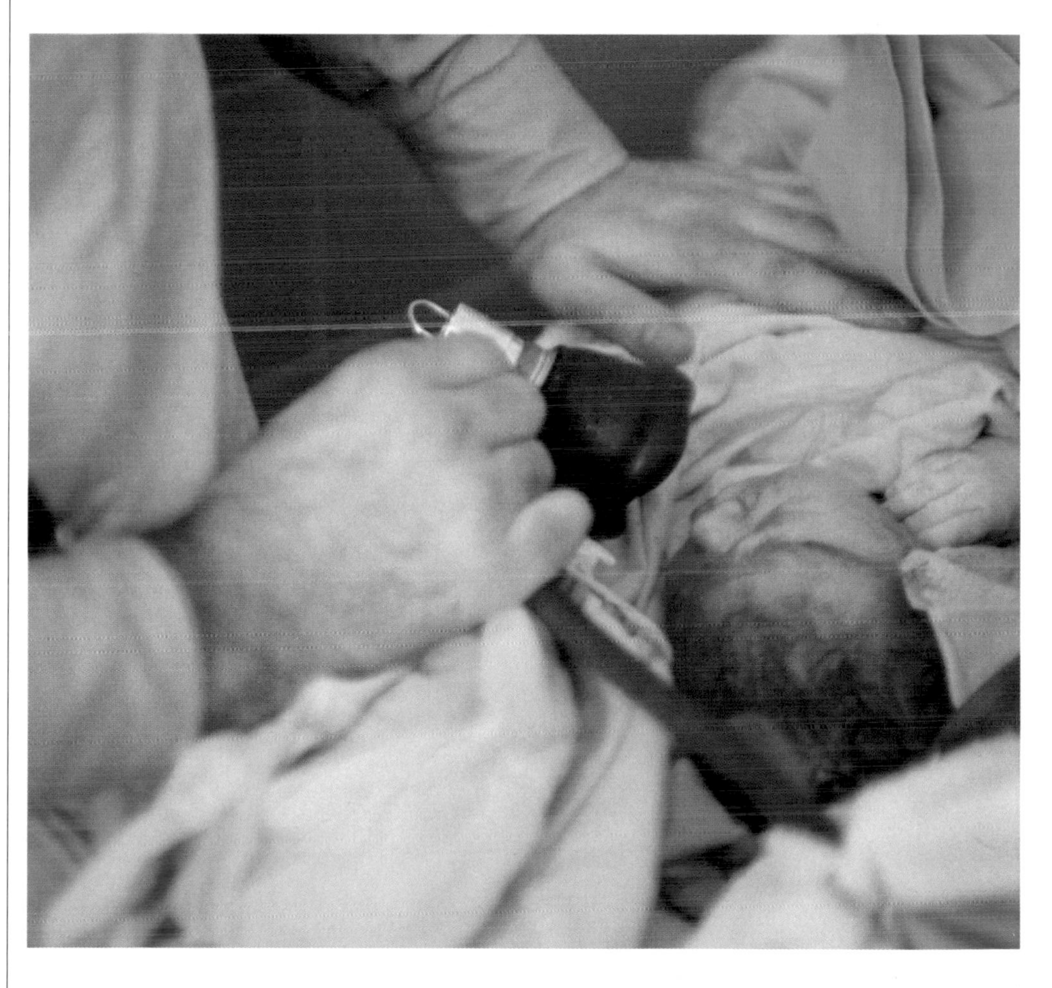

▲ *This obstetrician is assisting the breathing of, and giving oxygen to, a baby who has been delivered by a cesarean section.*

Questions and Answers

Does the obstetrician deal with any serious problems a baby may have at birth, or is he or she only concerned with the health and safety of the mother?

Once the baby has been safely delivered, the obstetrician usually arranges for him or her to be examined by a pediatrician, who specializes in the care of babies and children. If problems arise, the pediatrician will continue to supervise the baby's medical care. The obstetrician continues to care for the mother after the birth.

How early in my pregnancy should I arrange to see an obstetrician?

If you have any medical problem, such as diabetes, it is wise to see an obstetrician as soon as your pregnancy is confirmed. When an expectant mother has an illness, the medical treatment will probably need to be altered to enable her body to cope with the additional stress of pregnancy.

If you are healthy it is advisable to see an obstetrician by the time you are 12 weeks pregnant. You should definitely see him or her before you are 16 weeks pregnant. During this period a blood test should be performed to exclude some serious abnormalities of the baby's spinal cord and brain.

I have been told that my baby can be delivered by a nurse-midwife. Would it be better if the baby was delivered by an obstetrician?

Your question suggests that your doctor expects the delivery to be perfectly normal. Obstetricians are more skilled than nurse-midwives at conducting deliveries when help is needed to assist the birth by artificial means—such as by forceps or by cesarean section. If you are worried, talk to your obstetrician; he or she will be able to set your mind at ease.

OBSTETRICAL DUTIES

From the time her pregnancy is confirmed, an obstetrician ensures that the expectant mother and developing fetus are healthy.

A pregnant woman should visit her obstetrician once a month during the first trimester, then once every two weeks until the ninth month, when she should visit every week until her due date. The obstetrician will check her blood pressure and estimate the size of the baby.

During the birth the obstetrician will take over from the nurse-midwife if, for example, a forceps delivery is required. After the birth, the nurse-midwife checks that the uterus is returning to normal and has no signs of infection, and may give advice on feeding and bathing the baby. Some midwives are trained nurses, but all obstetricians must be trained doctors. Many women choose to have their baby in a hospital; here, whenever the mother's health is in question, an obstetrican will be close by.

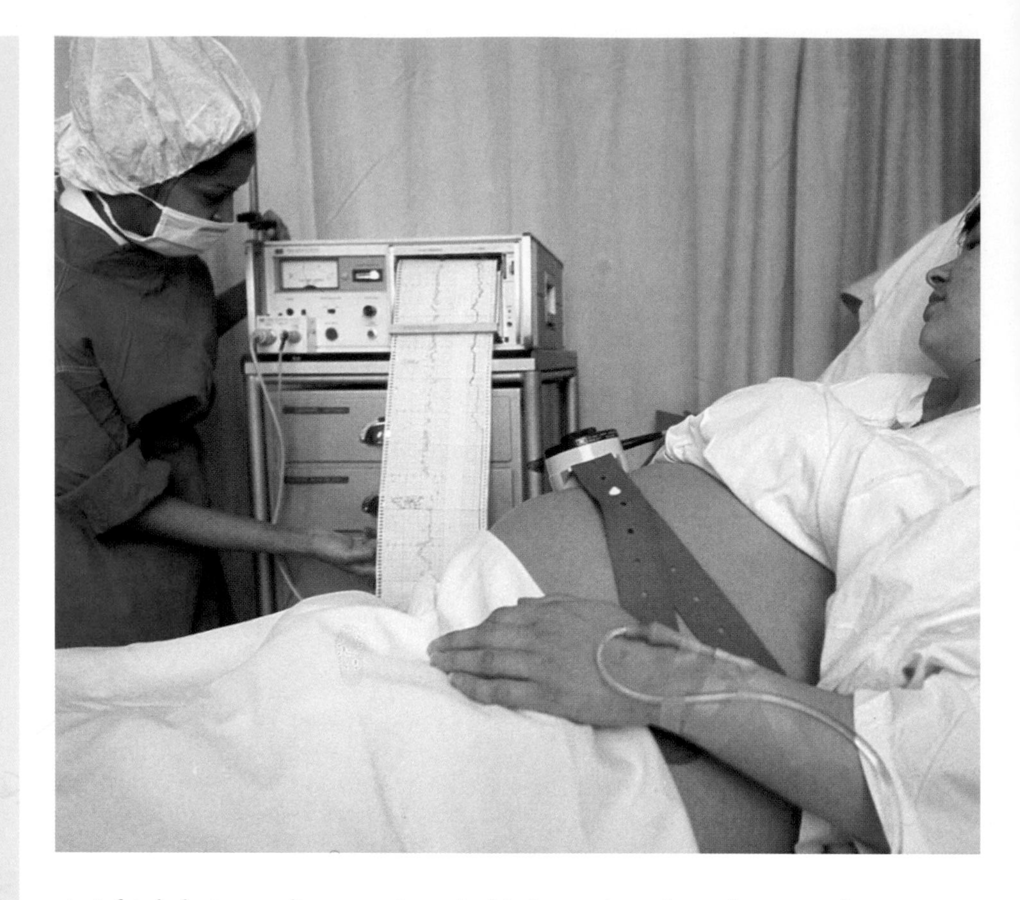

▲ *A fetal electrocardiogram gives vital information about the state of a pregnancy by measuring the baby's heartbeat.*

supplements that she may require. They also teach her about care of the baby and make arrangements for her to attend classes on the process of labor and any special techniques—such as breathing exercises—that will help her during labor and delivery.

Any woman attending a prenatal clinic will usually see an obstetrician during her first visit. During later visits, a doctor or a nurse-midwife may examine her. However, the obstetrician will need to examine her when she is 36 weeks pregnant and again if she passes the estimated date of delivery—usually around 40 weeks—without going into labor.

During the first visit the obstetrician will discuss the progress of the pregnancy, and there will be an opportunity for the expectant mother to discuss any anxieties she may have. The obstetrician will then examine her to check that she is in good health.

This first examination includes an internal, or pelvic, examination to make certain that the uterus has enlarged to the correct size for the length of the pregnancy. The obstetrician will also be able to see whether the woman's reproductive organs are healthy and whether the bones of her pelvis are wide enough to allow the baby to pass through. Blood tests are taken to ensure that the woman is not anemic and that there is no possibility of her having syphilis, which she could pass on to the baby. They will also indicate her blood group and whether or not she is immune to rubella (German measles).

At 36 weeks, the obstetrician palpates (examines by feeling and touching) the woman's abdomen carefully to see if the baby is growing well and is lying in the correct position for a normal delivery. For a normal birth the baby's head should occupy the lower part of the uterus at this stage. If the baby is too large to be delivered normally, or if the mother's bones are too narrow, the baby may need to be delivered by a cesarean section (see Cesarean Birth). Once a pregnancy has continued for longer than 41 weeks, the placenta may become less efficient at providing the baby with oxygen and nourishment. At that time, the obstetrician and mother must decide whether or not to start labor artificially (see Induction of Labor).

Labor

During labor any woman who has chosen to have a normal hospital birth will have the constant companionship of the hospital staff. If during this time there is any indication that artificial intervention may be needed, the advice of an obstetrician will be sought. Most women in the United States are seen by an obstetrician even when there are no problems; he or she will also deliver the baby in most cases. European babies are often delivered by nurse-midwives.

Puerperium

The time from the birth of the baby until the woman has returned to her normal pre-pregnant state is called the puerperium—it lasts about six weeks. During the first 10 days she is usually visited by an obstetrician or nurse-midwife. If the new mother shows signs of infection or other medical problems, she will be treated. At the end of the puerperium period most women are seen by their obstetrician or a family doctor to ensure that they have adapted both physically and emotionally to the new child.

See also: **Birth; Fetus; Natural childbirth; Pregnancy; Prenatal care**

Occupational hazards

Every year, occupational hazards result in disease, injury, and sometimes even death. People encounter a variety of potential problems in the workplace, and many of these can be prevented.

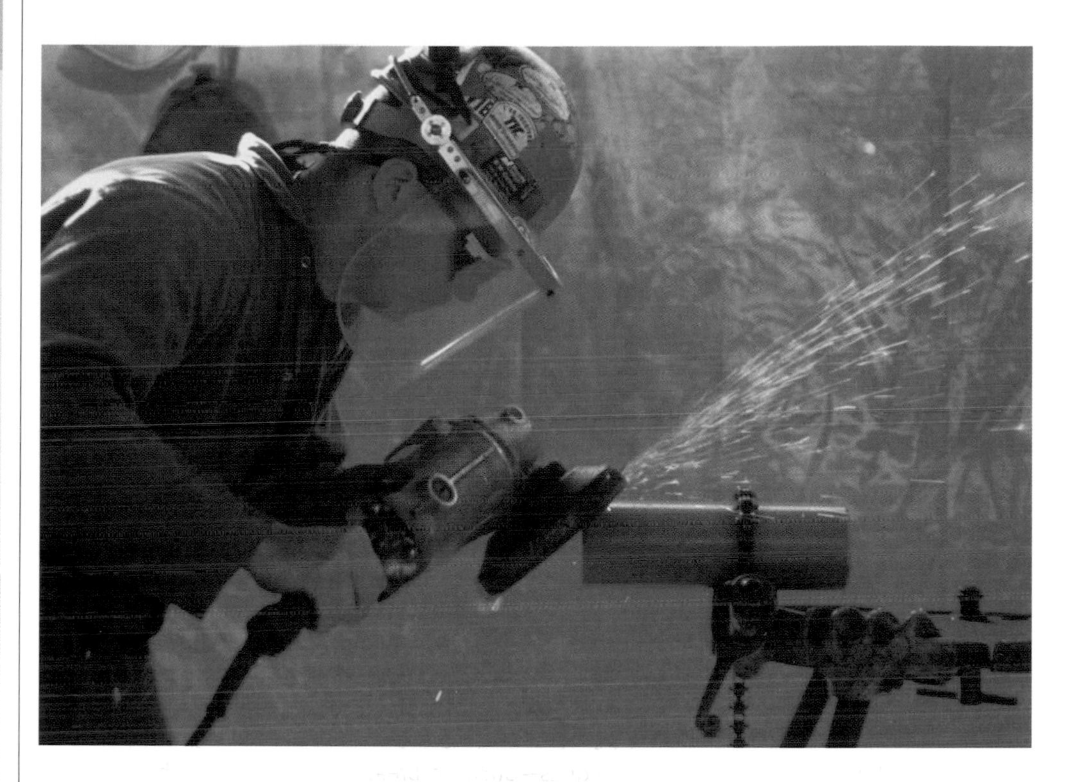

▲ *This industrial worker wears a special helmet with a visor to protect his face from the dangerously sharp bits of metal that are flying off the metal tube he is grinding.*

Health hazards associated with work have existed for centuries. In the last few hundred years, with the development of industrialization, very specific occupational hazards have been recognized. While industry was slow to acknowledge and deal with the problems, safety measures are now regarded as a high priority by many employers and labor unions.

Apart from the personal toll that such occupational disease and injury can bring, there is a heavy economic price to pay. Millions of working days are lost each year in the United States through work-related health problems.

Many of the most serious occupational hazards have been brought under control by legislation. However, the risks can never be eliminated completely as new products and working methods are devised and tried. There is also the reality that accidents with machinery can never be totally eliminated, because of human error. However, these accidents can be minimized. Employers should ensure that safety standards are maintained, and staff members should always adhere to safety regulations (see Accident Prevention).

Hazardous materials

Occupational hazards may arise with the use of gases, liquids, or solids. Substances can enter the body through the lungs.

One dangerous metal is lead, a toxic substance that has been used in the manufacture of batteries, rubber, paint, roofing, and soldering material. It can enter the body through the inhalation of small dust particles and fumes or by ingestion. The earliest symptoms may include fatigue, headache, loss of appetite, constipation, and mild abdominal pain. Acute poisoning can result in severe abdominal pain, muscle weakness, kidney damage, convulsions, coma, and death.

Questions and Answers

I read that inhaling some kinds of dusts found at work can be dangerous. Why is this?

Although it is not desirable to have any foreign particles enter the lungs, some dusts are more harmful than others. A stonecutter who works only with marble and inhales its dust has practically no chance of getting lung disease. Yet if he were working on sandstone, the risk of lung disease and death caused by the dust would be high. The reason for these differences is not fully understood. Many dusts, such as asbestos, are a special danger and can cause cancer of the lung and the pleura (lining of the lung), as well as the disabling disease asbestosis.

I have heard mixed reports about whether computer screens are safe to use. What are the health risks?

Reports on the risks to health from radiation as a result of using computers are very mixed, but prolonged use of terminals may cause physical problems such as eyestrain; headaches; pain in the back, neck, arms, and fingers (carpal tunnel syndrome); and more general stress. Some of these ailments can be avoided if the terminal is set in a properly designed workstation. Regular breaks should be taken away from the computer screen, with at least 10 minutes' rest every hour.

We have a representative in our office whose sole concern is health and safety. Why do we need one?

Every year thousands of office staffers are injured at work. Half of the injuries are caused by falls, such as tripping over carelessly placed wires or objects. These accidents can be easily prevented, and a safety representative is very helpful in assessing the potential dangers to the staff and advising the management accordingly.

Questions and Answers

I often have to work night shifts. Will this affect my health?

About 20 percent of people enjoy working nights; another 20 percent dislike it intensely and have to quit. No studies have shown any difference in causes of death between day and night workers, but if you have been working during the day and then are put onto a night shift, it can take time for your body to adapt. Research shows that there is a slightly higher incidence of cancer in people who are not exposed to normal diurnal and nocturnal light and dark cycles.

I work near a hot furnace. Will the high temperatures harm me?

The body can usually adapt to raised temperatures, but if physical labor is involved, and if the salt and water lost during sweating are not replaced, you may suffer from heatstroke or heat syncope, leading to unconsciousness. Treatment involves cooling the body and rest. If you become used to high temperatures, heat tolerance is likely to be greater and the chance of problems reduced.

I am a smoker. Can smoking increase the risk of my getting a work-related disease?

Yes. Smoking is likely to increase your risk of developing a number of health problems. One problem is that smoking damages the airways, undermining the natural defense of the lungs and allowing harmful substances easier access into your body.

Why are substances thought to cause cancer still used in industry?

It is not possible to eliminate these substances entirely from many industrial processes. However, the Occupational Health and Safety Administration constantly studies these substances to establish safe levels and safeguards to protect workers. Companies that do not follow these guidelines risk legal action.

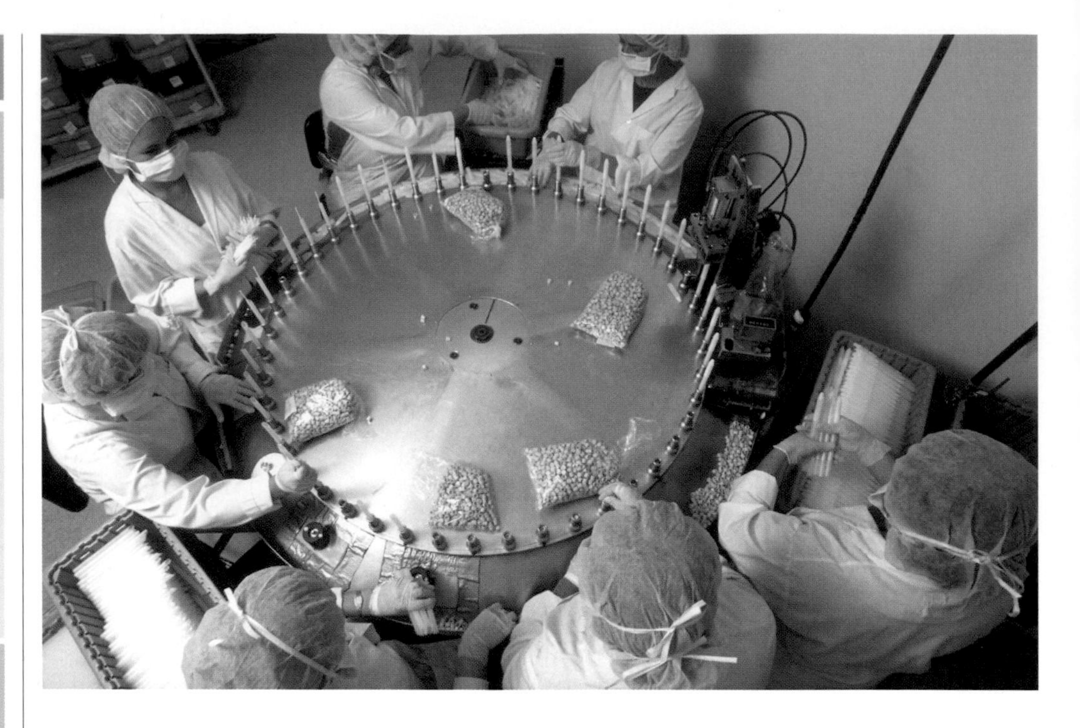

▲ *These pharmaceutical workers packaging pills are wearing sterilized gowns, masks, and gloves to prevent any diseases or infections from reaching the consumer.*

Mercury, a silver-colored liquid that has been used in some thermometers, is another hazardous metal. It has been used in the electrical industry to manufacture fluorescent lamps and precision instruments, as well as in dentistry.

Mercury poisoning causes jerky movements starting in the fingers, irritability, and drowsiness. In the final stage, the person becomes mentally disturbed. Other symptoms include sore throat and gums, vomiting, and diarrhea. Compounds from mercury can also be dangerous when they occur in the form of industrial effluents. The effluents are absorbed by fish, which are then eaten by people (see Pollution). The poisoning results in blindness, mental deterioration, lack of coordination, birth defects, and even death (see Birth Defects).

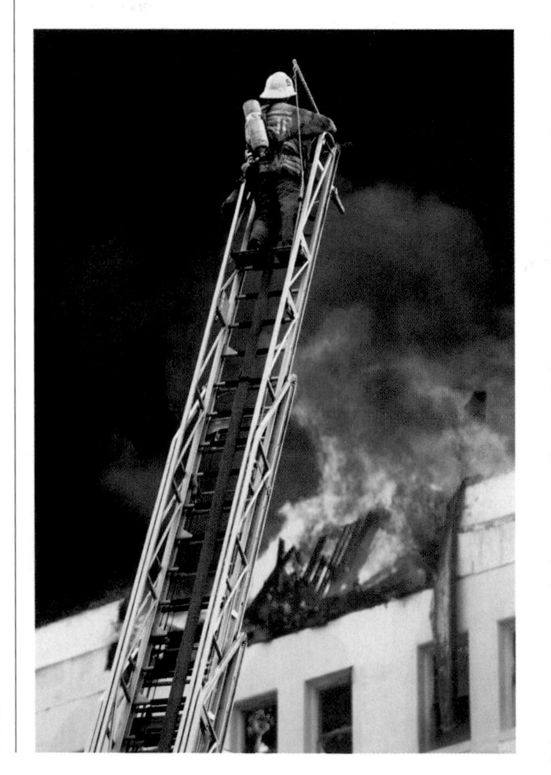

Cadmium, a soft metal that is used for increasing the hardness of copper, and as a protective plating for other metals, is particularly dangerous. Once a person has inhaled or ingested a certain amount, there is no known cure. Poisoning can be gradual because the amount of metal in the body builds up slowly. However, at a critical point the lungs and the kidneys will cease to function properly, causing death.

Chromium, a silver-white, hard, brittle metal, is used to make various types of steel, including stainless steel, and high-speed tools. Its compounds are used in chrome plating as well as the production of pigments in paints and inks. It is also used in leather tanning, in timber preservation, and in photography and dyestuffs. The major danger of chromium is that even slight contact with dilute solutions can cause skin ulcers (see Ulcers).

◄ *Firefighters face many occupational hazards that can result in injury or death from falls, burns, and smoke inhalation.*

The inhalation of fine droplets or mist containing chromium salts can cause ulcers inside the nose. Although lung cancer has not been associated with chrome plating, it has been linked with the manufacture of chromates. Asthmatic symptoms can occur, as can sensitivity to chrome—a strong reaction to chrome following symptoms of exposure (see Asthma).

Many liquids are classed as solvents, and employees in nearly all occupations are exposed to them. Solvents evaporate very quickly, and the vapors can enter the body by inhalation through the lungs, the skin, and, more rarely, the digestive system. Once they enter the body, they can attack the liver, the heart, the lungs, and the nervous system (see Solvent Abuse).

Solvents are found in inks, varnishes, glues, cleaners, dry-cleaning fluids, and many other substances. Some of the most dangerous ones may be pleasant to smell, while others that are foul-smelling can be quite harmless.

Trichlorethylene smells good, but it can cause loss of consciousness and death. Benzene is another pleasant-smelling solvent, used in the manufacture of artificial leather, some detergents, pesticides, and paint removers. It can cause dizziness and coma. When poisoning is chronic, leukemia may result (see Leukemia).

Because of the dissolving properties of solvents, they can attack the skin and cause skin inflammation (dermatitis). Contact with solvents should be strictly limited.

All isocyanates are dangerous. They are used in the manufacture of a variety of polyurethanes that are used to make foams, adhesives, lacquers, and paints. Overexposure to isocyanates that are in the air can lead to painful skin inflammation, eye irritation, and breathing difficulties, including severe asthma. Some people can also develop sensitivity to isocyanate.

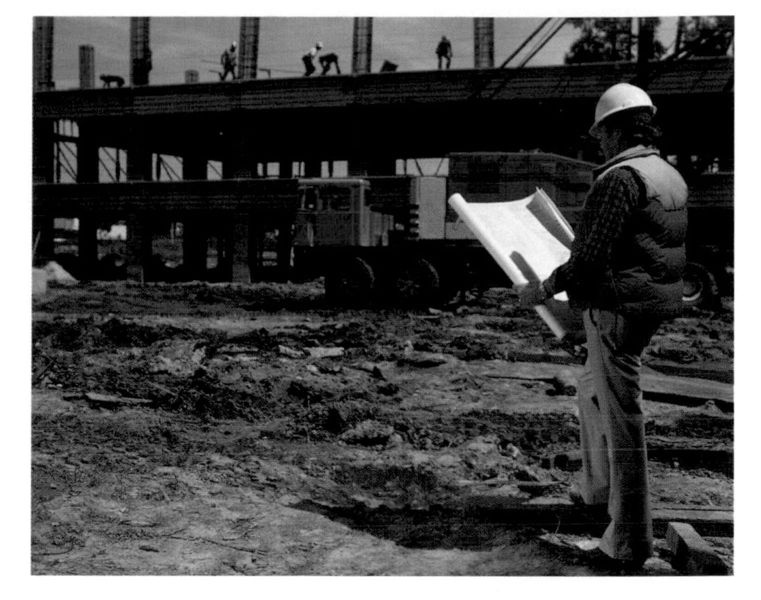

▲ *Thousands of construction workers are injured or killed in accidents on construction sites each year, most commonly from falls, but also from electric shocks, collapsing structures, fires, explosions, welding, and machinery.*

Dust is the biggest killer in industry. Some dusts are relatively harmless, but others are deadly. There are four basic categories. The

Emergency first aid

To give first aid in an emergency, first see if the patient is breathing. If breathing has stopped, either start mouth-to-mouth resuscitation, or if the patient's mouth is burned with chemicals, start cardiac compression. Next, check for serious bleeding. Control bleeding by pressing at the site of the wound with a sterilized pad or with your fingers. Raise the injured limb, if possible, to help slow the blood flow. If the patient is unconscious, make sure that he or she can breathe and the throat is not obstructed. Place the person in the recovery position; get expert help immediately.

OTHER INJURIES	TREATMENT
Burns and scalds	Cool the area by flushing with plenty of clean, cool water. Then cover with a sterile dressing or clean material. Do not apply any ointment, or burst any blisters, or remove any clothing sticking to burns.
Chemical burns	Remove contaminated clothing, taking care that you do not contaminate yourself, and dilute the chemical by flushing with plenty of water. Then apply a dry dressing.
Chemical in the eye	Quickly flush the open eye with clean, cool water and continue for at least 10 minutes.
Foreign body in the eye	If the object cannot be removed easily with the corner of a clean piece of material or by flushing with water, send the patient to the hospital.
Broken bones	Unless there is a danger of further injury, do not move the patient until expert help arrives.
Electric shock	Do not touch the patient until the current has been switched off. If breathing has stopped, give mouth-to-mouth resuscitation or cardiac compression and call for expert help.
Gas inhalation	Move the patient into fresh air, but wear suitable breathing equipment so that you do not become a victim yourself. If breathing has stopped, give mouth-to-mouth resuscitation or cardiac compression.
Amputation of finger	Keep pressure over the stump to prevent arterial bleeding. Wrap the finger in an ice pack. Rush the patient and the protected dismembered finger to the hospital.

Questions and Answers

I've heard that if a man works with dangerous substances his wife can be affected. Is this true?

Yes. This can happen if proper precautions and hygiene are not followed. Cases of lead poisoning have been seen among families of lead workers who went home without changing their work clothes. Employees can also carry contaminating fibers home on their clothing. However, strict regulations are ensuring that such risks are a thing of the past.

I work in industry and am planning to have a baby. Are there any health risks that could affect my pregnancy?

There are laws to protect women from most dangerous hazards, such as lead. Other risks can include waste anesthetic gases to which operating room staff members can be exposed; these gases can cause miscarriages and birth defects. Radiation is a danger, and a fetus is 10 times as vulnerable as an adult. Mercury and its compounds, which can produce mental abnormalities in children, are a potential problem. It should be remembered that the fetus is at risk from all toxic substances that are transferred via the mother. Therefore, smoking and drinking alcohol in pregnancy are not recommended.

I use a pneumatic drill whose noise level is controlled. Could the vibrations affect my body?

The major hazard for people using vibration tools is vibration white finger; the blood supply to the fingers is impeded and the fingers appear pale and can tingle and feel numb. At a certain stage, the tissue damage becomes permanent. People with poor circulation should not do this sort of job. Others should wear warm clothing and padded gloves when using the tools. Where possible, employees should be in a warm environment to ensure good circulation in the extremities. Hours for this type of work should be strictly limited.

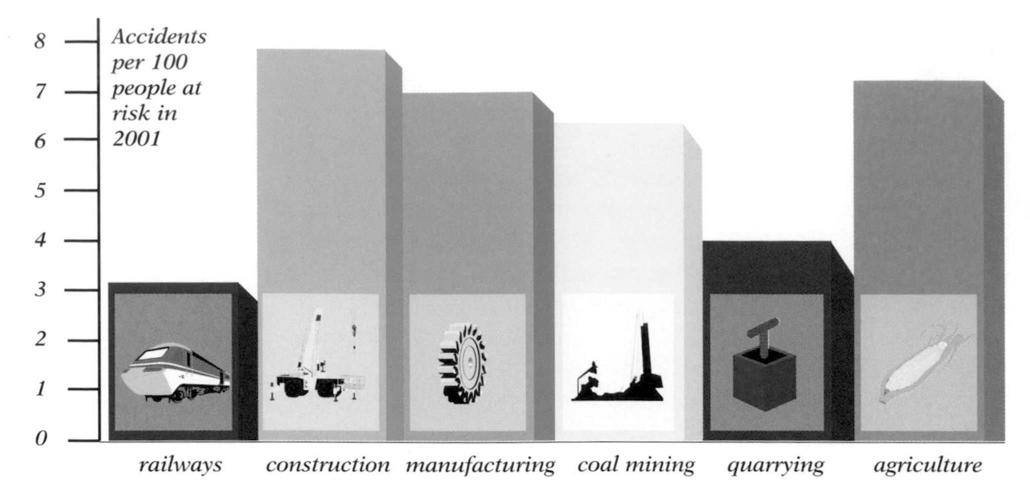

▲ *The graph shows hazardous occupations, as measured by the number of accidents recorded at work. Many other jobs also involve health hazards for workers.*

first category is nuisance or inert dust such as plaster of paris, starch, and portland cement. Such dusts can accumulate in the body without producing a serious reaction. Second, toxic dusts include lead and chromium compounds. They can have serious effects on specific organs in the body such as the kidneys and the nervous system. Third, dusts that produce allergic reactions, such as some wood dusts and fungus spores from grain, can cause eczema and asthma (see Eczema). Fourth, there are some dusts, like asbestos and coal dust, that alter the lung tissue, making the lungs inefficient. These cause death and serious disability in hundreds of people.

The danger of dusts depends not only on the type of dust but on the amount and the time over which it is breathed in. It is often more dangerous to inhale small quantities of dust repeatedly over a long period than to inhale a large amount of dust in a short period.

Healthy lungs can cope with a certain amount of some dust and fumes without any ill effects. However, the body's defense mechanisms may be unable to cope with the onslaught of dangerous or excessive dusts. This is why elimination of dust in the working atmosphere is so important, and why protective clothing and respiratory equipment must be used.

In many industries, working with deafening noise used to be accepted as part of the job. However, it is now a hazard for which there are controls and preventive measures (see Noise).

Basic preventive measures are to deaden the noise of machinery, and instruct workers to wear earmuffs or plugs that reduce sound levels (see Hearing).

Occupational injuries

Every year, some people employed in manufacturing jobs die as a result of an occupational accident or disease. Some jobs have a notoriously high risk of death, such as lumberjacking or working on oil rigs. Other jobs are not dangerous in themselves, but they involve machinery that can give rise to accidents if misused.

A number of accidents occur through the use of unguarded machinery. Laws declare that all machinery must be safeguarded, but some employers try to cut corners and do not always ensure that these safeguards are taken. Moreover, some employees believe that

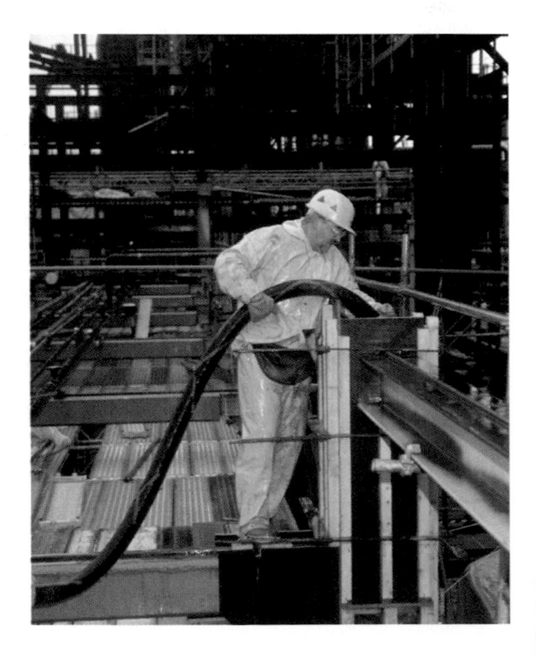

► *Factory workers at oil refineries risk injury or death from accidents involving gas leakages or explosions.*

Occupational hazards

HAZARD	INDUSTRY	ENTRY MODE	SYMPTOMS	TREATMENT	PREVENTION
AIDS	Doctors, dentists	Needle-stick injuries	Fever, fatigue, attacks of shingles or herpes	Anti-HIV drugs but no cure	Care with needles, proper disposal of blood-associated equipment
Asbestos	Many, including shipbuilding, pipe and boiler lagging, building	Inhalation	Breathlessness, dry cough, cancer of the lung or pleura (lining of thorax and lungs)	Remove from further exposure to inhalation and relieve symptoms	Enclosing dust-producing process, wearing masks and gloves, using substitute materials
Cadmium	Plating on metals; production of alloys, paints, enamel, and pigments	Inhalation or ingestion	Irritation of eyes and nose, breathlessness, coughing, vomiting, headache, diarrhea, colic, kidney damage	Symptomatic only	Enclosing process, wearing masks and gloves, monitoring of the environment
Chromium	Auto industry, steel, pigments, leather tanning, photography	Inhalation	Ulcers on skin, especially nasal membranes; asthmatic symptoms	Ointment and local treatment of ulcers	Enclosing process, environmental monitoring, wearing masks and gloves
Hepatitis	Laboratory and hospital workers	Contact with infected blood or excreta	Weakness, loss of appetite, malaise, jaundice	No specific treatment; hepatitis A often self-limiting	Safety clothing and protocols to avoid contamination
Isocyanates	Manufacture of foams, adhesives, synthetic rubbers, paints, polyurethane	Vapor inhalation or skin contact	Dermatitis, coughing, eye irritation, asthma, and breathlessness	Removal from contact, symptomatic treatment	Exhaust ventilation, wearing masks and gloves
Lead	Batteries, rubber, paint, roofing, and soldering	Ingestion, inhalation	Headache, convulsions, constipation, coma, abdominal pain, muscle weakness, kidney damage	Removal from exposure, chelation to remove lead and change properties, oral penicillamine	Exhaust ventilation, personal hygiene, regular analysis of blood and urine, environmental monitoring
Mercury	Electrical industry, fluorescent lamps, dentistry	Inhalation, ingestion, absorption through skin	Jerky movements, irritability, drowsiness, bleeding gums	Removal from source of contact	Enclosing process, exhaust ventilation, wearing masks and gloves
Noise	Boilermaking, drop-forging, shipbuilding	Ears	Deafness	Remove from further exposure	Reducing machinery noise, wearing earplugs
Radiation	Medicine, luminous dials, atomic energy and weapons, welding checks	Irradiation, ingestion of contaminated particles	Burns, scaling of skin, loss of hair, cancer, cataracts, dermatitis, genetic damage	Symptomatic; immediate removal from contamination	Screening from source; monitoring; wearing masks, gloves, and protective clothing
Silicosis	Pottery, mining, quarrying, sandblasting	Inhalation	Dry cough, bronchitis, breathlessness, severe respiratory disablement	Remove from further exposure, treat symptoms	Wearing masks and gloves, damping dust, enclosing process
Solvents	Inks, glues, varnishes, paints, degreasing and dry-cleaning agents	Inhalation, skin contact, ingestion	Many, due to damage to nervous system, liver, heart, lungs; dermatitis	Various; remove from exposure	Exhaust ventilation, monitoring environment, wearing masks and gloves
Vibration	Building, welding, forestry	Contact with tool	Pale, numb fingers	Removal from contact	Warm environment, wearing masks and padded gloves
Wood dust	Lumberyards, wood polishers, furniture	Inhalation and skin contact	Dermatitis, respiratory irritation, nasal cancer	Symptomatic	Dust extraction, wearing masks and gloves

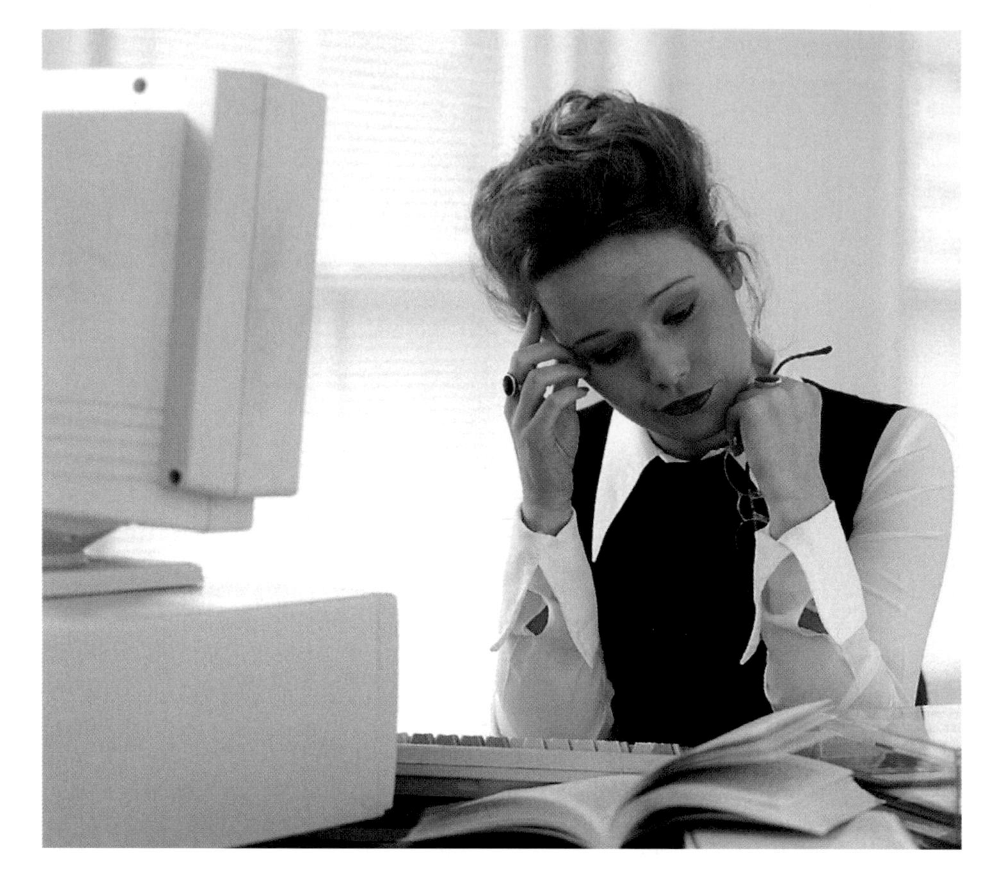

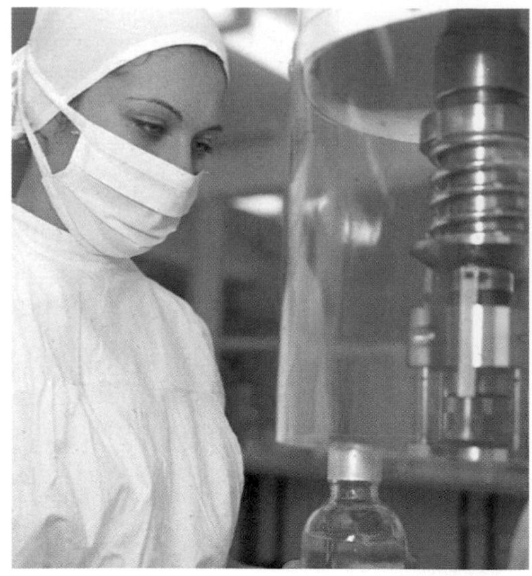

▲ *Laboratory accidents that may lead to contamination can be avoided by following safety procedures.*

◄ *It is important for computer workers to ensure that they are sitting correctly when they are working at a computer screen, and take regular breaks to rest their eyes.*

certain safeguards are slowing their output and costing them pay. Such people may deliberately remove the safeguards and so risk losing a limb.

Machinery maintenance is especially hazardous because safeguards often have to be removed for access. Unfortunate mistakes, such as failing to switch off the power supply, can be the cause of other serious injuries. Many injuries in factories are caused through the misuse of hand tools. Eye injuries from fragments of metal flying off drills, or chips of stone or metal split off in hammering, are common. Employees do not always like wearing eye protection, but such a basic precaution prevents minor eye injuries.

Certain types of hand tools such as chain saws can cause a condition that is known as "vibration white finger." The symptoms are pale or blue tingling fingers. This can progress to pain, or loss of sensation. There is no known cure for white finger. Because the injury causes a cold-sensitive spasm of the arteries, employees who must use vibration tools should wear padded gloves and keep their hands as warm as possible.

Falls in factories account for another high proportion of occupational injuries. Many of these falls occur on a level floor and are a result of clutter from boxes and various other items left lying around. Spilled liquids and general untidiness can also cause falls. Trailing wires, filing cabinet drawers left open, and poorly lit stairs are other avoidable traps that can cause accidents.

An increase in the use of computers has brought about a new set of work-related injuries, which can be divided into three basic groups: repetitive strain injury (RSI), back and neck problems, and eyestrain.

RSI is a disorder that results from performing repetitive tasks over a prolonged period of time (see Repetitive Strain Injury). Although RSI disorders such as "writer's cramp" were reported among clerks as an epidemic in London in the 19th century, the term "repetitive stress injury" originated in the 1970s when video display units (VDUs) were introduced in the workplace. The most common forms of RSI are carpal tunnel syndrome (caused by irritation and compression of the median nerve at the wrist, which results in numbness, pins and needles, pain, and lack of mobility in the wrist; see Carpal Tunnel Syndrome) and tendon injuries (caused by inflammation of the tendons, as in tendonitis, or the tendon sheaths, as in tenosynovitis, both of which result in pain in the hands and fingers; see Tendons).

The most common types of computer-related disorders are back and neck problems, with the accompanying pain. Such disorders often develop when workers remain in a sedentary position for long periods. Eyestrain also affects people who sit for long hours in front of a computer screen; it can lead to headaches and migraines.

Preventing injury

Many occupational injuries can be prevented by following safety regulations. Employers should actively enforce these regulations, and employees should make sure that they wear any safety equipment their employer provides for them. Employees also have a responsibility to encourage better office and factory maintenance. To help prevent computer-related disorders, workers should correctly position their chairs and screens in their work stations, check their posture, try not to remain in the same position for too long, and take breaks. Although occupational hazards will always exist, simple precautions can reduce the various risks that people encounter as part of their job.

See also: **Asbestosis; Burns; Chelation therapy; Dermatitis; Electric shocks; Hepatitis; Lead poisoning; Lung and lung diseases; Poisoning; Radiation sickness; Silicosis**

Occupational therapy

Occupational therapy involves the use of activities that can help people with some kind of impairment reach their maximum level of functioning and independence. The therapy can help people cope with all aspects of daily life.

Occupational therapy has a role complementary to physical therapy. Physical therapists work to improve any physical impairment by mobilizing stiff joints, strengthening weak muscles, improving coordination, and so on. They may use activities such as planing wood to exercise a weak back, a treadmill to exercise the legs, or weights to strengthen arms.

Occupational therapists help patients who are having problems performing everyday tasks. For example, they will teach someone with one arm how to dress him- or herself or cut up his or her food. They may have special tools that they can teach patients to use. Most occupational therapy departments will have a kitchen, bathroom, and bedroom section where patients can try out aids and practice new techniques.

Occupational therapists can also treat people with intellectual impairment or with a psychiatric illness. Therapists use activities like painting and music that provide opportunities for self-expression. They also use discussion and social activities to help shy and withdrawn patients express themselves and relate better to others, and they often work in centers where such patients can meet other patients and enjoy a pleasant change in their surroundings.

Occupational therapists can also help people with an impairment to live at home. This can mean arranging for the provision of aids such as extended legs to raise an armchair. They may work with architects to plan major alterations, such as a downstairs bathroom that is suitable for someone who uses a wheelchair. Shopping, cooking, and work activities help patients cope with daily living.

Benefits of therapy

Patients with a temporary problem, such as a hand injury, will need some physical therapy: in this case, to get the hand moving again as quickly as possible.

▼ *Older people find companionship and mental stimulation in an art therapy session.*

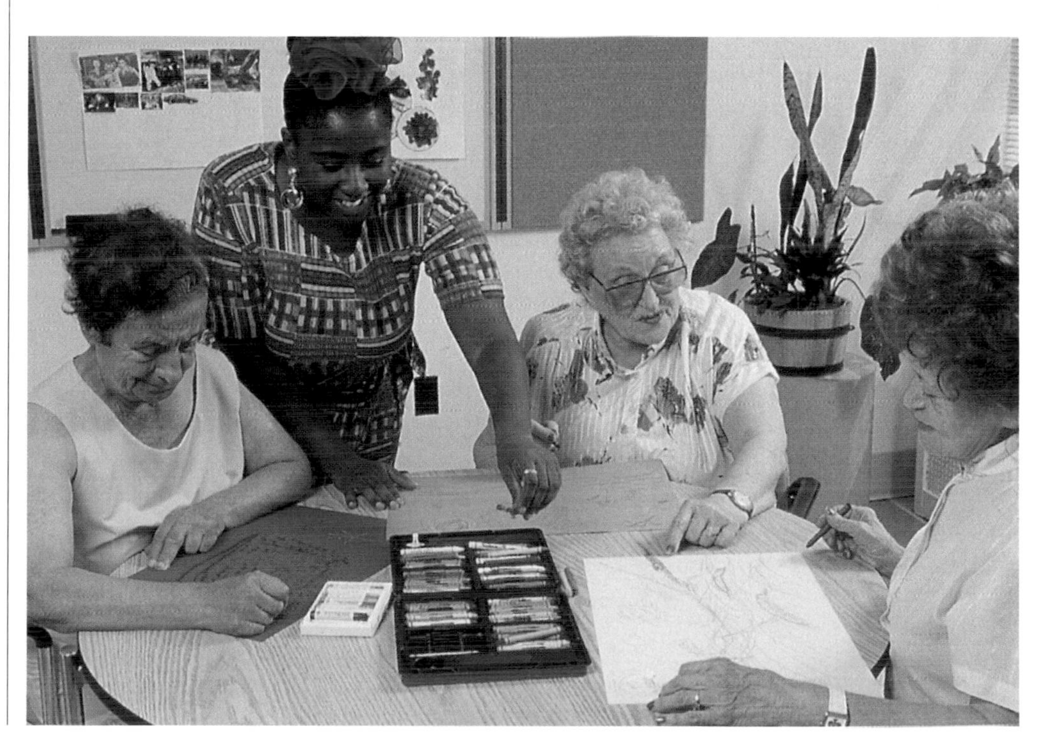

Questions and Answers

Since my wife had a stroke, her right arm has become almost useless. She wants to carry on cooking and cleaning, but finds it frustrating and slow with only one hand. Can anyone help her?

Physical therapists can help her rebuild muscle strength. Occupational therapists can teach her how to perform any physical movements she finds difficult. They will also teach her how to use special tools to make household tasks easier.

My son has had major depression. Will he need occupational therapy?

Depression often happens when people are unable to cope with stress. Therapy can help people become more resilient. They learn exercises that encourage self-confidence and social skills, like talking in front of others. Those who have been unemployed for a while may find it helpful to work with other people and accept responsibilities again.

I am afraid to take a bath because I find it difficult to get out of the tub. What kind of help can I get?

An occupational therapist can visit you who will analyze the problem and may suggest aids that can help, such as a nonslip mat, a bath seat, and a rail on the wall above the bathtub. He or she can help arrange for you to get these and teach you how to use them.

Why did my child get occupational therapy in the hospital when he was recovering from pneumonia?

Long hospital stays can be boring and demoralizing, especially for children. A depressed child will not recover as quickly. If your child is active and happy, he will readjust to the outside world much more easily when he is well again.

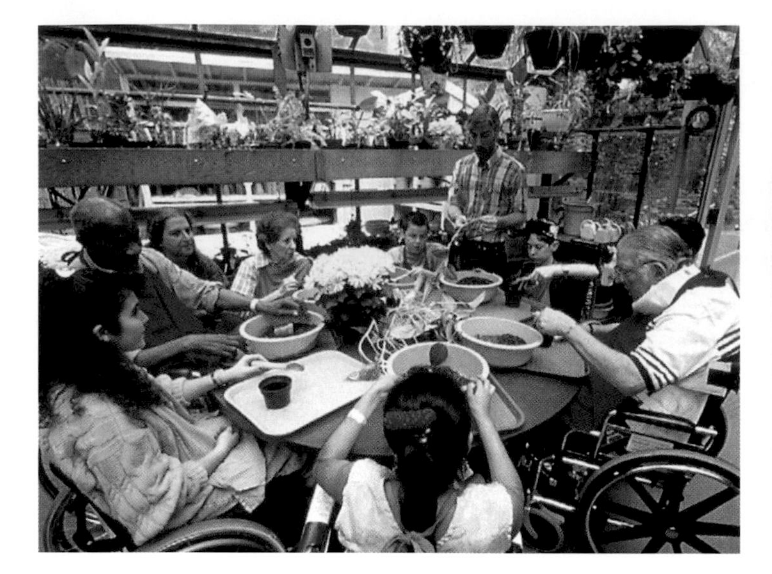

▲ *At a group horticultural therapy session patients practice potting plant cuttings. This activity is designed to improve perceptual and social skills, as well as skills relating to coordination and movement.*

People with a long-term illness, such as arthritis, need occupational therapy in the form of special exercises or instruction to show them how to use adapted household tools to help them cope with the practical and psychological problems that they face.

Patients who have been in a psychiatric facility because of depression, schizophrenia, or anxiety will need the support of occupational therapy in the form of "talk out" therapy or social involvement sessions as part of their treatment (see Anxiety).

Older people who tend to sit at home doing very little may begin to lose their ability to do the things they could manage before. These people can also benefit from therapy. It can stimulate them into wanting to do more for themselves and show them easier ways of doing tasks around the house.

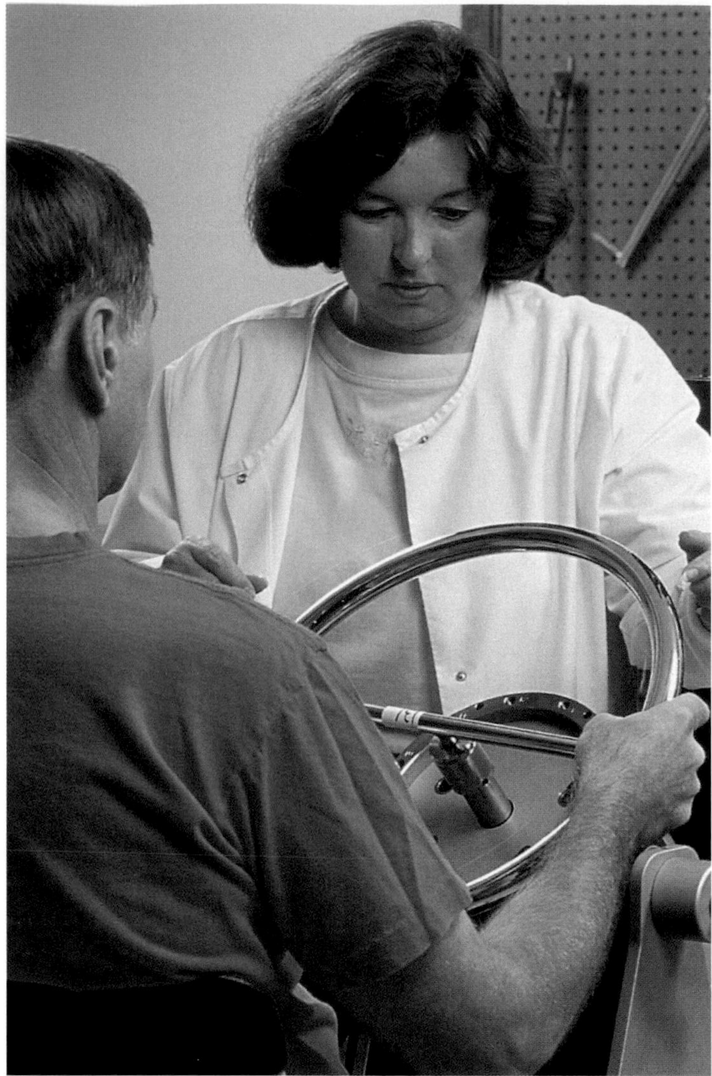

▲ *A male patient uses a steering wheel in a therapy session to test the strength of his arms.*

How therapists work

In the hospital, occupational therapists work as part of a team alongside doctors, nurses, and physical therapists. Therapists may initially see patients in their rooms but usually continue treatment in the hospital occupational therapy unit. The therapists often make home visits with patients before they are discharged to find out if people will be able to manage. If there are problems, the occupational therapist can arrange for appropriate help to be offered. Some outpatients may be advised to continue occupational therapy at the hospital, or they may have access to treatment at home.

Various forms of treatment are available in special units. Among these are centers where intensive daily treatment is available. There are also children's units, hospitals offering special day treatment for the aged, stroke units, spinal injury units, and burns units. An occupational therapist is usually part of a team that offers treatment at all these facilities. Therapists are also beginning to work in special schools that cater specifically to children with physical impairments.

In psychiatric facilities occupational therapists work with both psychiatrists and psychologists. Large outdated hospitals usually rely on a number of occupational therapy departments that can serve different types of patients. In the smaller, modern units that are now attached to regular hospitals, occupational therapists may work either in their own department or on the floors. They may also work in special units that are designed to treat patients who have drug and alcohol dependencies.

Alternatively, therapists may work outside the hospital in a special community setting. Specific techniques such as behavior modification may be used for patients who need to overcome psychological problems. In hospitals for the intellectually impaired, occupational therapists are especially concerned with helping patients to develop everyday social skills (see Behavior Therapy). In the community, occupational therapists may be part of a team with other types of workers. The therapists usually take a special responsibility for people with impairments. Some occupational therapists either work in or run day centers created especially for such people.

See also: **Arthritis; Depression; Exercise; Outpatients; Physical therapy; Psychiatry; Psychology; Psychotherapy; Schizophrenia; Stroke**

Oncology

Questions and Answers

What is psycho-oncology?

Psycho-oncology deals with the psychological impact of cancer on the patient and the patient's relatives and friends. In the past, doctors often withheld a diagnosis of cancer, since it meant certain death, but survival rates are improving all the time and people are more informed about the condition. Studies have shown that a patient's psychological health can influence the progression of a tumor, the outcome of treatment, and subsequent quality of life. Thus most modern cancer units employ psychiatrists and other professionals qualified in this area.

Why do cancer rates keep rising?

In April 2003, the World Health Organization (WHO) reported that cancer rates were set to increase from 10 million new cases each year to 20 million cases by 2020. It said the main causes in developed countries were high levels of smoking, unhealthy lifestyles, and exposure to occupational carcinogens. In developing countries up to a quarter of cancers were caused by diseases such as hepatitis B, and by afflatoxins from mold growing on damp grain and peanuts—a potent cause of primary liver cancer. WHO called for more preventive measures such as a healthy diet, quitting smoking, and access to immunizations.

What is integrative oncology?

This term is used to describe a holistic approach to treating cancer. Complementary therapies such as nutritional counseling, acupuncture, herbal supplements, and craniosacral therapy are used to boost a patient's overall health and well-being. These have no direct effect on the progress of the cancer but can help to reduce the symptoms, alleviate pain, and improve the patient's quality of life.

Oncology is the branch of medicine that deals with cancers of all types, including diagnosis, assessment of degree of malignancy and stage of spread, and the determination of the best form of treatment.

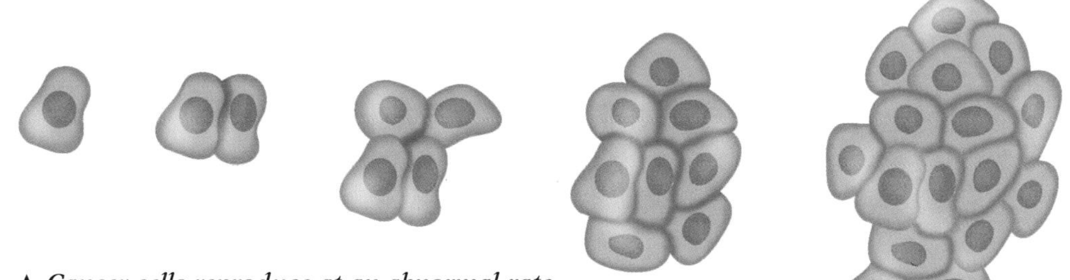

▲ *Cancer cells reproduce at an abnormal rate, making them susceptible to treatment that threatens DNA replication.*

In 2000, cancer was the leading cause of death in the United States, followed by heart disease, and caused one in four deaths. Approximately 15 million new cases of cancer have been diagnosed since 1990. Cancer is thus an increasing financial burden to the country, with an estimated $180 billion annual expenditure, including direct medical costs and loss of productivity due to illness and premature death (see Cancer). According to a report by the National Cancer Institute and the American Cancer Society in 2000, the overall rate of new cancer cases and cancer deaths declined by an average of 0.8 percent a year between 1990 and 1997 (although the decline in the death rate from heart disease was greater). The decline is due partly to advances in oncology.

In 2001 there were 1,268,000 new cases of cancer in the United States (625,000 women and 643,000 men), and 553,400 deaths (267,300 men and 286,100 women). Lung cancer was the leading cancer, with 169,500 new cases (90,700 men and 78,800 women) and 157,400 deaths (90,100 men and 67,300 women). In 2003, the American Cancer Society estimated that about 172,000 new cases of lung cancer would be reported, and about 157,000 deaths.

After lung cancer, breast cancer is the second biggest cause of cancer death in women. In 2001, 40,200 women and 400 men died from breast cancer; and more than 211,000 new cases were expected in 2003, resulting in about 40,000 deaths. In American men, prostate cancer accounts for about 10 percent of cancer deaths, with 198,100 cases in 2001, and 31,500 deaths.

History of oncology

Much was recorded about cancers throughout history, and for many centuries people believed in the "four humors," attributing cancer to an accumulation of black bile. The lymphatic spread of cancer began to be understood in the early 17th century, when the anatomist Hieronymus Fabricius recommended the removal of lymph nodes at the time of mastectomy (see Lymphoma); however, cancer was still considered to be a result of inflammation until 1802, when the French anatomist Marie Francois Xavier Bichat asserted that tumors were an overgrowth of cellular tissue (see Tumors). After 1830, when microscopes began to be used, cells were shown to be the basic unit of tumors. In 1867, Wilhelm Waldeyer published papers describing how cancers developed from cells that had started to reproduce abnormally; he also described local spread and metastases and distinguished benign from malignant tumors. His ideas remain current.

Radiation, which affects cells indiscriminately, was found to be a cause of cancer within a few years of the discovery of X rays in 1895. Radiotherapy treatment, which targets cancer cells, began in 1904, and statistics about cancer began to be compiled. It soon became clear than many industrial chemicals could cause cancer, and after World War II cancer chemotherapy began to develop. In 1964, the U.S. surgeon general reported on the link between cigarette smoking and lung cancer. In 1971, the United States committed itself to curing cancer. Since then, treatments have improved tremendously, as have methods of cancer screening and education about cancer prevention.

HOW CANCER SPREADS IN THE LYMPHATIC SYSTEM

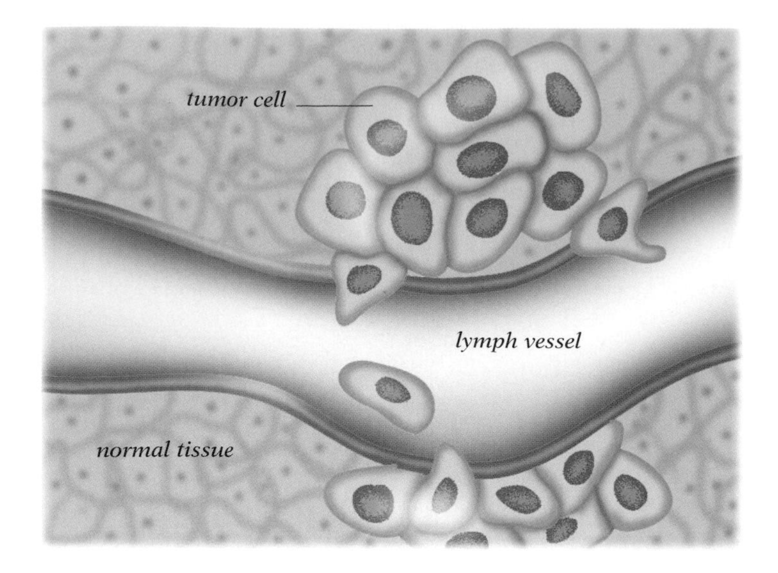

▲ *If a growing tumor invades a lymph vessel, cancerous cells may detach themselves and be carried away in the lymph.*

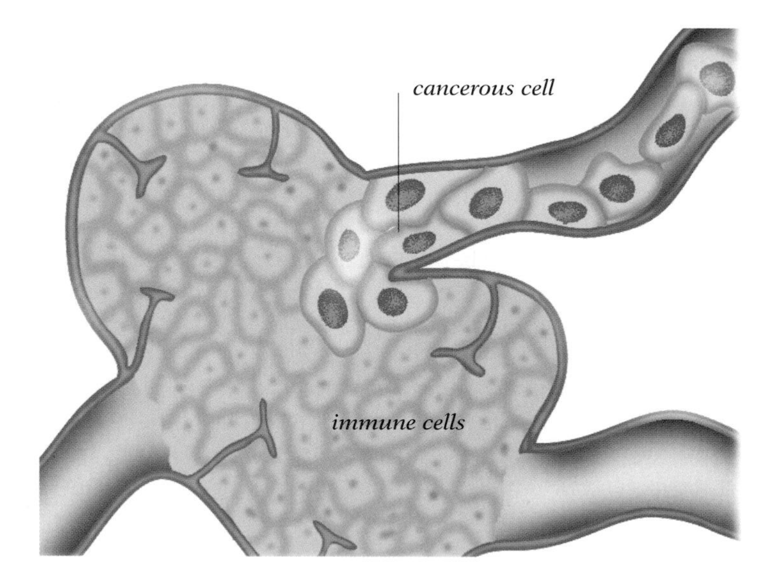

▲ *When the cancerous cell enters a lymph node, it may start dividing to form a tumor. The immune cells may then temporarily stop the cancer from spreading beyond the node.*

Who treats cancer?

An oncologist is a doctor specializing in the management of cancer patients, who either carries out cancer surgery or works in close association with a cancer surgeon. Some oncologists specialize in one type of cancer, while others treat various types. Usually cancer treatment requires the expertise of a number of health care professionals, including surgeons, radiation oncologists, medical oncologists (who specialize in the use of cancer medications), nurses, dieticians, and psychologists.

Cancer treatments

There are five modalities of cancer treatment: surgery, radiotherapy, chemotherapy, immunotherapy, and gene therapy. All of these, apart from surgery, depend on the fact that cancer cells reproduce at an abnormal rate, making them more susceptible than normal cells to treatments that threaten DNA replication. Different treatments may be combined, depending on the type and stage of the cancer.

Radiation oncology: Advanced physics, radiobiology, dosimetry (the science of calculating and optimizing the dose of radiation), and collaboration with surgeons and medical oncologists have made modern radiation therapy an effective and much safer method of treating cancer. Radioactive materials, X rays, gamma rays, and proton beams are all used, and techniques have been developed that focus beams of radiation on the tumor from several different directions, delivering a heavy combined dosage to the tumor while the surrounding healthy tissues receive a fraction of the total dosage. Brachytherapy is an advanced form of radiation oncology in which radioactive seeds or sources are placed in or near the tumor, to deliver a high radiation dose to the tumor, so that exposure in the surrounding tissues is reduced (see Radiotherapy).

Chemotherapy: Many less common cancers are treated by chemotherapy, which involves administering drugs that either kill the cancer cells or arrest their growth by targeting specific stages of the cell growth cycle. The drugs also tend to damage normal cells and cause various side effects. Numerous classes of anticancer drugs have been developed, all working in different ways to delay cell reproduction, and these are commonly used in various combinations. The newer therapies target growth pathways found only in cancer cells, and may be more effective and less toxic.

Immunotherapy: Immunology has developed greatly since the advent of AIDS in the early 1980s. The BCG vaccine has been used to stimulate the immune system to act against cancers; interleukins, especially Interleukin-2, have been used effectively against certain cancers; interferons can be helpful; and injections of pure tumor antigen have been used to stimulate the immune system to attack cancers (see Immunization). Scientists are also developing cancer treatments that involve biologically manipulating a patient's cells. For example, doctors may remove some tumor tissue and extract the patient's natural killer cells to be cloned. These cells are enhanced with substances that make them more capable of killing the cancer cells, and they are infused back into the patient by the billion.

Gene therapy: Gene therapy has been used to block oncogene (cancer-causing gene) activity, correct gene mutations, and enhance chemotherapy (see Genetics). Mapping the human genome (identifying all human genes) will accelerate the discovery of cancer-related genes, helping doctors to fight cancer more effectively.

What about prevention?

Two branches of oncology deal with prevention. Predictive oncology promotes primary cancer prevention by assessing people's susceptibility to cancer, and by controlling their exposure to carcinogens and other factors that encourage tumors to develop. It tries to identify cancer-prone individuals and to evaluate how tumors will develop and progress. Secondary prevention focuses on routine clinical and laboratory procedures that enable the early detection and treatment of cancers, on managing curable cancer lesions, and on general education and lifestyle modification.

See also: **Breasts; Cells and chromosomes; Genetic engineering; Lung and lung diseases; Prostate gland; X rays**

Open-heart surgery

Modern heart surgeons can perform operations that were previously impossible—for example, heart transplants—because the patient's heart can now be stopped during surgery and the blood circulated by a machine.

The term "open-heart surgery" describes surgery on the heart when the chest is opened, the function of the heart is taken over by a machine, and the heart is operated on directly. Before this technique was developed, any heart surgery was performed through a small incision in the chest. Instruments were passed into the heart through the incision, and surgery was performed while the heart was still beating.

In the 1950s a machine was devised that could pump blood without unduly damaging the red blood cells and at the same time saturate the blood with oxygen (see Blood). This meant that the patient's heart could be allowed to stop beating temporarily so that surgery could be performed inside it.

Before surgery

Before undergoing open-heart surgery for any type of heart disease, the patient will have had several tests, and the doctors will try to treat the condition with medicines if possible. However, if the disease does not respond well to treatment, surgery may be recommended. In the early days of open-heart surgery, the patient was often so ill by the time he or she came to have surgery that the results were poor. Nowadays, heart surgery is recommended much earlier in the progress of a disease, when the patient is relatively fit and able to withstand a major operation.

To diagnose the exact nature of the heart disease, patients have a cardiac catheterization. A fine tube 0.04 inch (1 mm) in diameter is passed into a blood vessel in the arm or leg and fed into the heart. X rays can then be taken of the heart, and an exact diagnosis is made by injecting a special kind of dye that is opaque to X rays. The tube can also be used to measure blood pressure and can be passed into the coronary arteries to show up a narrowing or blockage of the arteries.

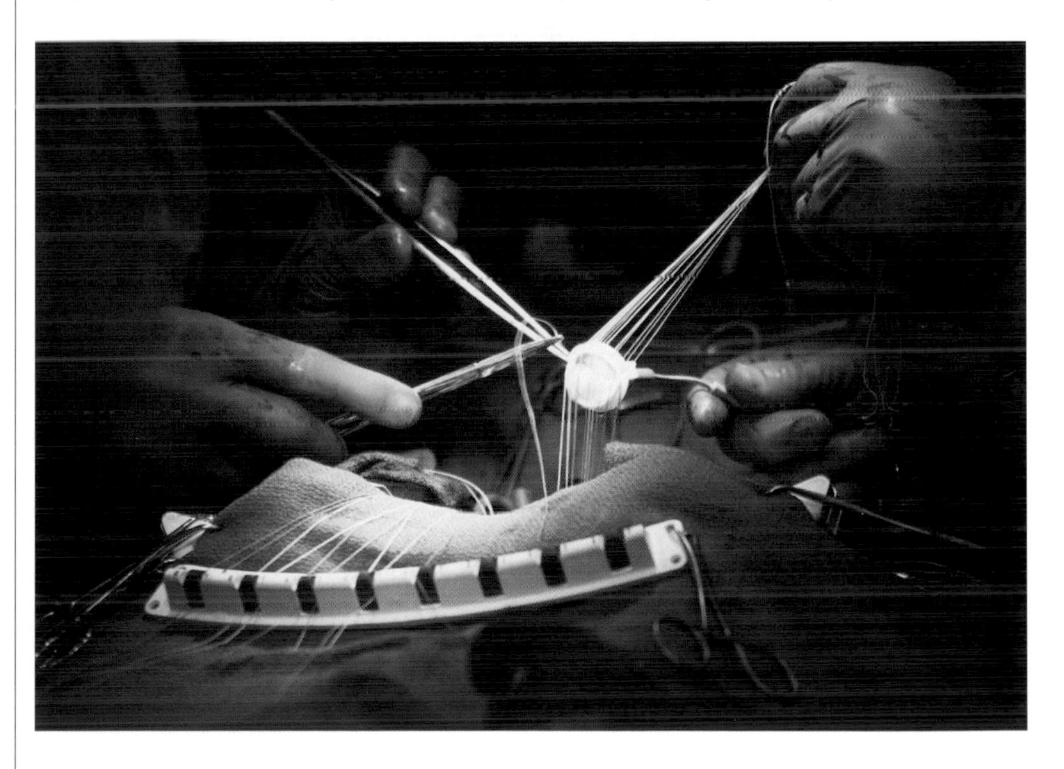

▲ *In this open-heart surgery, known as a valve replacement operation, surgeons sew in a new artificial heart valve (center) after removing the patient's original faulty valve.*

Questions and Answers

My son has a hole in the heart but the doctor does not advise surgery. Why is this?

There are many degrees of holes in the heart, and usually the ones that need treatment are the large ones that affect the functioning of the heart. A small hole should not prevent your son from leading a perfectly normal life.

My wife has just had open-heart surgery, and she was in the intensive care unit for three days afterward. Does this mean that there were problems?

No. It is routine for patients who have had open-heart surgery to spend the next few days in the intensive care unit to receive the specialized nursing care they need.

I have been told that I need to have a valve in my heart replaced. Isn't this a rather risky operation?

In the early days of open-heart surgery, there was a moderate degree of risk, but now the risk is small and the chances of success are much greater.

What does an artificial heart valve look like, and how does it work?

The most common valves are either a ball of plastic about the size of a small marble (that sits inside a metal cage), or something that resembles a trapdoor that opens and shuts a small way. Both allow blood to flow in one direction only. Sometimes, specially prepared pig's heart valves are used instead.

What are the most common and least common reasons for performing open-heart surgery?

The most common reason is to replace a heart valve. The least common is heart transplantation.

FUNCTION OF THE BYPASS MACHINE

► *Open-heart surgery is made possible by the use of a heart-lung bypass machine, which temporarily takes over the heart's function. Tubes are inserted into the patient: one into the aorta and two into the vena cavae. These are connected to the bypass machine, which takes over the pumping and oxygenating of the blood.*

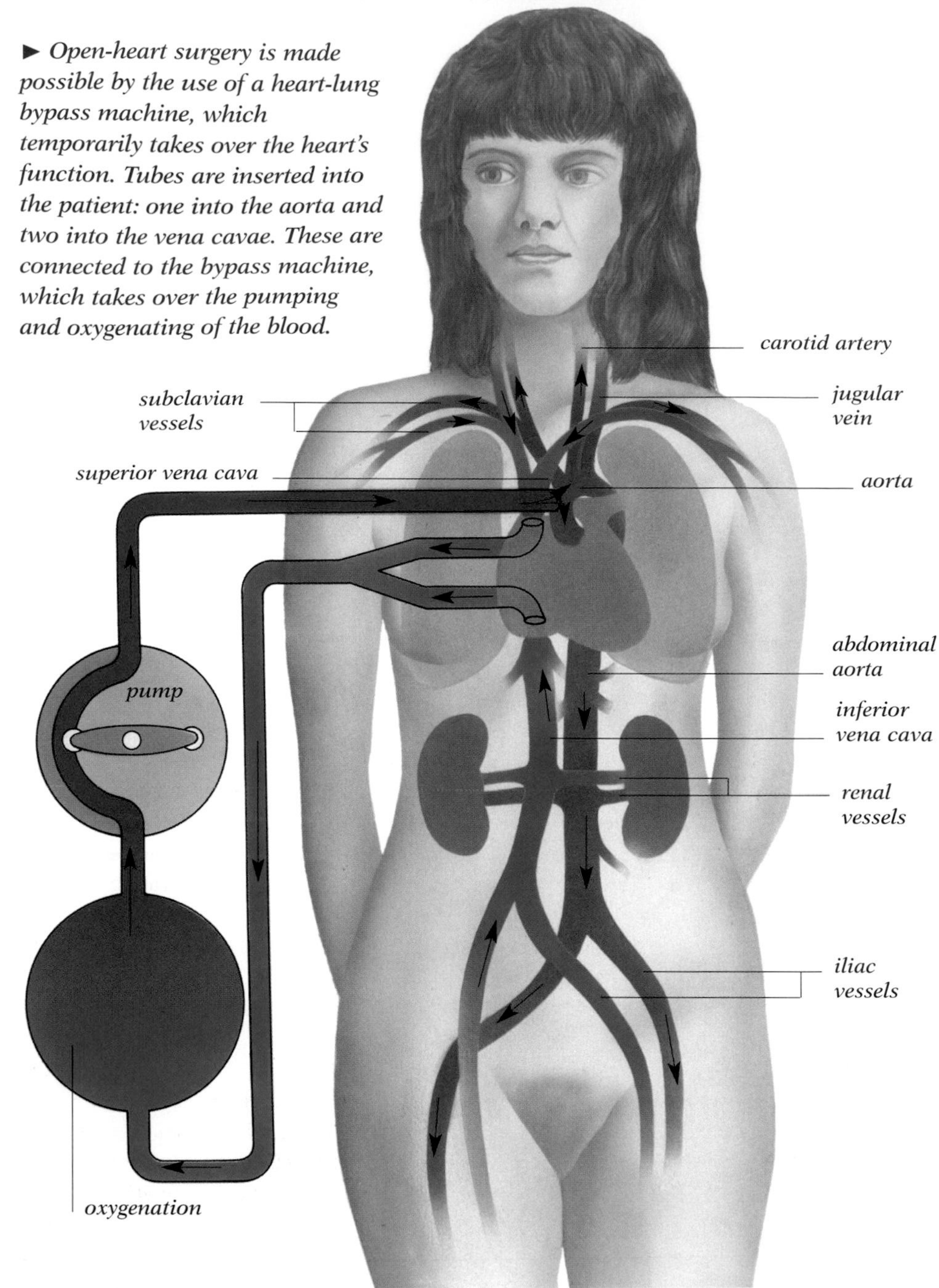

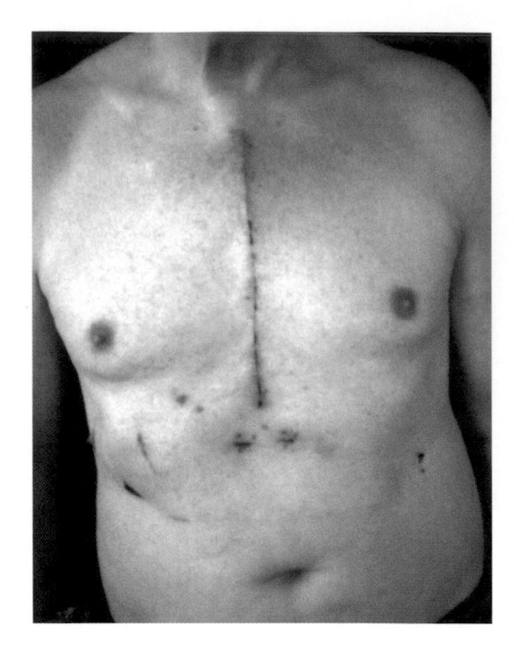

▲ *After open-heart surgery, the patient is left with a neat scar where the incision was made.*

The operation

The patient is first injected with an anesthetic drug and maintained with gases that are delivered through a mask (see Anesthetics). While the patient is still in the anesthetic room, he or she will be given an an infusion into a vein, called an IV (see Intravenous Infusion), together with needles in an artery and a vein to measure the arterial and venous pressure both during and after the operation.

The patient is then taken into the operating room, and the operation begins (see Operating Room). First the skin over the breastbone (sternum) is cut, and then the bone itself is divided by an electric saw. The division is widened with special instruments called retractors, and the heart is then exposed.

Then the patient is transferred onto the bypass machine. This has to be done very carefully, to avoid serious damage to the brain from lack of oxygen. At this stage the pressure in the arteries is continuously shown on a video monitor. First, a large tube is inserted into the aorta—the main artery leading out of the heart. Large tubes are also inserted into the venae cavae, which are the two main veins that bring blood back to the heart (see Veins). These tubes are connected to the bypass machine, which consists of a pump and an oxygenator. The oxygenator allows oxygen to diffuse across a membrane and into the patient's blood as it is pumped through the bypass machine. The machine is operated by a trained technician who monitors the pressure of the blood and the speed of its flow. The blood passes out of the patient's venae cavae, travels along a tube to the bypass machine, passes through the machine, and then passes back into the patient via another tube. The patient's heart, which is now empty of blood, usually stops spontaneously; or it can be stopped by an electric shock, special drugs, or cold fluid (cold cardioplegia). The heart can now be operated on, since its function has been taken over by the bypass machine.

Types of operations

Hole in the heart: In a hole-in-the-heart operation, a cut is made through the heart muscle to reveal the defect. This is repaired sometimes by sewing the edges of the hole together, or sometimes by sewing a patch of artificial material, or a portion of the heart's fibrous covering (the pericardium), over the defect. The cut in the heart muscle is then sewn up.

Valve replacement: There are four valves in the heart that allow blood to flow in one direction only, so that when the heart contracts

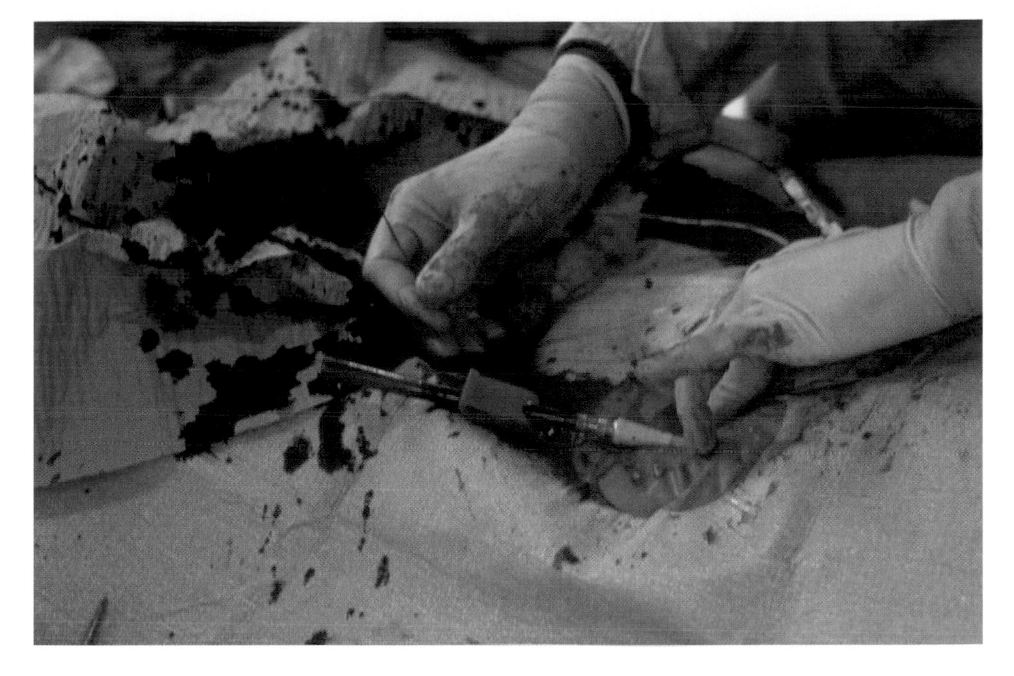

► *In a revolutionary alternative to open-heart surgery, Dr. Fayaz Shawl is performing mechanical percutaneous myocardial revascularization (MPMR)—a surgical bypass procedure to treat patients suffering from angina. A catheter is threaded through the femoral artery in the thigh and up into the heart. Then a needle is inserted into the catheter to drill tiny holes in the heart muscle that serve as channels for blood to flow around clogged arteries and through the heart.*

blood is forced into the arteries, and when the heart relaxes blood enters the heart from the veins. The valves can become faulty by becoming either leaky (insufficiency) or constricted (stenosis), so blood has difficulty in passing through them.

In a valve replacement operation, the old valve is cut out and a new one is sewn in position. The replacement valve may be made from metal and plastic, or a specially prepared natural valve from a pig's heart may be used. The valve is sewn in place with many fine stitches to ensure that there is no leak between the valve and the heart muscle.

Coronary artery surgery: Coronary arteries can become narrowed by the arterial disease atherosclerosis, and if this happens, the blood supply to a particular part of the heart becomes inadequate. If it occurs suddenly, the patient has a heart attack, but if it is gradual, the patient suffers from angina pectoris (choking and suffocating chest pains). If an X ray of the coronary arteries shows a localized blockage, surgery may be desirable.

Although it is not strictly open heart surgery, the most common procedure in coronary artery surgery is a coronary artery bypass graft, in which the blockage is bypassed using a piece of vein (see Grafting). A length of vein is taken from the patient's leg and cut to the right length. Most often, the vein graft is used to bypass the coronary artery blockage by carrying blood from the aorta just above the heart to a point on the coronary artery below the blockage. Alternatively, a chest wall artery—the mammary artery—can be stitched into the coronary artery. Mammary artery grafts are now preferred, as vein grafts are likely to become arterialized and then to develop atherosclerosis. This type of surgery has become more common, and it is most often performed on patients who suffer from severe chest pain that begins after exertion. Not all patients with coronary artery narrowing require bypass surgery. Most can be effectively treated by coronary angioplasty using an inflatable catheter.

After surgery

Once surgery has been completed, the patient is taken off the bypass machine and his or her heart is restarted. This is done by stimulating the heart electrically and gradually phasing out the bypass machine, while carefully monitoring arterial pressure. Sometimes, drugs have to be injected directly into the heart to stimulate it to contract forcefully.

A fine wire is placed in the heart muscle, and it is left sticking out through the chest wall, so that if the heart starts beating irregularly in the immediate postoperative period, the wire can be connected to a pacemaker immediately (see Pacemaker). The bypass tubes are removed, and the breastbone is stitched together with wire stitches. Several drainage tubes are generally left in for a few days following surgery, and the arterial and venous pressure monitoring lines are also left in until the patient's condition is considered to be stable.

Recovery time from surgery varies, depending on the type of operation and how ill the patient was beforehand (see Convalescence). Most people take about three months to recover completely. If a patient has had an artificial valve inserted in the heart, he or she will be given anticoagulant drugs to prevent blood clots in the valve.

Outlook

The advent of open-heart surgery in the 1950s was a major step forward in the treatment of many heart conditions. Before these operations were available, many people died who would otherwise have survived for years. This applied especially to people with valve disease and to children who were born with various heart defects. In the days before operations for a hole in the heart, if the defect was serious, for many affected children there was very little chance of surviving into adulthood. There is also evidence suggesting that coronary artery surgery prolongs life in many cases.

It is probably fair to say that the outlook after surgery depends very much on the medical care given before surgery, assuming that the surgery goes well and that there are no complications. The risks of surgery have now been reduced to such a low level that the outlook may well be determined by how long the patient had the heart disease before he or she sought medical help. If the condition is diagnosed before the disease has progressed too far, and if the surgery is performed promptly, the long-term outlook is very positive. Many people with artificial valves are able to lead full lives.

See also: **Arteries and artery disease; Chelation therapy; Chest; Coronary arteries and thrombosis; Heart; Heart disease; Stenosis; Surgery; Sutures; Valves**

Operating room

Questions and Answers

How many people are on the team that helps the surgeon with the operation, and what do they do?

The number of people in the surgeon's team varies according to the type of operation being performed. For a major operation there will be the surgeon, one or two assistants (usually doctors, medical students, or other surgeons), and the nursing staff. The operating room nurse gets all the instruments ready for the operation, hands the appropriate ones to the surgeon, and makes sure all the instruments are accounted for after surgery.

My husband had surgery on his stomach and was in the recovery room for about four hours. Does this mean that the operation went wrong or was very difficult?

Not necessarily. Patients are kept in the recovery room after surgery until they are awake. They are then sent back to their own rooms, where they are attended to by staff members who are specially trained in postoperative care. Your husband may have taken a while to come around after surgery, but this is normal.

Is anything done to reduce the risk of surgeons' eye fatigue during long surgical procedures?

The drapes covering the area around the operation are usually a restful color, such as green or gray, and the surgeon will occasionally focus on them. The light used does not cast shadows, thus enabling clear vision.

Do operation wounds get infected?

No matter what precautions are taken, any surgery carries a slight risk of infection. However, modern sterilization methods are highly effective and the risk is very small.

The operating room is a high-tech environment where surgical procedures are performed. It has all the equipment that will be needed for the surgery itself, and for any emergencies that may arise.

An operating room (OR) is the area in a hospital where patients are prepared for an operation, the surgery is carried out, and the patient then recovers before being taken back to his or her room. Within the same complex are scrubbing and preparation rooms where the surgical team gets ready and where the instruments are laid out on special carts after being sterilized. Administration of the operating room is carried out in adjoining offices. In a big hospital there may be a dozen operating rooms, each with its own surgery list.

Sterilization

In the 19th century, it was discovered that infection in a surgical wound could be prevented by using certain techniques to destroy bacteria on the instruments, on the surgeon's hands, and in the air. Before this, virtually every wound became infected, and a patient was very likely to die from the infection even if the operation was successful. Modern sterilization methods make wound infection very unusual.

The air in the operating room is cleaned through filters that remove bacteria, and it is then pumped through vents directly into the OR itself. The pressure maintained inside the OR ensures that air is then swept out of the various exits. Therefore, all the air in the OR remains clean, and there is no need for an air-lock system when a person enters or leaves the OR.

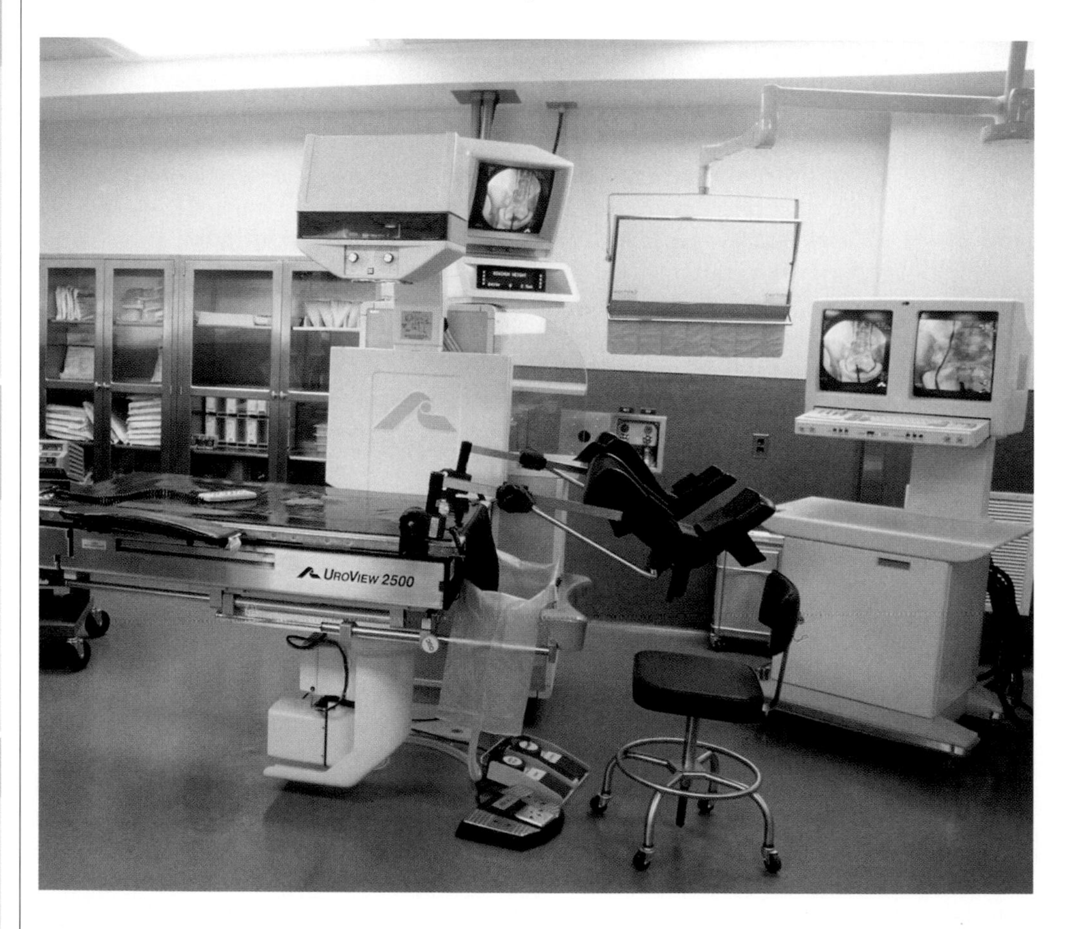

▲ *This operating room is ready for the next operation. The room has a state-of-the-art operating table and an array of sophisticated computers, equipment, and lighting.*

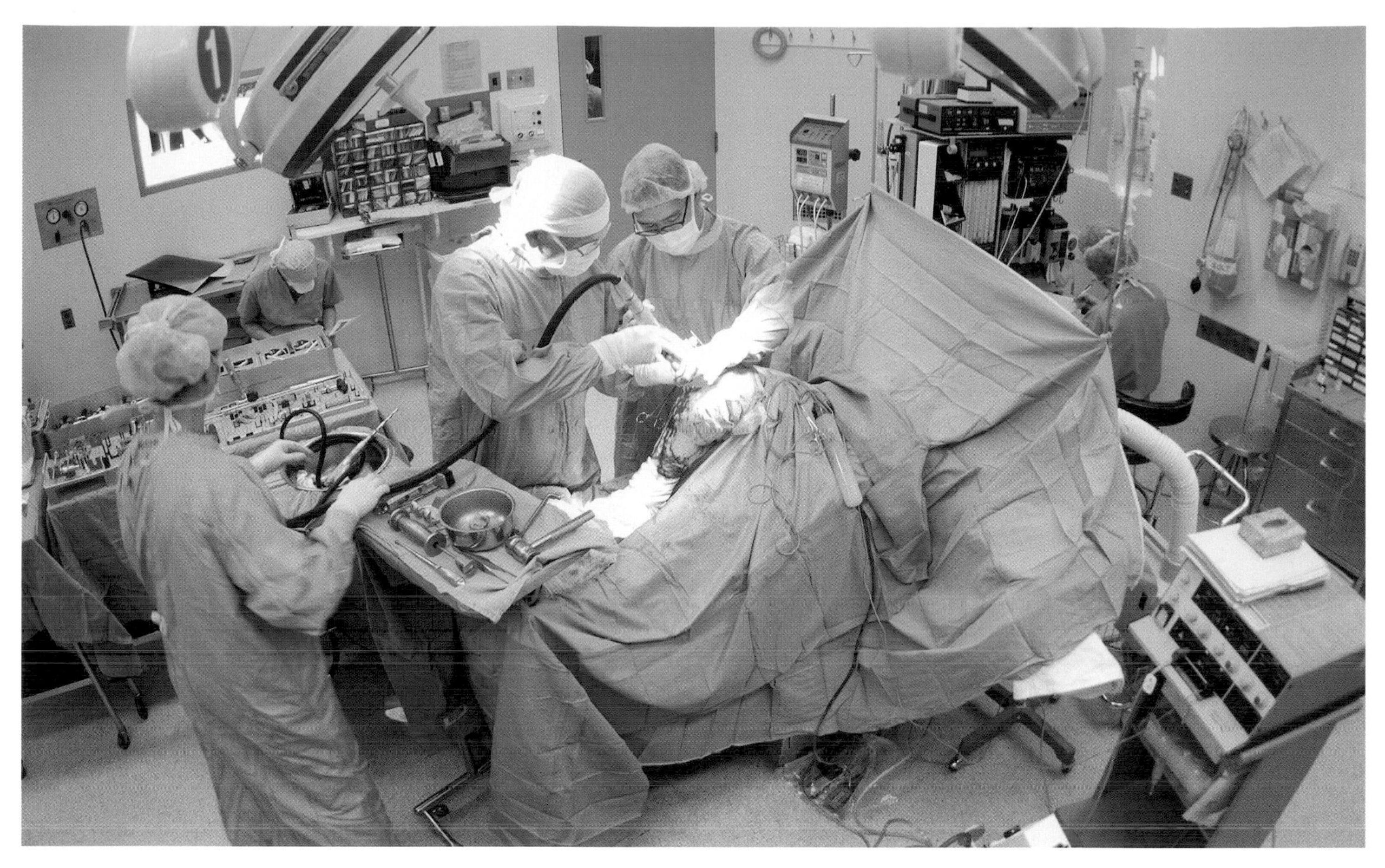

▲ *The operating team performs knee surgery wearing sterilized gowns, caps, masks, and gloves.*

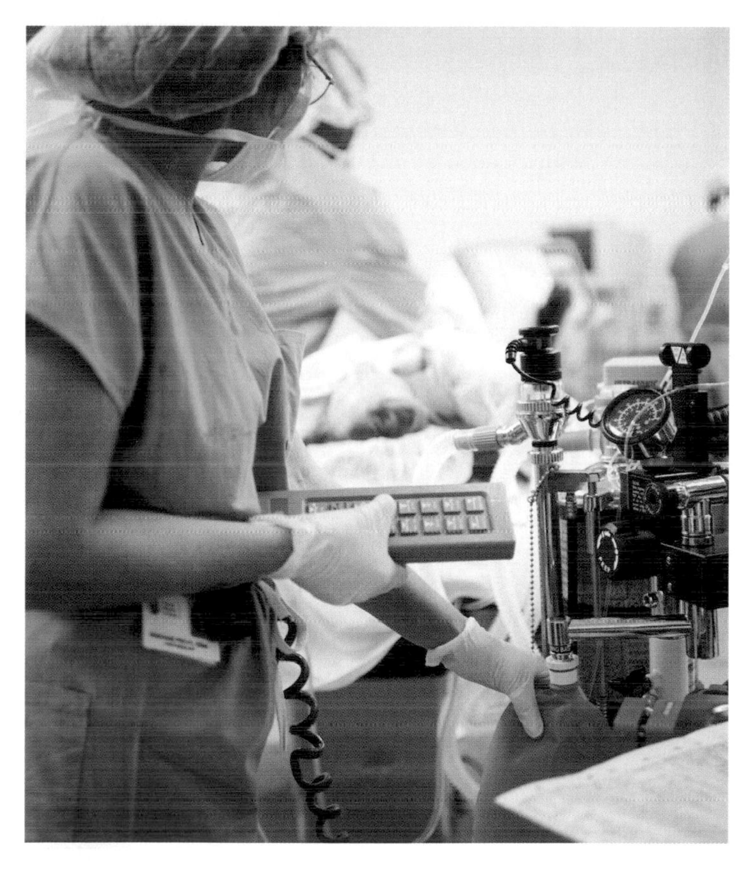

▲ *An anesthesiologist must be highly trained in order to use the sophisticated equipment that administers the anesthesia.*

All instruments, sutures, and anything that comes into contact with the wound during the operation will be sterilized (see Sutures). They may be heated in a device called an autoclave, which is a pressurized chamber capable of delivering superheated steam. Disposable equipment is usually sterilized by gamma irradiation at the place of manufacture; those instruments that would be damaged by the heating process are chemically disinfected.

Everyone who enters the OR area has to change into special clothes, including shoes. The surgeon and assistants clean their arms and hands by prolonged and careful scrubbing with antibacterial soap or solution and running water, and they wear sterile gowns and rubber gloves. All members of the team wear masks to prevent germs from being breathed into the wound.

The patient's skin in the area of the proposed surgery is disinfected, and once surgery is in progress, nobody except the surgeon and his or her assistants may touch the operating field. The surgeon must not touch anything that has not been sterilized. However, there will be several other assistants in the OR, such as the anesthetist and nurses, who are free to move around provided they do not handle any sterile items.

Anesthesia

Modern anesthesia requires highly sophisticated equipment. A patient undergoing major surgery is usually given an intravenous injection of an anesthetic drug that puts him or her to sleep within seconds. This takes place in the anesthetic room, which is

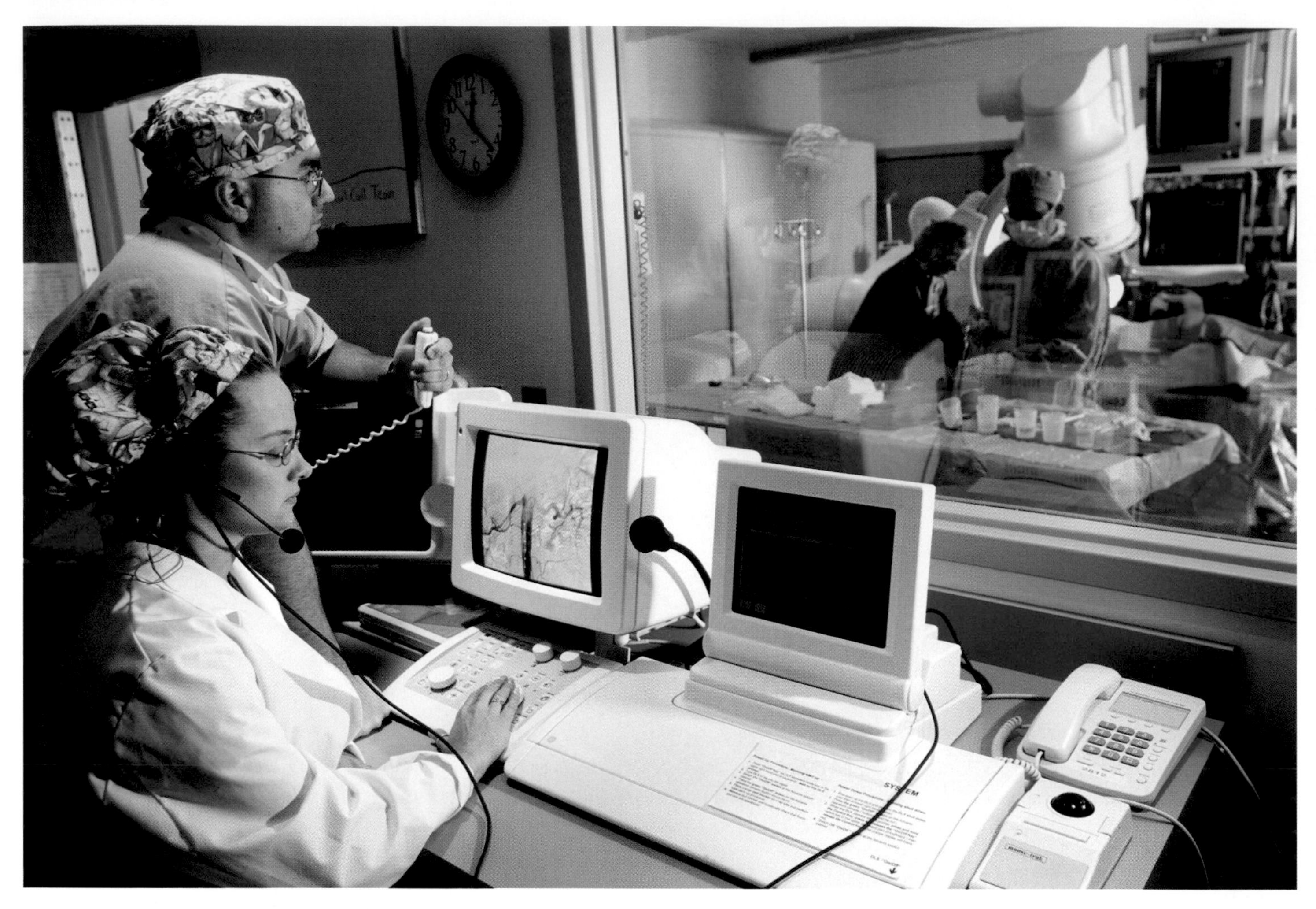

▲ *Technicians in the viewing room are able to watch surgical procedures in the operating room both on computer monitors and through a viewing window. The surgeons and technicians can also communicate with each other if need be.*

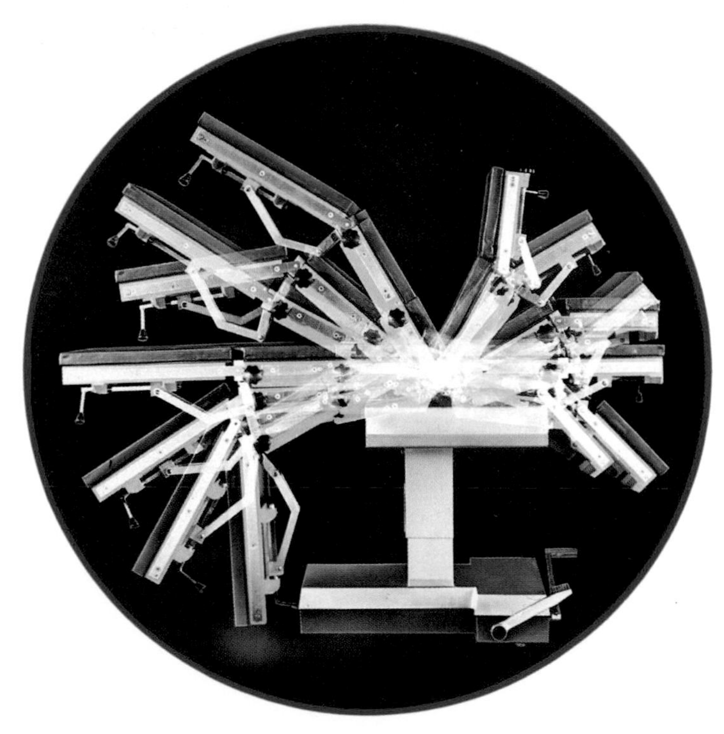

▲ *The operating table has to be extremely versatile to cope with different surgical positions and to provide constant support for the patient's body.*

immediately adjoining the OR. The patient is wheeled into the OR and is kept asleep during the operation by gas and oxygen that carries a volatile anesthetic drug such as isoflurane or sevoflurane.

A machine administers the correct amount of gas and oxygen through either a mask or a tube connected to the windpipe (trachea). In many cases a respirator is also used. This acts as a pump, pushing gas and oxygen into and out of the lungs. This may be necessary because the patient may receive a muscle relaxant at the same time as the anesthetic to make it easier for the surgeon to work, and this also tends to affect the muscles of breathing.

Modern developments

Recent innovations include a sophisticated type of sealed unit with air locks, used in the operating room, and "space suits" worn by the surgeons that prevent any expired air from reaching the patient. The risk that a patient's wound will become infected is thereby reduced even further (see Wounds).

See also: **Anesthetics; Bacteria; Hospitals; Hygiene; Infection and infectious diseases; Oxygen; Postoperative care; Respirators; Surgery**

Ophthalmology

Questions and Answers

If I need surgery on my eye, will it be performed by a general surgeon or by an ophthalmologist?

In the United States, all eye surgery is done by specialist eye surgeons called ophthalmologists. They use special instruments—many of which are scaled-down versions of the type of medical instruments used in operating rooms, or in a surgery—to examine the eyes and perform eye operations.

At what age should children first have their eyes tested?

All babies should have their sight tested regularly from the age of six months onward. One of the most important functions of child health clinics is to look for cross-eye, so that it can be treated in the early stages to avoid the suppression of sight in the affected eye. It is actually normal for babies to look cross-eyed soon after birth, but it should disappear by the age of three months. A baby with cross-eye after this age should be taken to the doctor or child health clinic to be examined. When the child begins school, the school health service will make regular checkups.

During an ordinary medical examination, does the doctor check your eyes or do you have to see an ophthalmologist?

Most medical examinations test your visual acuity (that is, the ability to see objects without blurring). The doctor will also use an ophthalmoscope to examine the inside of the eye, including the retina—the only place in the body where blood vessels can be seen clearly. If your doctor suspects that you might need glasses, he or she will send you to an optometrist; if he or she thinks that you have an eye disease, and that you need to be examined by someone with more specialist knowledge, you will be referred to an ophthalmologist.

Doctors who specialize in the field of ophthalmology are equipped to diagnose and deal with all aspects of eye disease, and they can perform intricate surgery to save a patient's sight.

Ophthalmology is the study of eye diseases. It is an unusual area of medicine in that nearly all the doctors who specialize in it are experts in two fields: not only are they eye specialists, but they are also highly skilled surgeons.

The ophthalmologist performs complicated tests on the eye, detects problems, and prescribes treatment; as a surgeon, he or she performs intricate and delicate surgery to improve, and often save or restore, eyesight.

Treating eye problems

Most people have had their eyes tested, either because they think they may need to wear glasses or as part of a general medical checkup. However, only people with more serious problems need to see an ophthalmologist.

If a person goes to his or her doctor with some deterioration in vision, the doctor will examine his or her eyes. If the problem is a refractive error (an inability to focus properly), the doctor will advise the patient to have his or her eyes tested for glasses by an optometrist. If the person needs specialized corrective treatment, he or she may be sent to an ophthalmic practitioner (a doctor who specializes in eye problems but does not do any surgery). Only a small proportion of people actually have symptoms like the clouding of vision caused by cataracts, that would make referral to an ophthalmologist necessary.

Ophthalmologists also deal with cases of trauma (accidental damage) to the eyes. Despite the eye's vulnerability to certain types of injury, many people fail to wear protective goggles when working with industrial equipment, such as grinding wheels or jackhammers, or even when they are riding on motorcycles (see Accident Prevention). As a result, ophthalmologists often have to perform intricate surgery to remove chips and splinters that have penetrated the cornea (the transparent front to the eye) and have lodged within the eye.

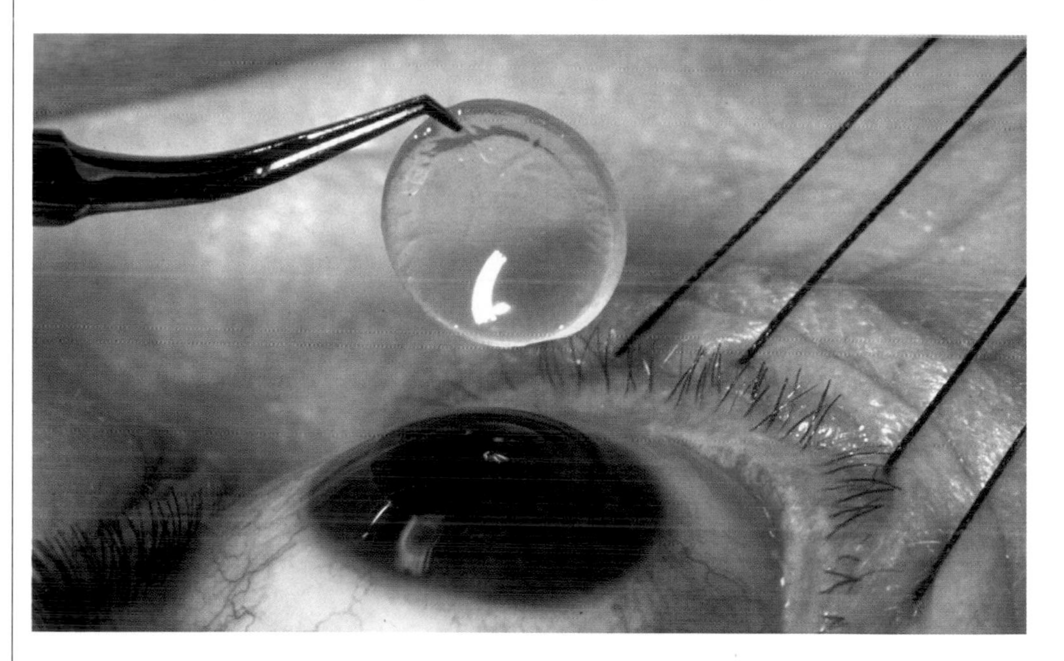

▲ *For a corneal transplant operation, the patient is usually given a local anesthetic to numb the eye. The ophthalmologist then removes the diseased or injured cornea and replaces it with a donor's cornea, which is sewn into place.*

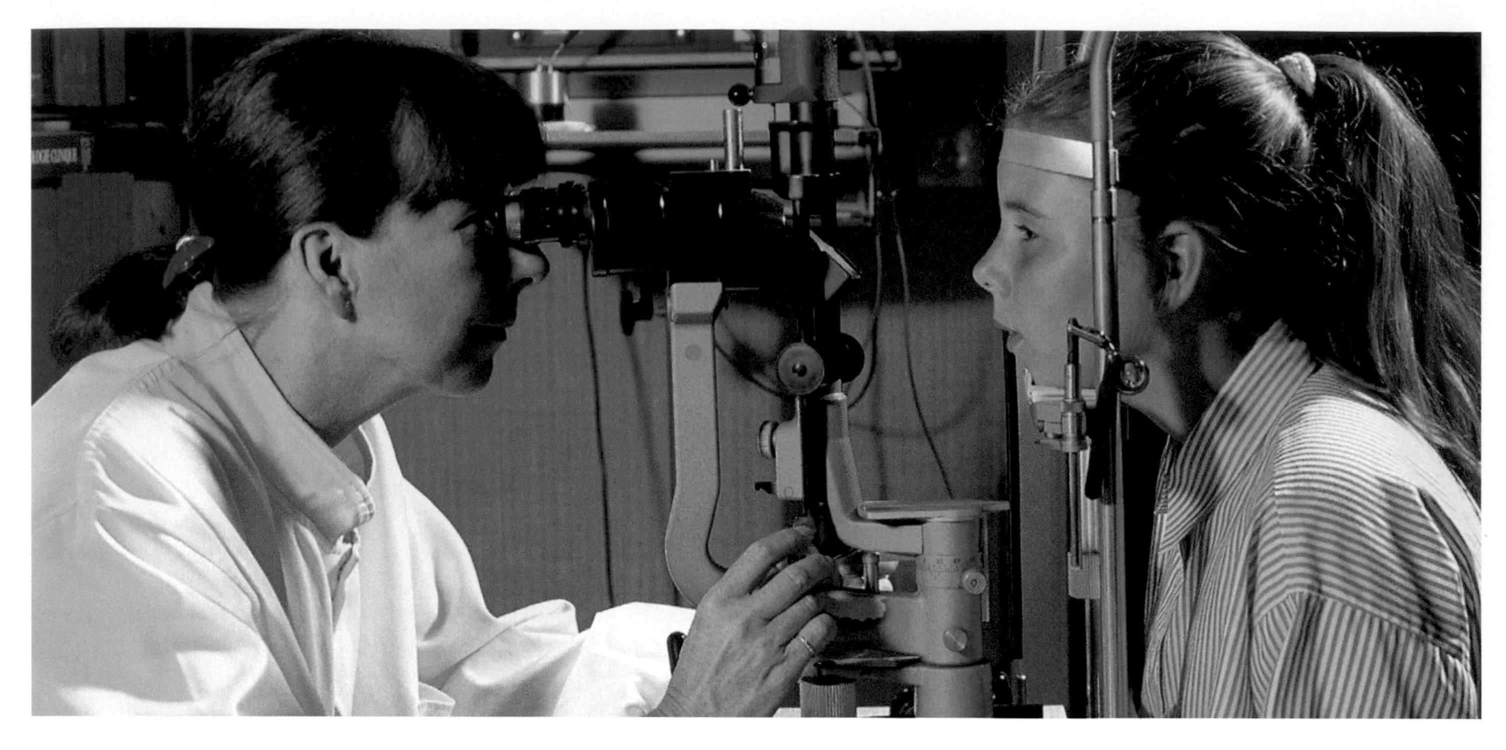

▲ *A slit lamp ophthalmoscope (above) is used by the ophthalmologist if a more detailed look at the eye is needed.*

Ophthalmic equipment

One of the basic tools of the ophthalmic profession is the ophthalmoscope, which is used by all doctors and optometrists, not just eye specialists. The ophthalmoscope shines a thin pencil of light into the eye and enables the doctor to look along the beam at the retina, the light-sensitive surface at the back of the eye. The ophthalmoscope has a number of lenses so that other parts of the eye can be examined.

When a more detailed look at the front of the cornea, the anterior chamber, or the iris is needed, an instrument called a slit lamp ophthalmoscope is used. The ophthalmologist may put drops of a fluorescent dye into the eye to make scratches or abrasions on the cornea show up more clearly. The slit lamp is also used in conjunction with a tonometer to measure the pressure in the eye. Raised pressure is indication of glaucoma.

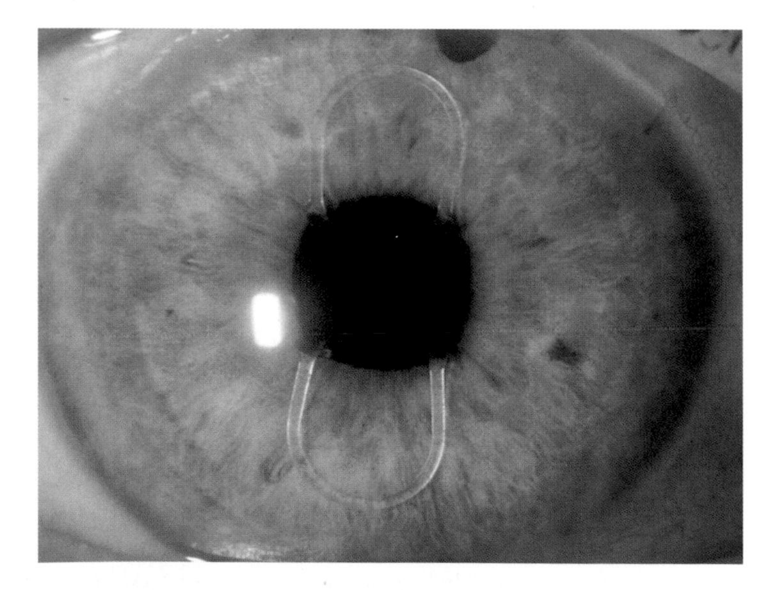

▲ *A tiny plastic lens must be inserted after cataract extraction to restore the focus of the eye. This photograph shows an early type of iris clip lens implant.*

Eye surgery

Although the ophthalmologist spends much of his or her time in the eye clinic testing different aspects of people's vision, perhaps the most exciting part of the job is in the operating room (OR). All of the many surgical procedures that are performed on the eye require great skill and precision. The size of the structures involved is so very small that the surgeon uses a special surgical microscope.

One of the most common procedures is the removal of a cataract. The diseased lens is replaced by a plastic intraocular lens. Supplementary reading glasses may be necessary. Surgical treatment may also be necessary to prevent loss of sight due to glaucoma. By operating on the iris and sclera and allowing fluid to drain from the anterior chamber of the eye, the ophthalmologist can relieve the high pressure in the eyeball that is causing poor vision.

When damage to the cornea results in scar formation, it may become opaque, making the eye effectively blind. A surgeon can help restore sight by cutting out a central disk of cornea and replacing it with a corneal transplant (see Donors). Laser surgery can help with some of the complications caused by diabetes by discouraging the growth of abnormal blood vessels in the retina (see Diabetes). Ophthalmologists can also reattach a detached retina. LASIK surgery can carve the cornea and alter its curve to correct refractice errors. Surgery can be performed on the structures surrounding the eye, to adjust the eye muscles to correct cross-eye, or to treat very watery eyes by clearing the tear ducts that drain into the nose.

See also: **Cataracts; Cornea; Eyes and eyesight; Glaucoma; Lasers; Lazy Eye; Optometrist; Retina and retinal disorders**

Opportunistic infection

Questions and Answers

Does opportunistic infection have anything to do with infections you can get in a hospital?

No. Opportunistic infections are mainly caused by germs that are easily overcome by a healthy immune system and thus don't ordinarily cause disease, except in those with immune deficiency problems like AIDS.

If opportunistic infections are caused by germs that don't usually cause disease, are the infections less serious than common ones?

No, they are usually more serious. In healthy people the immune system prevents these germs from spreading widely throughout the body, but with immune deficiency the immune system cannot combat the germs. Opportunistic infections can also involve common germs that normally cause minor effects. For example, in the case of herpes simplex, a healthy person might get an occasional cold sore; but in a person with immune deficiency the virus may cause herpes throughout the whole respiratory and intestinal tracts and may even spread to the brain, causing a dangerous encephalitis.

My son has AIDS and wants to join a protest rally in Times Square. I have a vague recollection that this may endanger his condition in some way. Is there any risk?

Yes, and from an unexpected source. Pigeon droppings contain the fungal germ *Cryptococcus;* in areas of high pigeon density like Times Square, it is present in high concentrations in the dust and is easily inhaled. It is usually harmless to healthy people, but people with immune deficiency can get a lung infection that leads to cryptococcal meningitis—an inflammation of the membranes surrounding the brain. Your son should try to keep well away from pigeons.

An opportunistic infection is one in which microorganisms that do not normally infect the human body take advantage of a deficiency in the immune system in order to spread infection.

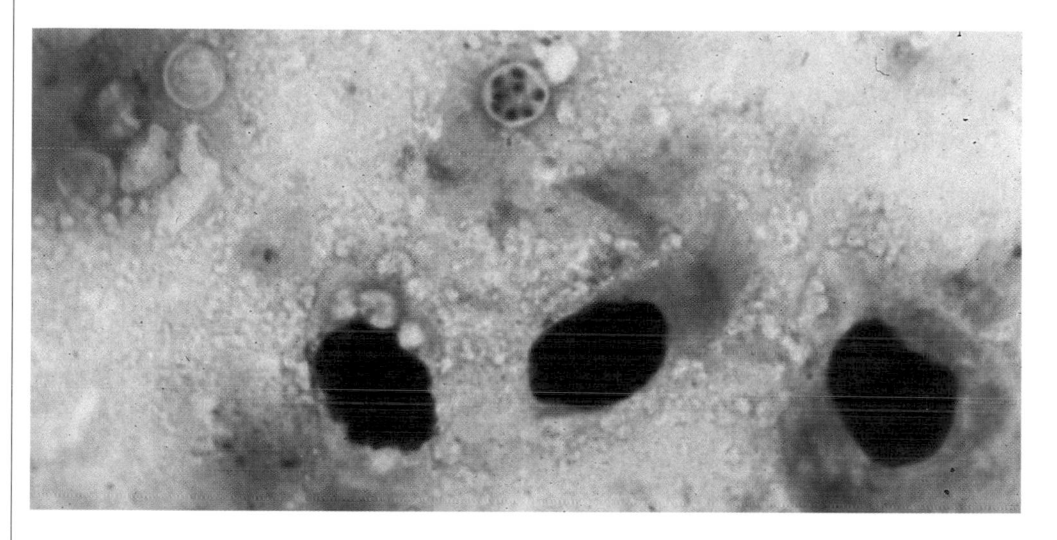

▲ *The germ* Pneumocystis jiroveci *(stained purple in this lung smear) causes pneumonia.*

People are constantly in contact with many forms of microscopic life ranging from viruses through bacteria, fungi, and protozoa. Most of these organisms are harmless, and only a small proportion will cause disease, because of the human immune system's efficiency in combating them. Some organisms, such as the herpes simplex virus or the thrush fungus *Candida albicans*, commonly cause minor external infections but are prevented by the immune system from spreading widely throughout the body (see Herpes). If, for whatever reason, however, the body's immune defenses are less efficient than normal, two things can happen: germs that never cause infections in healthy people begin to do so, and those that normally cause only superficial infections begin to spread widely within the body, affecting the internal organs. These are known as opportunistic infections.

The germs most likely to take opportunistic advantage of immune deficiency are a fungus *Cryptococcus*, causing brain infections with seizures and visual loss; the fungus *Candida albicans*, causing widespread thrush; *Cytomegalovirus*, causing severe pneumonia and damage to the retinas, resulting in blindness; *Pneumocystis jiroveci*, causing a dangerous form of pneumonia; *Toxoplasma gondii*, affecting the eyes and the brain; *Mycobacterium tuberculosis*, causing a severe tuberculous infection of the lungs and elsewhere; and herpes simplex and herpes zoster viruses. The term "opportunistic infection" is used for any common infective organism that, in the presence of immune deficiency, mounts a far more serious, widespread, and dangerous infection than usual.

Causes of immune deficiency

The most common cause of immune deficiency and the resulting opportunistic infections is acquired immunodeficiency syndrome (AIDS). Many of the severe conditions that affect people with AIDS—pneumonia, cytomegalovirus infections, atypical *Mycobacterium* infections, cryptococcosis, and histoplasmosis—are rare except in AIDS victims. However, immune deficiency can also occur naturally in old people or result from a genetic defect, prolonged alcohol abuse, or the use of strong antibiotics over a long period or immunosuppressive drugs to prevent rejection of transplanted organs. It may also be a feature of diseases involving the white cells of the immune system, such as chronic lymphocytic leukemia, macroglobulinemia, multiple myelomatosis, Hodgkin's disease, and other lymphomas.

See also: AIDS; Bacteria; Immune system; Infection and infectious diseases; Viruses

Optic nerve

Questions and Answers

What is my doctor looking for when he shines a light in my eye?

He is looking at the light reflex. An early sign of damage to the optic nerve is a failure of the pupils to constrict when a light shines on them. Other problems in the brain or eye can also interfere with this reflex.

My sister has multiple sclerosis, and she lost all vision in her right eye for six weeks. Her vision then recovered. How can this be?

Multiple sclerosis commonly affects an optic nerve. The initial inflammation can block impulses from passing along the nerve, but it is unlikely to destroy more than a proportion of the million or so separate fibers that it contains. Vision usually returns, although special testing may show reduced resolution and color perception.

What is the blind spot, and what effect does it have on sight?

The blind spot is the point at which the optic nerve enters the eye. At this point there are no rods or cones—the cells that enable us to see movement and color. It doesn't affect our sight, because when we look at something the image falls on a sensitive part of the retina called the macula.

Since the optic nerves from the two eyes cross, if one of them is damaged, can the other one still channel the necessary information?

Not quite, because only half of the information from one eye passes across to the other side of the brain. However, all the information from the left side of each eye goes, via nerve fibers, to the brain, where the images are interpreted, so even if half of the visual field is lost, the patient can still read.

The optic nerve is a bundle of nerve fibers that carries impulses from the retina—the light-sensitive lining of the eye—to the back of the brain. Some of these nerve fibers cross over to the other side of the brain at the optic chiasma.

The back of the eye behind the lens is called the retina, and it is made up of a layer of light-sensitive cells. Each of these cells is connected by a nerve to the brain, where vital information about pattern, colors, and shapes is computed.

All the nerve fibers collect together at the back of the eye to form a single cable, which is known as the optic nerve. This runs from the eyeball, through a bony tunnel in the skull, to emerge inside the skull bone just beneath the brain, in the region of the pituitary gland; here it is joined by the optic nerve from the other eye.

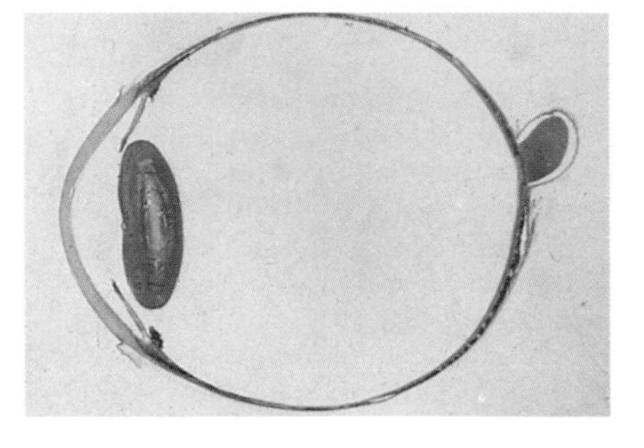

▲ *A vertical section through a human eye shows the optic nerve (the protrusion on the right).*

Half of the nerve fibers from each side then cross over so that some information from the left eye is passed to the right side of the brain and vice versa. Nerves from the temporal (side) part of each retina stay on the same side of the brain, whereas the fibers from the central part of the eye—the part that does most of the seeing—run to the opposite side of the brain. This crossover point is called the optic chiasma (see Eyes and Eyesight).

Structure of the optic nerve

Each optic nerve consists of a bundle of tiny nerve fibers that carry minute electrical impulses. Each fiber is insulated from the next by a fatty layer called myelin. At the center of the optic nerve, running its entire length, is a small artery called the central retinal artery. This emerges at the back of the eye, where vessels from it spread over the surface of the retina. A corresponding vein that drains the retina runs back down the optic nerve alongside the central retinal artery.

Nerve pathways

Nerves emerging from the retina are sensory. Unlike the nerves that supply muscle (motor neurons), which make only one connection on their way to the brain, optic neurons make more than one connection (see Nervous System). The first connection or cell station is in the lateral geniculate body, which lies just behind the optic chiasma (where the sensory information from each eye swaps over). Here some information from the left and right eyes is swapped again across the midline. The function of this connection is linked with the reflexes of the pupils.

From the lateral geniculate body, the nerves fan out on each side around the temporal (side) area of the brain to form the optic radiation. They then turn slightly and meet to pass through the main exchange, the internal capsule, where all the motor and sensory information from the body is concentrated. From there the nerves pass to the visual cortex at the back of the brain.

Sensitive cells

There are two types of light-sensitive cells in the retina, the rods and the cones; and like photoelectric cells they convert light energy into electricity. The rods are used principally to detect objects in the dark—they are very sensitive to movement, so they register objects appearing from the extremes of the visual field in dim light. The cones are responsible for sharp color vision, and they are most plentiful at the fovea, the central point of the macula where the lens focuses light. However, there are no rods or cones at the point where the optic nerve enters the eye; this is known as the blind spot because light focused here is not perceived.

The diameter of the pupils is controlled in a way similar to the aperture in a camera. Light falling on the retina sends impulses up the optic nerve to the cell station behind the optic chiasma

THE MECHANICS OF SEEING

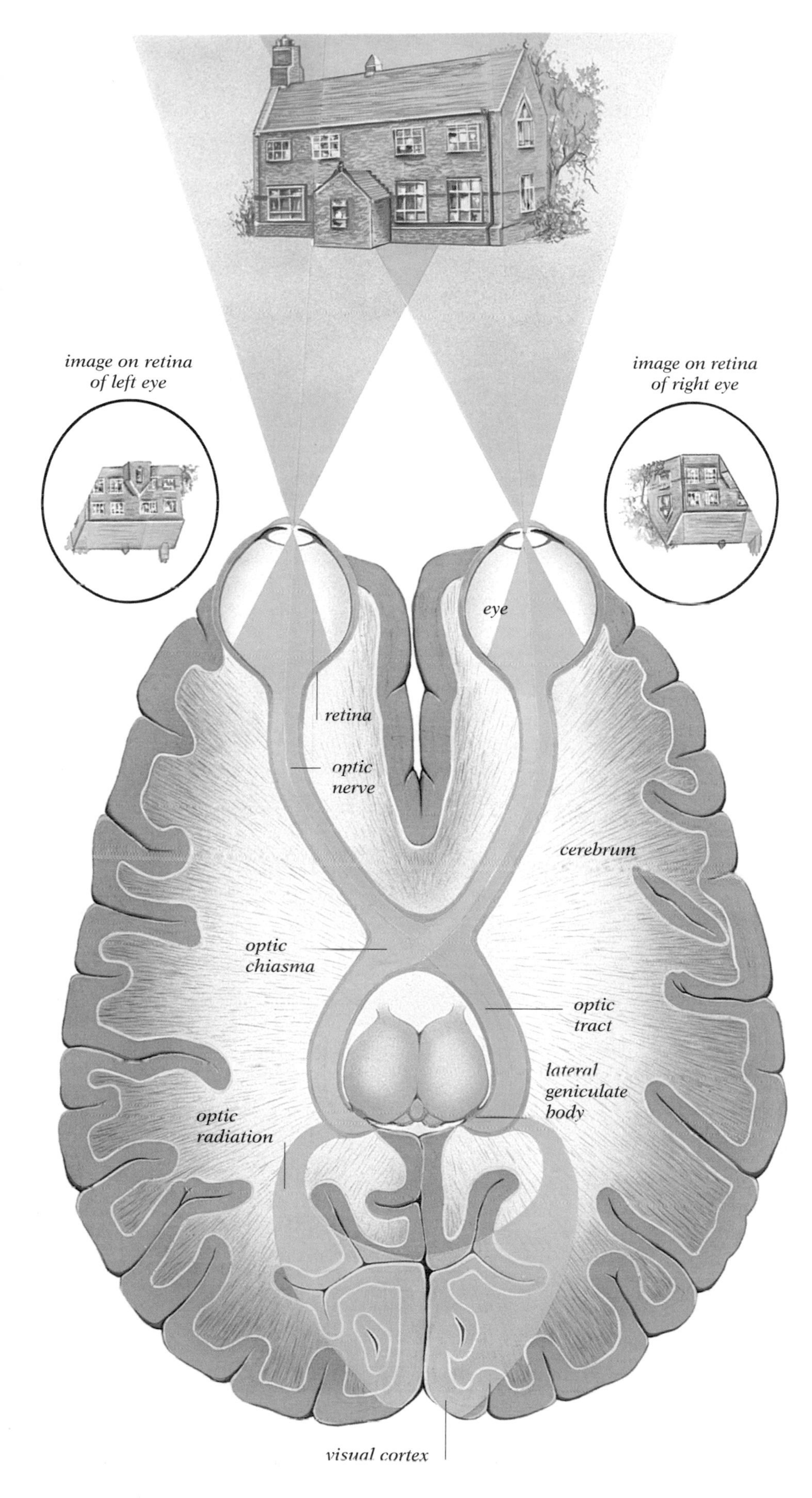

◄ *The right and left eyes have slightly different fields of vision, each split into a right and left side. When light rays reach the retinas, they are transposed and inverted. They then travel down the optic nerves to the optic chiasma, where a crossover takes place. All the information from the left side of each eye travels down the optic tract through the lateral geniculate body and the optic radiation to the right visual cortex, and vice versa. Later these images are combined and interpreted by the brain.*

and then back to a motor nerve supplying the muscle of the pupil. The brighter the light, the more tightly the pupil constricts.

What can go wrong

Obstruction of the central retinal artery causes sudden total blindness. Although this is rare, it may occur if the optic nerve swells in its bony tunnel through the skull and presses on the artery. Vision can also be affected if the blood vessels running over the top of the retina rupture and bleed over the surface, thereby cutting out the light, as can occur in people with diabetes.

Some toxins can affect the retina and optic nerve; the most common is methanol (wood alcohol), which can cause blindness.

Multiple sclerosis can cause inflammation of the optic nerve, and visual loss occurs as a large central blind spot called a scotoma. If the optic nerve is sufficiently inflamed, it turns pink and sticks out like the head of a thumbtack from the back of the eye; this condition is called papilledema. Tumors of the pituitary gland may press on the optic chiasma, producing visual abnormalities depending on which fibers they constrict.

Strokes commonly interfere with the blood supply to the nerves that pass through the internal capsule, the main exchange center of the brain. Damage to this area results in a total loss of movement and sensation on one side of the body and an inability to see objects moving in from that side—a paralysis called hemiplegia. Sight, movement, and sensation are quite normal on the opposite side.

Damage to the visual cortex at the back of the brain, for example as a result of a gunshot wound, may cause total blindness.

See also: **Brain; Diabetes; Multiple sclerosis; Poisoning; Reflexes; Stroke**

Optometrist

Optometrists are responsible for testing people's eyes and prescribing glasses when necessary. They are trained to detect eye defects but are not qualified to prescribe drugs or perform corrective surgery.

Three types of eye problems require the specialist services of an optometrist. The first is myopia (nearsightedness), which makes it difficult for a person to see objects in the distance. The second is hypermetropia (farsightedness). People with this condition have difficulty in reading small print and in focusing close up, although distant objects are usually well defined. Finally, there is presbyopia, which people develop as a natural consequence of aging: focusing close up becomes increasingly difficult, even if there has been no previous hypermetropia. Any of these problems can be complicated by the condition known as astigmatism, which causes blurring.

Vision

Sight depends on light, which should be thought of as individual rays traveling in straight lines. These rays can change direction only if they pass through certain materials, such as the glass of a camera lens or the transparent tissue of the eye. The bending of light rays is called refraction. By refraction, rays of light are concentrated in the chamber of the eye so that they cast an image on the light-sensitive area at the back of the eye known as the retina (see Eyes and Eyesight). Most of the refraction takes place at the front of the eye in the cornea, the eye's transparent

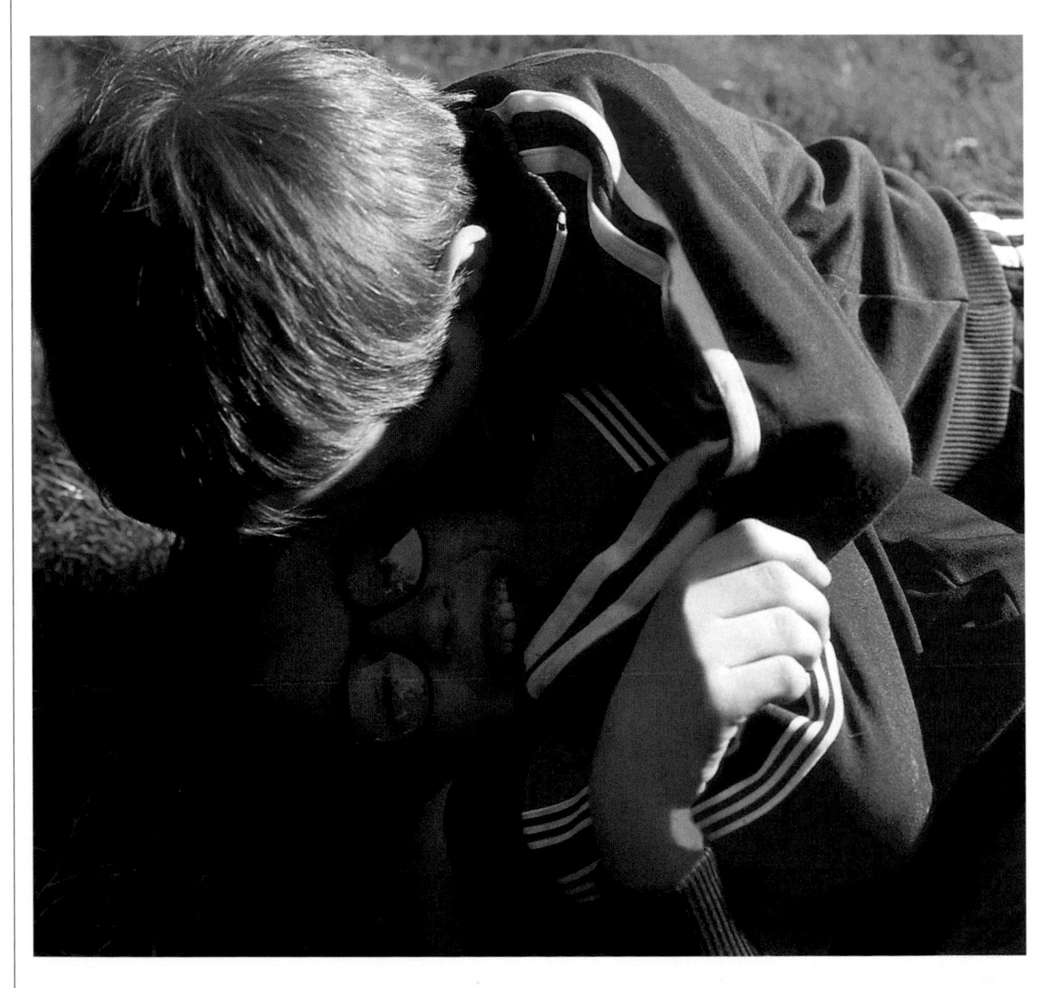

▲ *A child who wears glasses need not refrain from playing active games and sports. However, he or she will have to be a little more careful than other children.*

Questions and Answers

I've been having severe headaches recently, and I've heard they can be caused by defective eyesight. Should I visit an optometrist, or is it a medical problem?

Of all the thousands of people who go to their doctors each year complaining of headaches, only a minority are found to be suffering from defective eyesight. It is much more likely that you are having tension headaches or a severe type of headache called a migraine. However, if you also notice symptoms such as the blurring of objects in the distance, or if you have difficulty reading or feel that your eyes are tired and strained at the end of the day, it is worth having your vision tested. If defective sight is the cause of your headaches, wearing glasses will probably cure them.

Is it true that you can ruin your sight by wearing someone else's glasses, even if they do seem to improve your vision?

Never wear glasses that are not your own. Babies and young children can be seriously affected by wearing the wrong glasses, and an adult may experience a sense of strain or begin to get headaches. If you do have defective sight, an optometrist can give you the proper glasses to correct it completely.

My mother is in her seventies and has problems with deteriorating vision. Even her new glasses don't seem to help. Why is this?

Not all eyesight problems can be corrected by an optometrist. Cataracts—the clouding of the eye lens—require surgery, not glasses. Equally, the retina—the light-sensitive area at the back of the eye on which the image forms —can degenerate in old age. The latter is something neither glasses nor surgery will help.

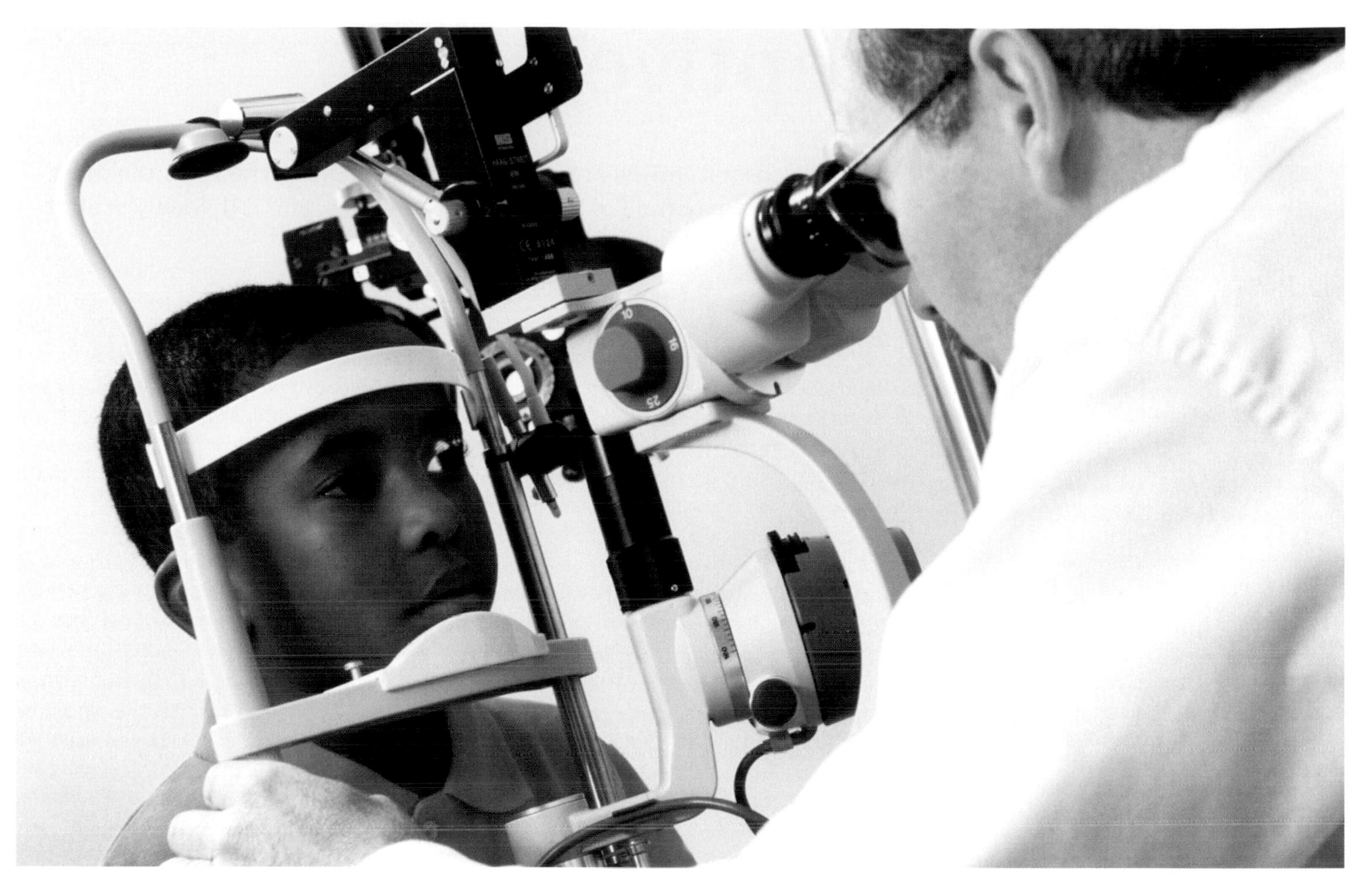

▲ *By examining the inside of each eye, an optometrist can tell whether someone is near- or farsighted.*

window (see Cornea). There is further refraction as light passes through the lens immediately behind the iris, although the main function of this lens is fine focusing, which is achieved by the circular ciliary muscle that surrounds the lens.

The main reason for poor eyesight, or imperfect refractive capacity, is not a fault in the lens's focusing power but a fault in the shape of the cornea and the length of the eyeball.

The ideal shape for the eyeball is spherical. If it is too long, the cornea tends to be too rounded. The rounder (stronger) the cornea, the more sharply it bends light rays, causing the image to focus in the space in front of the retina and leaving a blur on the retina itself. This is nearsightedness.

If the eyeball is too short, the cornea is too flat. Thus it does not bend the rays sharply enough and the image falls behind the retina, causing farsightedness. In youth, ciliary focusing (accommodation) can compensate for moderate degrees of farsightedness, but accommodation in short sight makes matters worse.

Astigmatism is caused by an imperfectly curved cornea, which causes the light rays to focus at different points (see Astigmatism).

Myopia, hypermetropia, and astigmatism are all hereditary.

Visiting the optometrist

Optometrists particularly look out for disorders of focusing. The basic item of equipment that they use is the test chart, which is usually positioned 20 feet (6 m) away from the person being tested. The letter at the top of the chart is a size that someone with normal sight can read easily at 197 feet (60 m). The next row down can be read at 118 feet (36 m) and each successive one at 80, 60, 40, 30, 20, and 16.5 feet (24, 18, 12, 9, 6, and 5 m) respectively. If a person can read the seventh row at 20 feet (6 m), his or her sight is considered normal. Normal vision is called 20/20 (6/6) vision: the first number refers to the person's distance from the chart and the second number refers to the distance of the row being read.

The optometrist will ask the person being tested to wear a special frame while looking at the chart. By fitting a combination of lenses into this and asking how clearly he or she can read the appropriate row of letters, the optometrist can determine the strength of the lens that is required to give the person 20/20 vision.

At the same time the optometrist will peer into each eye through a retinoscope. This enables him or her to see whether the person is near- or farsighted. It also shows when the correct strength or combination of lenses has been put into the frame. This is usually different for each eye.

If both tests indicate that the same strength of lens is necessary, the optometrist has confirmation of that person's requirement and can prescribe glasses.

The retinoscope is also needed to test for astigmatism. If a person has this defect, the glasses prescribed will be designed to correct it.

Finally, the optometrist will advise on whether contact lenses can be worn instead of ordinary glasses, and when the person should return to have his or her sight retested.

See also: **Aging; Contact lenses**

Oral contraceptives

A hormonal contraceptive is commonly called "the Pill." The Pill is the most reliable reversible method of birth control available, and it is widely used to prevent pregnancy.

Oral contraceptives are made of synthetic hormones similar to those that occur naturally in a woman's body. Hormones are the body's chemical messengers that influence or control the activity of body cells. When hormones are released into the bloodstream, they seek out particular cells and slowly stimulate or suppress these cells' activity. Some hormones govern sexuality and fertility; oral contraceptives contain synthetic versions of sex hormones that prevent conception. Some oral contraceptives work by stopping ovulation; others make it difficult for sperm to reach the egg or for a fertilized egg to implant in the wall of the uterus (see Sperm; Uterus).

The idea of chemically altering the body to prevent pregnancy is not new. Many cultures, such as the ancient Egyptians and Native American tribes, chewed certain leaves to increase or decrease their likelihood of fertility. Oral contraceptive pills were introduced in 1961 and became widely available during the 1960s. They have become linked with women's liberation, and the ability of women to control the functioning of their own bodies.

The first oral contraceptives were combined pills containing synthetic estrogen and progestogen. The second-generation pills contain progestogen alone and are often known as the mini-pill. None of the pills contain natural estrogen or progesterone. The substances used are synthetic analogues of the natural hormones. The estrogen most often used is ethinylestrodial, and the progestogen used is levonorgestrel, norgestrel, or norethisterone. More recently, third-generation progestogen-only pills contain desogestrel or gestodene, and a controversy has arisen as to whether these latest pills are more likely than second-generation pills to cause thrombosis in veins (see Thrombosis). This controversy continues, but the risks are still very low.

How oral contraceptives work

Different types of oral contraceptives work in different ways. The combined Pill contains hormones very much like those produced by the body during pregnancy. As a result, the pituitary gland, which normally sends a message to the ovaries to produce a monthly egg, acts as if the

▼ *It may be helpful to explain to a sexual partner about the use of oral contraceptives.*

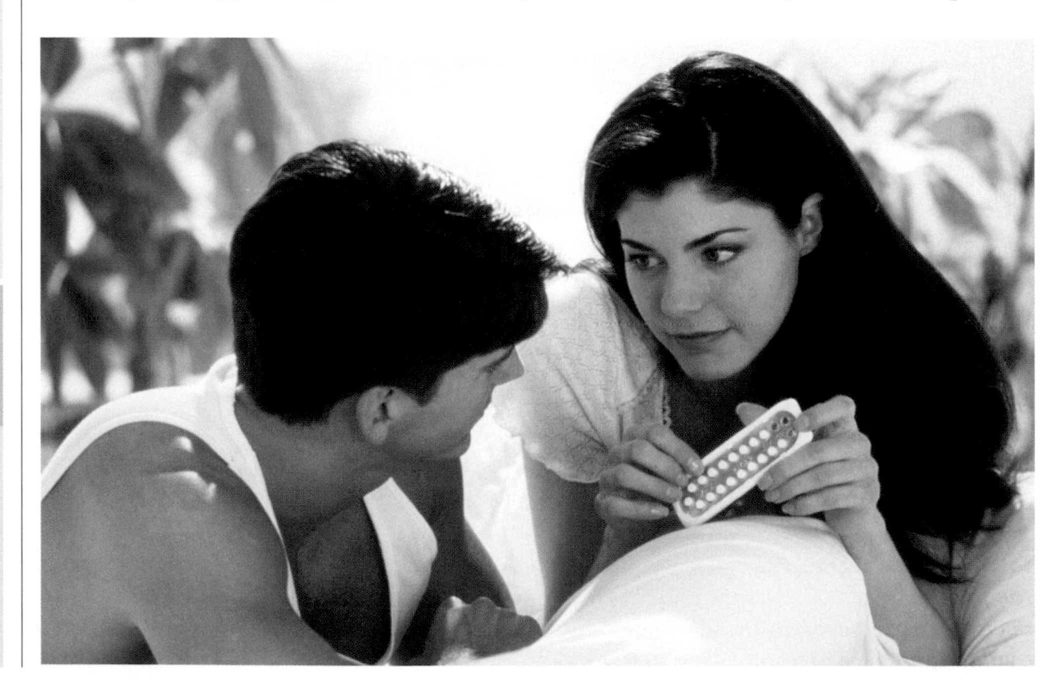

Questions and Answers

Can the Pill cause a loss of libido?

Some women do find that their interest in sex is decreased when they go on the Pill. However, this can often be corrected by a change of Pill. If you have this problem, and are concerned, it is worth seeing your doctor and getting a prescription for a Pill that contains a different balance of hormones.

I have varicose veins and I have heard that the Pill can make them worse. Is this true?

If your varicose veins are minor, and if you are not in a high-risk category for any other reason, such as your medical history or being a smoker, you will probably be able to take the Pill with no complication. Talk to your doctor before the Pill is prescribed.

Should I regularly take a break from the Pill in order to allow my body to get back into its normal menstrual cycle?

There is no need to do this frequently, although it was once considered necessary. Nor is there any indication that women who have irregular periods when they are off the Pill need to have extra breaks from it. It is now generally thought that, provided you are fit and healthy, the Pill can be taken continuously without a break. You should, however, have regular medical checkups.

Should I tell any doctor I see that I'm on the Pill, even if the consultation is about something entirely different?

Yes. A doctor knows which drugs interfere with each other, and can avoid prescribing those that will reduce the effectiveness of the Pill. He or she needs to know that you are taking it, because it can affect the results of any laboratory tests.

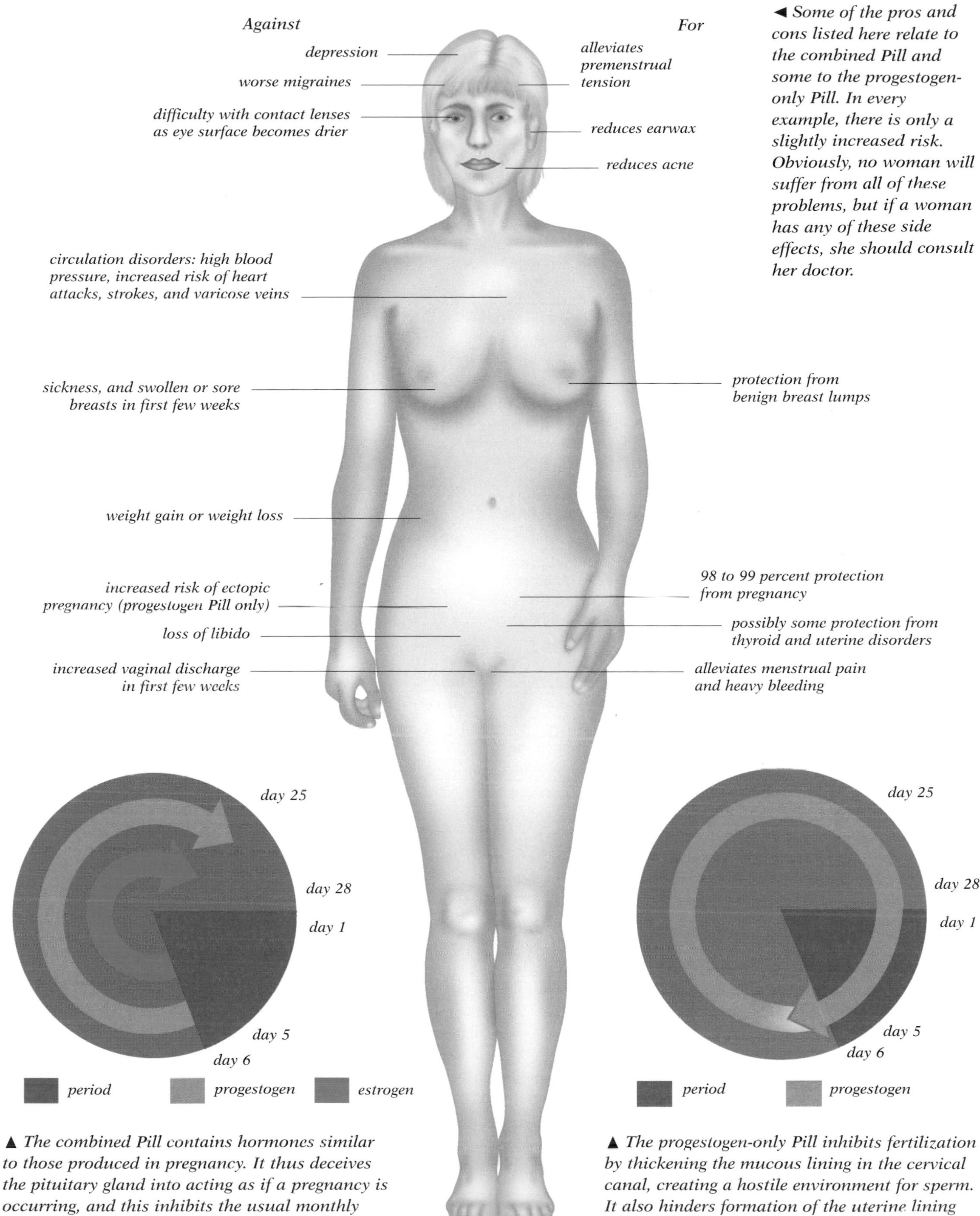

◀ *Some of the pros and cons listed here relate to the combined Pill and some to the progestogen-only Pill. In every example, there is only a slightly increased risk. Obviously, no woman will suffer from all of these problems, but if a woman has any of these side effects, she should consult her doctor.*

▲ *The combined Pill contains hormones similar to those produced in pregnancy. It thus deceives the pituitary gland into acting as if a pregnancy is occurring, and this inhibits the usual monthly ovulation by the ovaries.*

▲ *The progestogen-only Pill inhibits fertilization by thickening the mucous lining in the cervical canal, creating a hostile environment for sperm. It also hinders formation of the uterine lining that would support a fertilized egg.*

Questions and Answers

I have been on the Pill for five years, and I now want to become pregnant. When should I stop using the Pill?

It is worth coming off the Pill at once to give your body time to resume its normal menstrual cycle. You may find that there is a delay before regular periods return. You should use another method of contraception until you have had two periods, after which time you can try to become pregnant. The delay that sometimes happens between stopping the Pill and the hoped-for pregnancy may not be due to the Pill at all, or it may be that the body needs a little more time before ovulation begins again. If you fail to become pregnant after a year or more, a fertility clinic may be able to help you.

I became pregnant when I forgot to take two Pills, but I continued taking them for a while because I didn't know I was pregnant. Could this have harmed the baby?

Taking the Pill during the early weeks of pregnancy has not been shown to harm the developing fetus, but research into this area is continuing. Doctors advise any woman who suspects that she may be pregnant to stop taking the Pill and use another method of contraception until it has been confirmed whether or not she really is pregnant.

How often should I have a medical checkup when I'm on the Pill?

You should see your doctor after the first three months on the Pill, and thereafter have a checkup every six months. Your blood pressure should be checked, and if it is high, the doctor may prescribe a different type of Pill.

Am I likely to gain weight if I go on the Pill?

Not necessarily: on first taking the Pill, approximately one-third of women gain weight, one-third lose weight, and one-third stay the same weight.

Taking the Pill

Taking the combination Pill at the same time as part of a routine makes it easier to remember.

If you miss a day, take two pills the next day, then continue with the rest of the pack as normal.

If you miss two days, double up the dose for the next two days, and use additional contraception until your next period.

If you miss three days, throw out the pack and use alternative contraception until your next period. Then, start a new pack following the same procedure that you used when you first started taking the Pill.

After your first month on the Pill, if troublesome side effects do not disappear, contact your doctor.

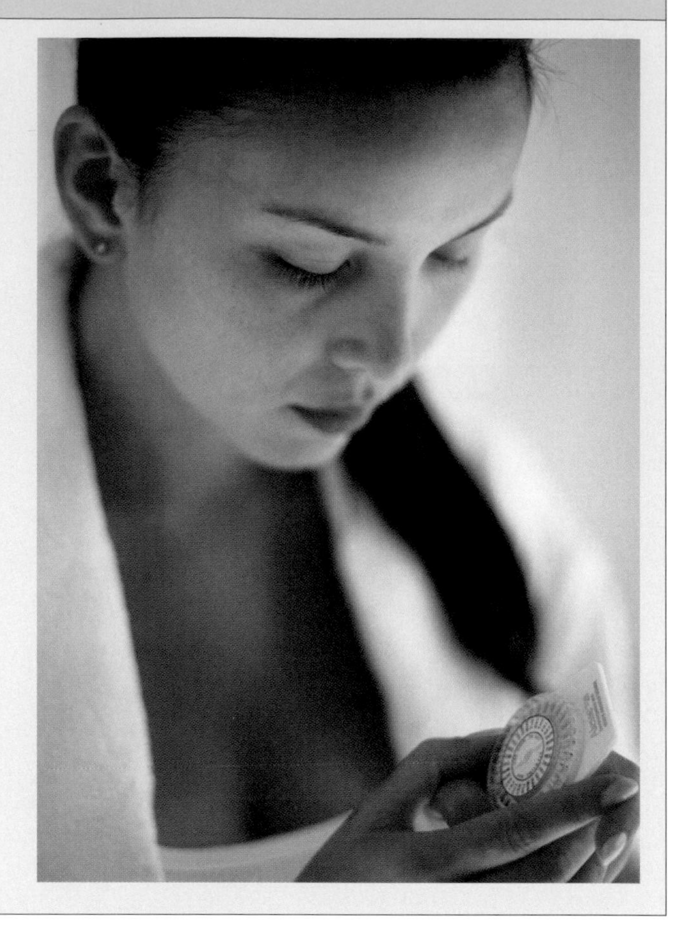

body is already pregnant. It does not send its egg-stimulating hormone to the ovaries, and therefore ovulation does not take place (see Pregnancy).

The progestogen-only Pill (the mini-pill) does not always prevent ovulation. It makes fertilization more difficult by thickening the mucus in the cervical canal (the passage that leads from the vagina to the uterus), and it inhibits the formation of the uterine lining (in which the fertilized egg must implant itself). As a result, implantation and pregnancy do not take place.

Different types of pill

A number of pharmaceutical companies make contraceptive pills. Although there are versions of the Pill that have different brand names, they are all made from the same hormones: the combination Pill with estrogen and progestogen, and the progestogen-only Pill as its name implies. However, different brands offer different synthesized versions of progestogen.

Triphasic pills contain the same two hormones found in the combination Pill, but in a different amount for each week of the cycle, in an attempt to mimic the menstrual cycle more effectively. Some women prefer to take a Pill every day because they find it easier to remember, so 21-day combination pills exist that include seven dummy pills to be taken in the fourth week.

The progestogen-only Pill must be taken every day, and it can cause changes in a woman's periods while she is taking it. Some women do not have any bleeding for several months; others have frequent breakthrough bleeding during the month. However, most women do not have any problems of this kind. Bleeding does not indicate that the Pill is not working properly, but women who find irregular bleeding troublesome should ask their doctor for advice. If a woman's period is more than two weeks overdue, she is probably not pregnant, but she should see her doctor. The type of Pill a woman takes will be decided by her and her doctor. The progestogen-only Pill is thought to involve less risk of circulatory problems, so it is often the Pill of choice for those who may be at risk from this kind of disease. Estrogen can cause blood clots in the veins and high blood pressure (see Blood Pressure; Veins).

There are many positive effects of the Pill, not least the protection from unwanted pregnancy. The reliability of the combined Pill is 99 percent, and that of the progestogen-only Pill is 98 percent. The Pill can also actively protect women from certain disorders, such as the formation of benign breast lumps. Since the body is no longer going through the menstrual cycle, many of the problems associated with periods (pain, heavy bleeding, and premenstrual tension) can be alleviated. Research suggests that it may also offer some protection against uterine cancer, but this has not yet been confirmed.

Side effects

Troublesome side effects may occur at the beginning of a course of pills. Some women find that when they first start taking the Pill they feel nauseated, gain weight, and get—or are cured of—acne, or their breasts become swollen and sore (see Breasts). Some women who suffer from migraines may find that the Pill makes their condition worse, although others find that their condition improves. The Pill can also affect a woman's ability to wear contact lenses, since the amount of fluid on the surface of the eye may be reduced.

The combination Pill can also cause depression and loss of libido (sex drive). Women who suffer from these symptoms should consider changing to an alternative type of pill (see Depression). The most dangerous side effect of the combination Pill is the increased likelihood of circulatory disorders such as high blood pressure, heart attacks, thrombosis, and strokes (see Heart Disease). For this reason, a doctor will check a patient's blood pressure while she is on the Pill. In rare cases, a blood clot in the veins may be fatal if part of the clot breaks off and travels to the lungs. Circulatory problems affect only a tiny minority of women on the Pill, and the risk has been greatly reduced by the introduction of pills containing lower doses of hormones. However, prospective users must be screened to see if they are at risk, and a doctor will need to study a woman's medical history and that of her family. Women who smoke, are overweight, or are over 35 years of age have an increased risk of circulatory disorders, so they are often advised not to use the combination Pill. For some users, there is also an increased risk of gallbladder disease.

The progestogen-only Pill does not seem to carry such risks, and it is the one most often prescribed for older women. The risk of vein thrombosis with the contraceptive pill is very low. For a woman not on the Pill, the risk is about five per 100,000 women per year. For the second-generation Pill it is about 15 per 100,000 women per year, and for the third-generation progestogen-only Pill it is about 25 per 100,000 women per year. Neither the second- nor the third-generation pills increase the risk of heart attacks in young women, and the risk of stroke is increased by about one in 24,000 regardless of the type of Pill taken. The risk of dying from a deep-vein thrombosis exists in 1 to 2 percent of all cases, so the risk of death from vein thrombosis caused by the third-generation Pill is very low indeed—less than three women in a million in a year.

The progestogen-only Pill is not quite as effective in preventing pregnancy as the combined Pill. Because it does not prevent ovulation, there is a small risk that an egg will be fertilized and, if so, that the egg will implant itself outside the uterus, since the uterine lining is not soft or spongy enough to receive it. This is called an ectopic pregnancy, and it can take place in one of the fallopian tubes (see Ectopic Pregnancy). The risk of ectopic pregnancy is small, but it is a dangerous condition that needs prompt treatment. Any persistent pain in the lower abdomen should be reported to a doctor.

Common problems and solutions

PROBLEM	SOLUTION
Missed one combination Pill	Take two pills at the usual time, and continue with the rest of the packet as normal.
Missed two combination pills	Double the dose for the next two days, then take the rest of the packet as normal. Protection may have stopped, so use an additional form of contraception until the end of the month.
Diarrhea or vomiting	Continue to take pills as normal if you are keeping them down.
No period in the pill-free week	Check with your doctor to see if you are pregnant and therefore whether or not to start the next packet of pills. Until you see your doctor, use a diaphragm or condom (both with spermicide).
Side effects at the beginning of a course of pills, such as nausea, depression, swollen breasts, weight gain or loss, and headaches	Wait to see if these symptoms gradually disappear over the first month. If they do not, go back to your doctor to discuss alternative pills or methods of contraception.

When a woman stops taking the pill, the return of her menstrual cycle may be delayed, but it is now thought that this does not affect fertility in the long term (see Endocrine System). The initial choice of Pill will be made by a doctor or gynecologist. Most women begin with a low-dose combination Pill, which the doctor will advise they start taking on day one of their next period. The combination Pill should be taken at the same time every day, at whatever time of day is best. Many women find that taking it before bedtime is easy to remember.

The effectiveness of the Pill may be affected by vomiting or diarrhea, because the chemicals in the Pill may not have had time to be absorbed into the body before the contents of the stomach are emptied (see Diarrhea). Other medication, including some antibiotics, drugs for epilepsy, and certain sedatives and painkillers, can also reduce the effectiveness of the Pill. Women should check with their doctor to make sure that there is no risk of this.

Coming off the Pill

Most women can remain on the Pill until they reach menopause (see Menopause). However, because there is an increased risk of clotting, if a woman is likely to be bedridden for several weeks or months, she may be advised to stop taking the Pill temporarily. Women coming off the Pill to become pregnant should use an alternative form of contraception for two months to allow the body to readjust.

See also: **Acne and pimples; Contraception; Estrogen; Hormones; Libido; Menstruation; Migraine; Ovaries; Premenstrual syndrome; Stroke**

Organic food

Questions and Answers

Can any food be certified organic?

Yes, if it has been grown and processed according to national organic standards. A wide range of organic products is now available: not just fruit, vegetables, and meat, but also pasta, milk, frozen meals, and baby food. Products not traditionally considered "healthy," such as chocolate, wine, and vodka, may also be certified "organic." There is also a wide range of organic fiber products available, including bed and bath linen, T-shirts and other clothes, hygiene products, and tablecloths.

Are all organic foods entirely free of pesticides?

No. If organic farmers are unable to control pests or weeds by using natural methods, they sometimes request permission from certifiers to use nonpersistent pesticides. Also, agricultural chemicals have been used for half a century, and pesticide residues are still present in rain and groundwater. It is sometimes impossible to prevent these residues from tainting organic crops. The shift toward farming organically, however, ensures that fewer of these pesticide residues will be present in our water in the future.

Why does organic food usually cost more?

The strict regulations governing organic food production raise the cost of the products. Production is more labor- and management-intensive, and organic farms tend to be smaller. All stages in organic food production—growing, harvesting, transportation, and storage—are strictly controlled and therefore more expensive. As bigger food manufacturers enter the market, however, prices are expected to drop and be more in line with conventional items.

Organic food is growing steadily in popularity, with the sale of organic products in the United States increasing 20 to 25 percent annually from the 1990s to the 21st century.

"Organic" generally refers to products, practices, and procedures that are seen as healthy for people, animals, and the environment. Organic farming is practiced all over the world and is now expanding beyond the major markets of Europe and North America. In the United States there are about 12,200 organic farms. To protect producers and consumers, strict laws have been introduced to govern the certification of food as "organic." In the United States the definition of what is organic may vary in common use, but in 1995 the U.S. National Organic Standards Board defined organic agriculture thus:

"Organic agriculture is an ecological production management system that promotes and enhances diversity, biological cycles, and soil biological activity. It is based on minimal use of off-farm inputs and on management practices that restore, maintain, and enhance ecological harmony. 'Organic' is a labeling term that denotes products produced under the authority of the Organic Food Production Act. The principal guidelines for organic production are to use materials and practices that enforce the ecological balance of natural systems and that integrate the parts of the farming system into an ecological whole. Organic agriculture practices cannot ensure that products are completely free of residues; organic growing methods are used to minimize pollution from air, soil, and water; organic food processors, handlers, and retailers adhere to standards that maintain the integrity of organic agriculture products. The primary goal of organic agriculture is to optimize the health and productivity of interdependent communities of soil life, plants, animals, and people."

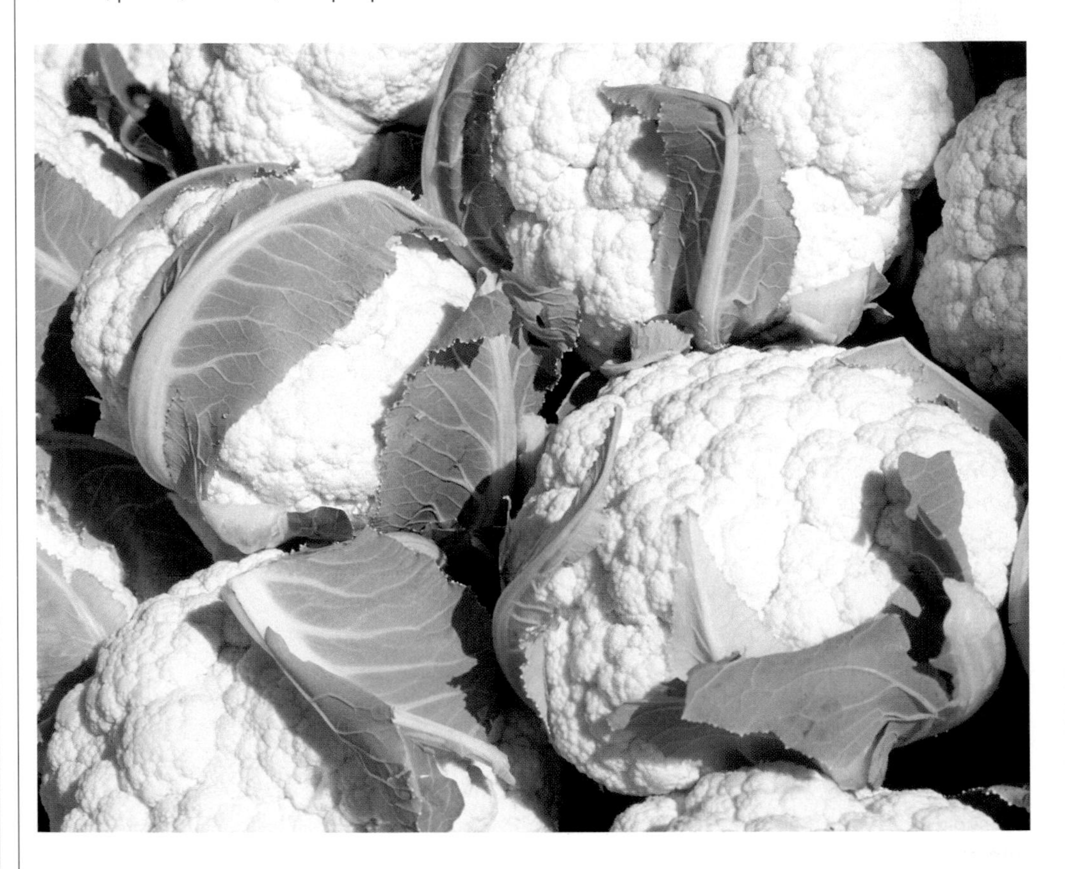

▲ *Cauliflower is a crop that can deliver a good yield without the use of chemicals or pesticides, and some people claim it has a better taste and texture when grown organically.*

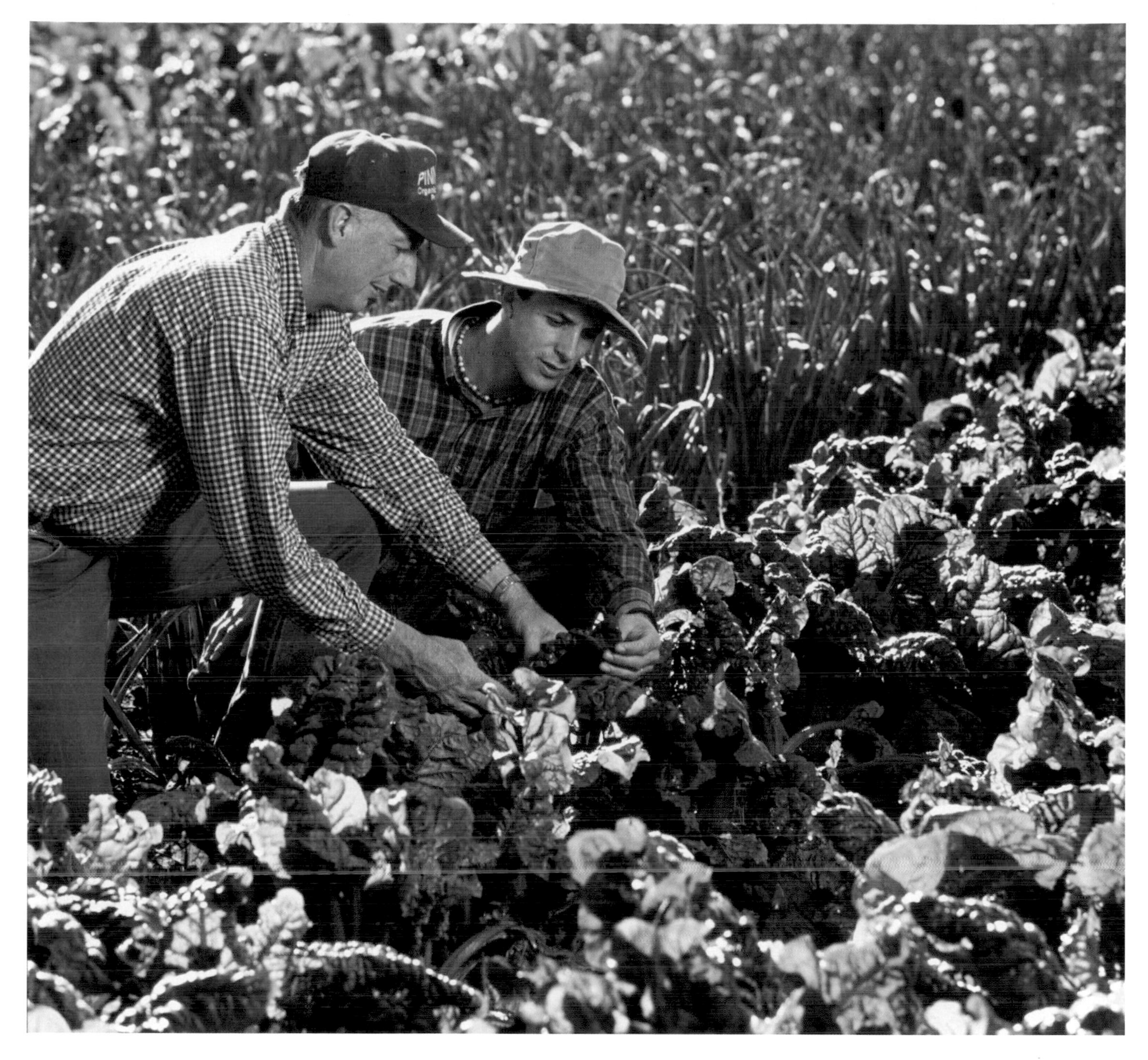

▲ *Organic farmers in San Juan Bautista, California, inspect their red chard. California is the leading state in organic acreage, with a total of about 190,000 acres in 2001. Vegetables, fruits, and nuts form 90 percent of California's organic revenue.*

What does it all mean?

To consumers: To consumers, if a food is labeled "organic," it was produced by a farmer using methods that aim for a balance with nature, and that have a low impact on the environment. Consumers can expect that "organic" food is of high quality and that its production has not involved the use of persistent pesticides. Consumers can expect that the food has been processed only minimally, and that it has not been enhanced by artificial ingredients. In the United States, organic food is sold at nearly 20,000 natural food stores, at farmers' markets, and at more than 73 percent of grocery stores. In 2002, sales of organic food and drink totaled more than $11 billion, and the market is expected to grow rapidly owing to new standards in certification.

To producers of grain, fruit and fiber: Organic crop farmers must avoid using toxic and persistent chemical fertilizers and pesticides on crops. They are urged to rotate crops (grow crops in different fields rather than the same field year after year) to preserve soil fertility, and to plant cover crops, such as clover, to add nutrients to the soil and prevent weeds. Organic farmers also release beneficial insects to prey on pests, helping to eliminate the need for chemical insecticides, and they add manure and plant wastes to the soil. The areas of the United States with the most organic cropland are North Dakota, Minnesota, Wisconsin, Iowa, California, Montana, and Colorado. United States-certified organic cropland increased by one million acres from 1997 to 2001.

To producers of livestock: To these farmers, regulations governing what constitutes "organic" require that eggs, poultry, and meat must be produced using organic animal feed and without using persistent pesticides, growth hormones, antibiotics, or parasiticides. Animals must have access to fresh air and sunlight. Montana and Texas are the states with the most organic pastureland.

Background

Prior to the introduction of synthetic pesticides in the 1940s almost all food was what we now describe as "organic." The first organic food company, Walnut Acres, appeared in 1946. When many farmers began turning to pesticides and other artificial methods of growing crops and raising livestock, the early supporters of organic farming looked instead to nature for methods of pest control.

In the next half century, different standards of organic agriculture developed around the country, and in the 1980s organic farmers began to demand a uniform standard nationwide. The Organic Food Production Act was introduced in 1990, but many farmers rejected its provisions because they said these did not go far enough to stop the production of genetically altered (GA) food or irradiation of food.

The U.S. Department of Agriculture (USDA) then set up the National Organic Program to revise these standards, and a uniform national standard eventually came into use, in June 2002. Under the new laws food can carry the label "100 percent organic," or "organic," which means that up to 95 percent of the ingredients must be organic; or "made with organic ingredients," which means that 70 percent of the ingredients must be organic. USDA certification is granted after a farm is inspected by an accredited USDA official.

In addition to specifications for producers outlined above, the laws include the following requirements: retail outlets are excluded from most of the act's requirements, as are food producers, when gross income from organic sales is less than $5,000 a year; immediate notification of a drift of a prohibited substance from one property to another; banning of pesticides on land designed for organic use for three years prior to planting; intervals to be established between application of raw manure to crops and harvesting them.

In 1999, the USDA lifted restrictions on organic meat labeling, and by 2001 many areas of the country had certified organic livestock. The United States Department of Agriculture certification is voluntary, but fraudulent labeling is punished with fines.

Obstacles to organic farming

Despite the growth in the organic food industry, however, still only 0.3 percent of all U.S. cropland, and 0.2 percent of all pastureland, is organic. In recent years, demand for organic food has steadily increased as a result of publicity surrounding its health benefits and the potential risks of eating genetically engineered food and eating produce that has been heavily treated with pesticides.

Although sales of organic beans, tomatoes, carrots, and other foodstuffs have been increasing rapidly, some U.S. farmers are still hesitant about switching to organic production. Analysts point to several reasons for this. Some growers fear that organic methods of farming involve higher costs and that organic farming is more labor-intensive. Many of the organic farms that are up and running tend to be small and locally run; this fact has implications for output and distribution. Some growers say they are put off switching to organic methods because their crops will be harmed in any case by lax laws governing genetically altered food. Nevertheless, it is estimated that organic products will account for 4 to 5 percent of all food output in the next few years, as bigger food manufacturers try to claim their place in the market.

Why choose organic food?

Groups and organizations that back organic farmers and their produce, such as the Organic Trade Association (OTA), say that organic food not only tastes better but has many other advantages. These include nutritional benefits: the OTA cites studies showing that organically grown fruit, vegetables, and grain are richer in many nutrients—including vitamin C, iron, and magnesium—than produce grown using synthetic pesticides and fertilizers (see Nutrition). In particular, the OTA says, it is important to provide children with organic food to reduce their exposure to harmful and toxic substances found in air, water, and soil.

Although there appears to be no conclusive evidence that organic food is nutritionally richer, it is clear that regular, high-level exposure to pesticides can have harmful consequences for health. Consumer health groups claim that most Americans eat a diet rich in persistent organic polluters (POPs), including dieldrin and dichlorodiphenyldichloroethylene. They cite studies showing that exposure to POPs has been linked to various cancers, nervous system disorders, reproductive damage, and disruption of hormonal systems (see Hormones).

Organic agriculture is considered to benefit the soil by helping to prevent the erosion of topsoil. Organic agriculture also safeguards the environment by promoting biodiversity and by protecting habitats. It reduces overall exposure to toxic chemicals from synthetic pesticides that can end up in the ground, air, water, and food supply. The only pesticides allowed in organic agriculture must be approved, and their use is restricted.

Many consider organic agriculture the only possible future model of farming that can guarantee the health and balance of the planet.

Arguments against organic food

Genetic alteration of food is a new science and the subject of much debate. It involves transferring genes from one plant to another, and thus modifying the DNA (deoxyribonucleic acid) of a plant. Many scientists and others who support GA food say that scientific manipulation of food offers the only solution to world hunger, and problems of pest control, weeds, and diseases. They say that organic food is too expensive to produce in large enough quantities to solve such problems, and criticize negative publicity surrounding GA food.

To some extent, the debate has been characterized as a battle between new, modern, efficient biotechnology and traditional, older methods of farming. However, new legislation introduced under the Farm Bill of 2002 should make it easier for organic farmers to increase productivity and efficiency by offering conservation support to organic farms, establishing organic research programs, and making provisions to share the cost of organic certification. In the future, organic farmers may benefit from financial incentives. In Germany, for example, the government pays farmers to switch to organic methods because this has proved more cost-effective than cleaning up chemicals in water supplies.

See also: **Environmental hazards; Genetically altered food; Irradiation; Pollution**

Organ removal

There are few better examples of the adaptability and strength of the human body than its capacity to survive, in good working order, after an organ has been removed.

It is common knowledge, even common sense, that a human body can survive with only one eye. What is less obvious is that it can even function well without one of its two lungs, kidneys, testicles, or ovaries.

In addition to this, the stomach, which is not duplicated, can be removed entirely, and provided that appropriate surgery is performed, the patient will be capable of normal digestion in the intestine. Likewise, the larynx (the voice box) can be removed, and the patient can learn to talk by burping air up through the esophagus. Some organs, especially the liver, do not have a twin but instead consist of several smaller units, one of which can be removed completely without endangering the whole. In the case of the liver, this is possible because of the liver's powers of regeneration (see Liver and Liver Diseases).

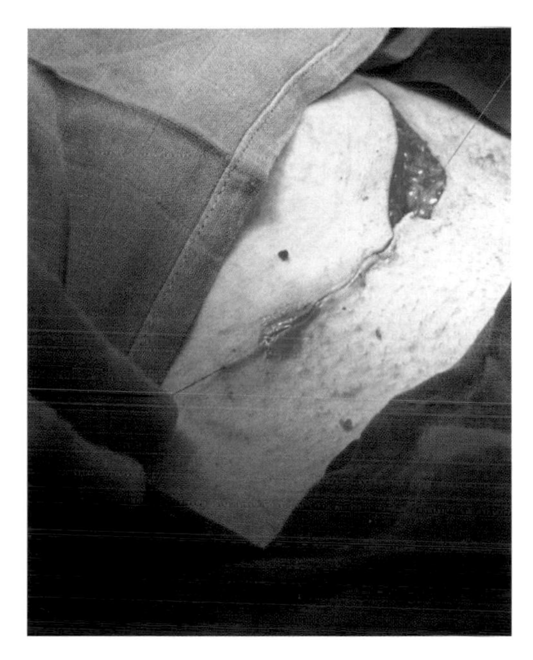

▲ *Surgeons stitch the incision after surgery for a hysterectomy.*

Why remove an organ?

One of the reasons for removing an organ is that it has become so diseased as to be a danger to the rest of the body. For example, a breast in which a cancerous tumor has developed must be removed, wholly or partially, as early as possible before the cancer spreads (see Tumors).

Accidents, particularly automobile accidents, account for a significant number of organ removals. A ruptured spleen or kidney that causes internal bleeding is the typical result of being thrown violently against the steering wheel (see Spleen).

What can and cannot be removed

People can survive the removal of any organ that is one of a pair, provided that the remaining organ is in good condition. They can also manage without an appendix, tonsils, adenoids, gallbladder, or spleen (see Appendicitis). These are not paired organs, but their function does not need to be maintained, because tens of thousands of years of changing living and eating habits have made them partially or wholly unnecessary to the survival of the individual. In the same way, the uterus is essential for reproduction but not for the individual's survival (see Uterus).

The decision to remove an organ

In spite of the body's ability to adapt, the decision to remove an organ is never taken lightly. One of the major considerations in deciding to carry out surgery will be whether to perform a partial or full removal. Whenever it is possible, the surgeon will opt for removal of only the unhealthy part, and will go to great lengths to preserve even the smallest area of healthy tissue.

The thyroid is an example of an organ that is seldom removed completely. It controls growth and metabolism, and for various reasons it can become overactive, with resulting ill effects on, for example, the heart. The surgeon's aim is to remove enough of the thyroid to put its hormone production back in balance (see Thyroid). The same applies to the ovaries: the surgeon tries to leave behind enough healthy tissue for them to continue to secrete hormones.

Questions and Answers

If one of my lungs is removed, will the space that it leaves make my chest collapse?

No. Your remaining lung will soon spread out to fill some of the cavity and increase in size, so that its air spaces will grow too. In turn, more oxygen will come into contact with the blood pumping through the lungs.

I have been told that after having one of my breasts removed I could have a silicone implant, but are these implants safe?

In addition to saline-filled breast implants, silicone implants have been used. However, concerns about possible health risks when silicone is used have led to many lawsuits, and the bankruptcy of one manufacturer. No scientific study has yet demonstrated a clear health risk, but silicone implants are no longer used, partly because of ongoing concern about possible health risks, but also because of the legal liabilities that are involved.

I am having one ovary removed. Will I still be able to get pregnant?

Probably, yes. Normally, each of the two ovaries releases an egg on alternate months. Therefore, after one ovary has been removed, it may take a little longer to become pregnant. Some women ovulate more from one ovary than from the other, in which case the chance of conception depends on which ovary is removed.

My husband had his prostate gland removed. Will it affect our sex life?

The prostate does not secrete sex hormones, so the gland's absence should not affect your husband's performance. However, depending on the type of operation used to remove the prostate, damage to the nerves can lead to impotence.

ORGANS THAT MAY BE REMOVED

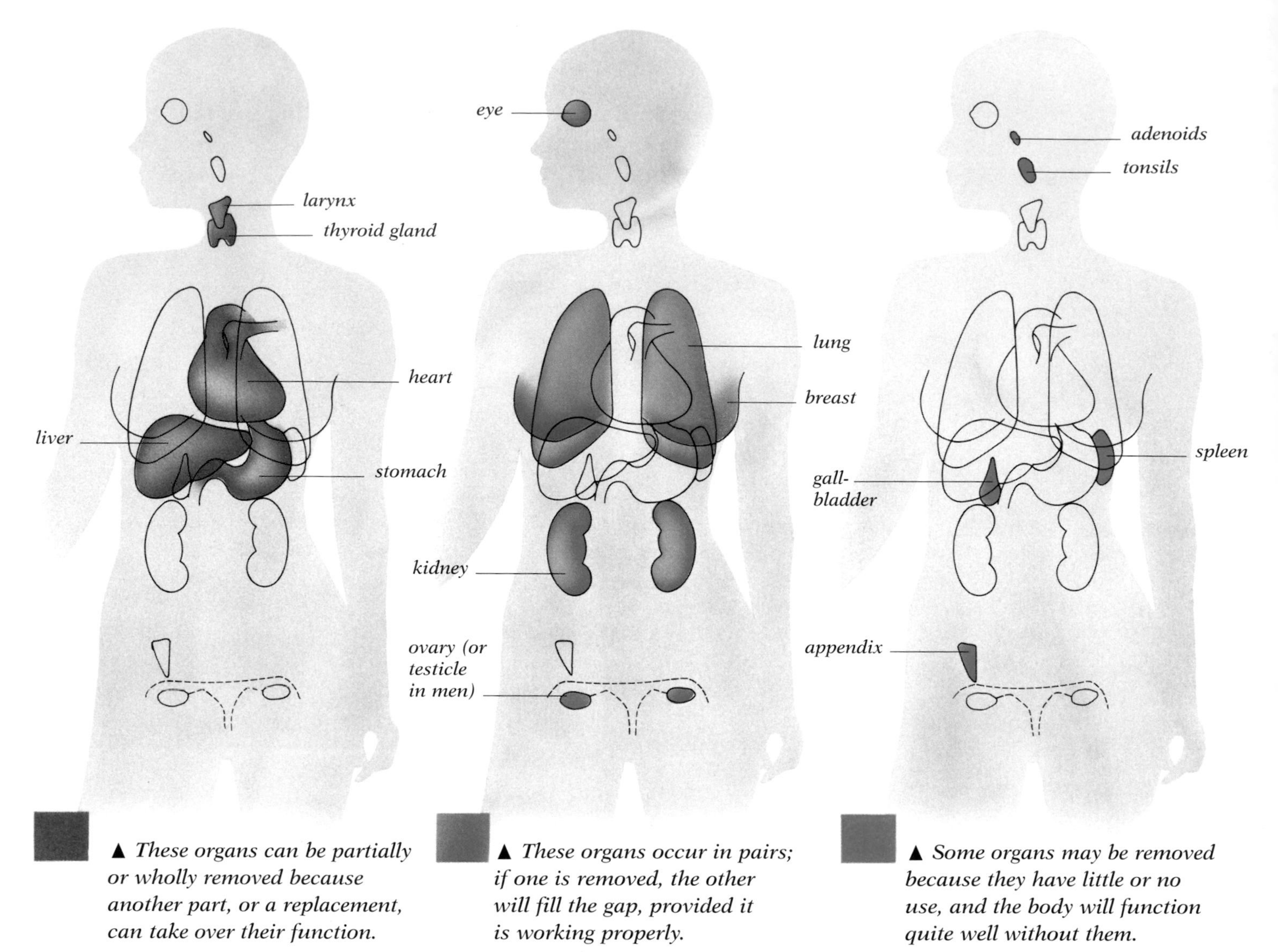

▲ *These organs can be partially or wholly removed because another part, or a replacement, can take over their function.*

▲ *These organs occur in pairs; if one is removed, the other will fill the gap, provided it is working properly.*

▲ *Some organs may be removed because they have little or no use, and the body will function quite well without them.*

Another consideration is how much additional surgery will be required. Considerable functional difficulties occur in removing some organs, aside from the obvious necessity of joining or tying up blood vessels. If the stomach is removed, for example, it becomes necessary to join the esophagus (down which food travels toward the stomach) to the intestine.

The heart and liver present more serious problems. A diseased heart can be removed and replaced with a donor heart, but the candidate for such a transplant needs to be psychologically and physically capable of undertaking the strict regimen of medication that follows (see Transplants). This can be difficult for someone who has been living for some time with serious heart disease.

Obviously, a surgeon wants to avoid an organ transplant if possible. It can be very successful, but the risk of rejection is unavoidable. In the case of a diseased liver, a transplant is sometimes possible, but the crucial question is how much of the organ has been affected, for example by malignant (spreading) cancer.

After surgery

Most of the problems associated with organ removal disappear as the body adapts to the loss. People who have a lung removed are breathless at first, but later recover some of their breathing capacity. Minor adjustments to the diet are necessary after removal of the stomach. Some discomfort under the arm is felt after removal of a breast, but it usually disappears with appropriate exercise.

If a hormone-secreting organ, such as a second ovary or the thyroid, is removed completely, it will be necessary to find an alternative way of controlling the hormone level. Usually, the patient must take hormones orally for the rest of his or her life (see Hormones).

However, the biggest problem is often psychological. Doctors should explain to their patients that one of the body's qualities is its ability to survive a loss and regenerate. In some cases the experience of organ removal can have positive advantages. After the removal of the uterus, for example, a woman's sex life can actually improve because she is no longer bothered by the pain and bleeding that accompany uterine disorders or by the risk of pregnancy.

See also: **Adenoids; Breasts; Gallbladder and stones; Hysterectomy; Kidneys and kidney diseases; Larynx and laryngitis; Ovaries; Stomach; Surgery; Testes; Tonsils**

Orgasm

Questions and Answers

My friend says that she often has multiple orgasms. Can this be true, and can any woman have them?

It may well be true, but not everyone has this experience, nor is it common. Each woman has a different threshold of sexual response, and this can vary during a lifetime. Some women may have a very intense orgasm; others may have a series of orgasms of varying intensity. If you are satisfied with the orgasms that you have, relax and enjoy them.

I am having prostate surgery. Will this affect my ability to have orgasms?

No. If the surgery and subsequent recovery are without problems, you should experience no difficulties. However, since there is a high incidence of impotence following certain types of prostate surgery, you may wish to discuss this issue with your doctor.

Is it true that a woman can have vaginal and clitoral orgasms?

No. All female orgasms depend on clitoral stimulation. This is achieved either indirectly or directly. Sexual intercourse provides indirect stimulation of the clitoris, since the movement of the penis inside the vagina results in friction on the vaginal lips, which are connected to the clitoral hood. Direct stimulation of the clitoris takes place when the clitoris is stimulated manually or during oral sex. Some women reach a climax easily from indirect stimulation; others need direct stimulation.

I think my wife fakes orgasm, but she denies it. What should I do?

Tell her your doubts make you feel insecure. More trust and less pressure will help you both relax.

Orgasm, the climax of sexual arousal, has been called the most exquisite of all physical sensations. What happens to the body during an orgasm, and how strongly does the mind govern human sexual response?

An orgasm is simply a reflex response to sexual stimulation. But even though physical stimulation is essential, the mind also plays a vital role. A lack of sexual attraction or emotional involvement, worries about sex, or tension in other areas of life can all affect the ability to reach orgasm (see Stress). Frank, open discussion can help partners to overcome any difficulties (see Intercourse).

Male orgasmic problems

Most men find that reaching orgasm is relatively easy. However, problems can stem from the inability to maintain the plateau phase, the second stage in the orgasmic cycle when the penis is erect (see Erection and Ejaculation). This can result in either premature ejaculation (a climax takes place very quickly after arousal has begun) or the loss of erection. In rare cases there is a physical reason for this. Other factors, such as the effect of drugs that treat depression or high blood pressure, or overindulgence in alcohol, can all make arousal or orgasm difficult. Medications to treat diabetes can cause impotence. A man experiencing problems should consult his doctor to rule out physical causes.

The most common reason for difficulty with orgasm is psychological. A man may find it easy to maintain an erection and have a satisfying climax by masturbating, but fail to do so when he is with a partner. Some men worry about their performance and fear failure; others find that lovemaking makes them feel so nervous and overexcited that they reach a climax before sexual intercourse begins. Both these problems can begin after an unsatisfactory experience, which leads to anxiety from then on.

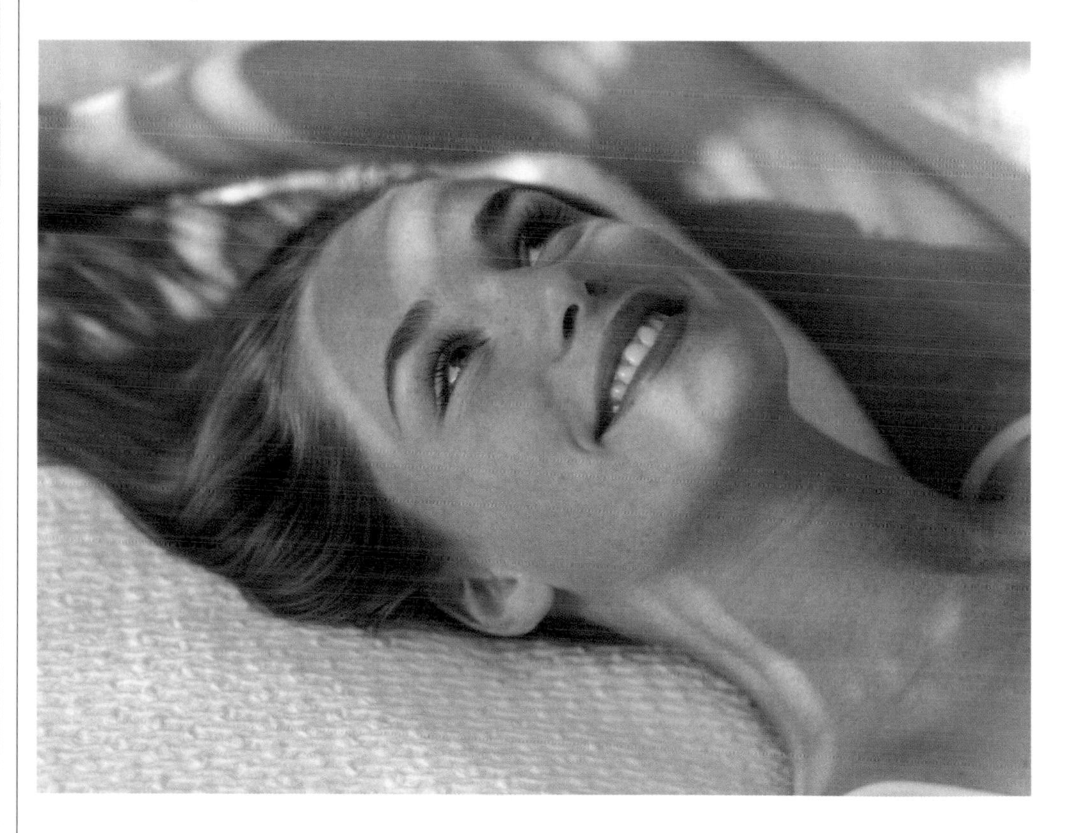

▲ *Mutual understanding and good communication between partners in a loving relationship can help them achieve sexual satisfaction.*

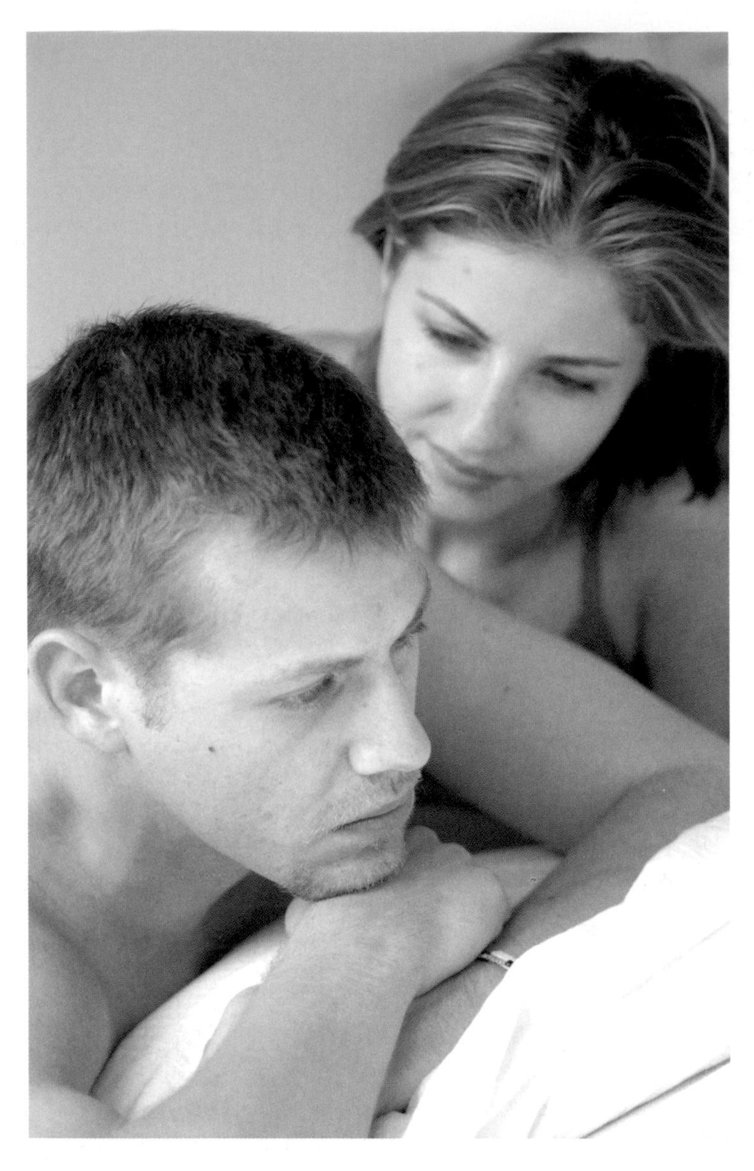

▲ *Many men have temporary problems with impotence. If the problem is persistent, there may be a psychological or physical reason, or a combination of both factors.*

Female orgasm

A female orgasm starts as a buildup of sensation around the genitals. Before orgasm there is a feeling of tension, when the pelvic muscles surrounding the vagina and uterus contract. The orgasm is felt as a series of rhythmic muscular contractions, first around the outer third of the vagina, then spreading upward to the uterus.

Male orgasm

During the male orgasm, the contraction of all the seminal ducts and vesicles forces the semen into the urethra. The muscles around the urethra give rapid involuntary contractions, which force the semen out of the penis at high pressure. Three or four major bursts of semen are followed by weaker, more irregular contractions.

Discussion with a partner is helpful so that the man does not feel under so much pressure to perform. Sex therapy can be very successful also, as it may give the man an opportunity to learn more about his sexuality and help him to feel more relaxed about his performance (see Sex).

Female orgasmic problems

Women often find it more difficult to have orgasms. Some women may have physical problems, such as an unusually overdeveloped hymen, inflammation of the vagina or bladder, or a shrinkage of the vaginal lining after menopause, all of which can produce pain during intercourse (dyspareunia). Sometimes the sex drive (see Libido) can be adversely affected by drugs the woman is taking, including the contraceptive pill. Women who are experiencing such difficulties should consult their doctor.

Many women are able to have orgasms through masturbation when they are alone, but find it impossible to reach a climax when they are with their partners. This may simply be a question of technique; the woman may need direct clitoral stimulation, but her partner may be willing to have only intercourse and nothing else.

Other women find it difficult to express their needs, so their partners are unaware that different techniques are required. An unvarying pattern of cursory foreplay followed by intercourse can also cause difficulties, since what a man may consider to be merely the preliminaries to real sex, that is, intercourse, may be what the woman finds most pleasurable and stimulating. She may be just about to reach climax, but because direct clitoral stimulation ceases, she is unable to do so. To overcome this problem, either the woman or her partner should continue to stimulate the clitoris manually during intercourse.

Some women have never had an orgasm, either alone or with a partner. The reasons for this are various and include simple lack of knowledge and a fear of asking for their partner's help to satisfy them. Therapists advise women who have never had an orgasm to explore their bodies and find out about their sexual response through masturbation, either manually or by using a vibrator (see Masturbation). Once they begin to have orgasms, they can communicate their desires and appropriate techniques to their partners. Almost every couple can achieve a satisfactory sex life once they are more relaxed, whether through therapy or just by discussing the subject.

Available help

Failure to achieve orgasm can usually be treated successfully. Because a sexual problem of one partner may be caused by the reaction or behavior of the other partner, sex therapists and doctors usually prefer to see both partners together, in an effort to ensure that each partner understands the other. Sex therapists may recommend exercises to be carried out at home by both partners. If the problem goes deeper—for example, back to childhood—some form of psychotherapy may be required. If the problem is due to drug treatment, alternative medication can be prescribed.

See also: **Psychotherapy**

Orthodontics

Uneven or protruding teeth can usually be corrected by orthodontic treatment, preventing various dental health problems and avoiding lifelong embarrassment. Treatment is most effective in children and adolescents.

Orthodontics is the branch of dentistry that is concerned with correcting the position of irregular or misplaced teeth, correcting faults in the way the upper and lower teeth come together, or adjusting the bite (see Teeth and Teething). By using orthodontic appliances such as braces and expanders, an orthodontist can gradually move the teeth into their correct position and even influence the way in which a child's jaws develop. If the teeth are too crowded, the orthodontist may also extract some of them to provide space for the others to grow normally.

The ideal position of teeth

Ideally, the upper and lower rows of teeth—the dental arches—should be symmetrical, with the teeth in even positions. There should be no overlapping (crowding) of the teeth, no spaces between them, and no tilting. The upper arch should be slightly larger than the lower one, so that when the teeth bite, the upper row fits just outside the lower one. However, this perfect arrangement is rarely found; just as people vary in their height and in other physical characteristics, so the position of their teeth and the structure of their jaws vary.

Slight variations from the ideal pattern do not affect the health of the teeth or a person's appearance. In fact, many people consider a minor degree of tooth irregularity attractive. Orthodontic treatment is necessary only when the teeth are so uneven that they spoil a person's appearance or cause dental problems, or when they do not bite together properly—a condition known as malocclusion. For instance, teeth that overlap are more difficult to clean, and this problem may result in gum disease and tooth decay (see Gums and Gum Diseases). Grossly irregular or spaced teeth may cause problems with speech, although this is unusual. In people with an incorrect bite—when misplaced teeth cause the person to bite to one side, when the teeth fail to meet properly (an open bite), or when the lower teeth bite outside the upper teeth

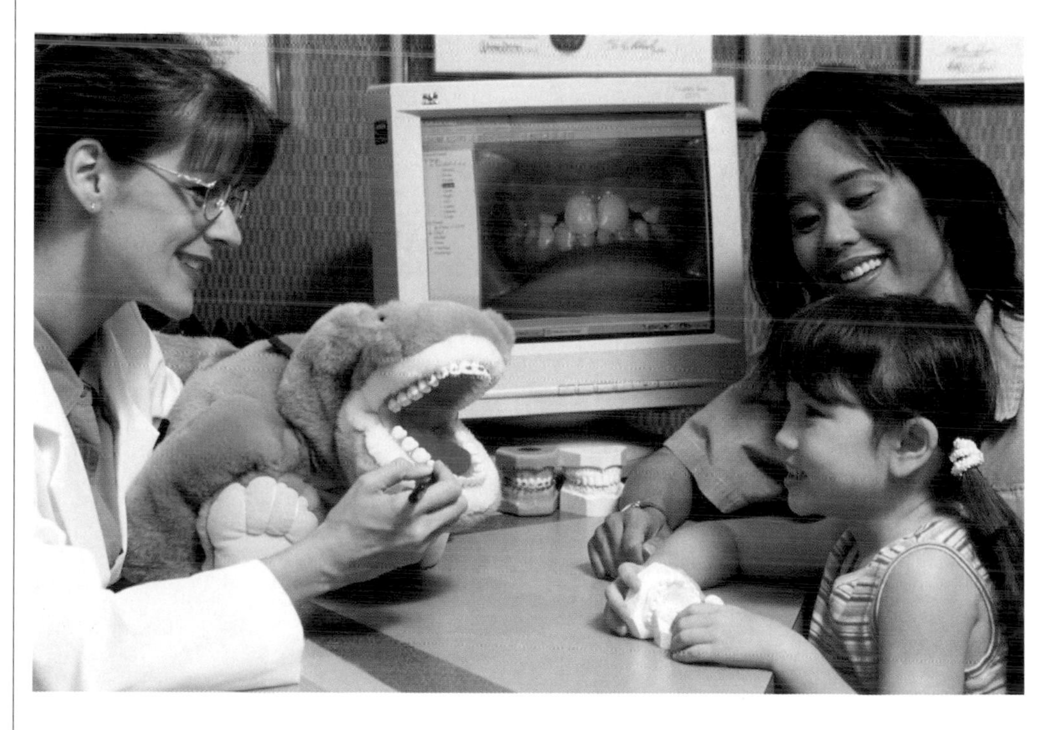

▲ *Children are often nervous about visiting the dentist, so if orthodontic treatment is required, using visual aids to explain the nature of the treatment can help put them at ease.*

Questions and Answers

I am 28 years old and I have overlapping front teeth. Am I too old to have them fixed?

No. Orthodontic treatment can still be carried out on adults, although it tends to take longer than when it is done in childhood. Provided you can accept the idea of wearing an appliance, it may still be possible to have your teeth corrected. However, severe discrepancies of tooth position are sometimes beyond the scope of orthodontics, even in childhood, and in these cases surgical treatment may be the only solution.

My daughter's teeth are very crooked and unsightly, but the dentist tells me that he will not consider giving her orthodontic treatment until she improves her oral hygiene. What should I do?

You should insist that your daughter cleans her teeth properly; otherwise, she will be susceptible to gum disease and tooth decay and may even lose her teeth when she is an adult. Your dentist is quite right to refuse orthodontic treatment without satisfactory oral hygiene, because wearing orthodontic appliances can make ordinary dental care more difficult and an existing oral hygiene problem even worse.

Is there any danger that wearing an orthodontic appliance will damage my teeth?

Provided that you clean your teeth and the appliance thoroughly to prevent any plaque from accumulating, the presence of bands or wires in the mouth should not cause any damage. However, if you do not clean the appliance properly, it will become a reservoir of bacterial plaque, and gum disease and tooth decay will inevitably result.

Questions and Answers

Is wearing an orthodontic appliance painful?

There may be some discomfort, depending on the appliance and the type of work being done.

What special precautions are required while a person is wearing an orthodontic appliance?

The most essential precaution is to maintain good oral hygiene. Teeth should be thoroughly cleaned with a toothbrush and dental floss, and removable appliances should be taken out at least twice a day and scrubbed using a toothbrush and toothpaste to keep them free from bacteria. Fixed appliances are more difficult and time-consuming to clean—the most effective way is to clean around them using a very small toothbrush.

If the gums begin to bleed on contact with the toothbrush, they may be inflamed, in which case even more thorough brushing is required. This may make the gum bleed at the time, but if thorough brushing is maintained, the gum will become firmer and will no longer bleed when brushed. If you continue to have problems with your gums, see your dentist.

Is it true that badly misplaced teeth can be transplanted?

It is possible to transplant buried teeth, but only if there is adequate space for them. This method of treatment is used mainly when upper canine teeth have failed to erupt; this occurs in about 2 percent of people, and the teeth concerned remain below the surface, usually in the palate. Such teeth can be removed surgically and then immediately inserted into a specially prepared socket. After the transplant it is necessary to hold the tooth in place with a splint, usually for about three weeks, while the healing process takes place.

Although most teeth that have been transplanted remain in good condition, a small number have to be removed subsequently, either because of infection or because the root has been reabsorbed.

(an underbite)—abnormal jaw movements can result in strain and damage to the jaw joints (temperomandibular joint disorder), leading to pain in the jaws, headaches, and even arthritis. If the lower incisor teeth bite against the roof of the mouth instead of against the upper teeth, this condition can also cause the palate to become inflamed (see Mouth).

Causes of irregularities

The size and position of a person's teeth, and the relative size of the jaws, are largely determined by that individual's genes—in other words, characteristics inherited from both parents affect the way in which the teeth and jaws develop (see Heredity). For example, a child who has a father with large teeth and a mother with small jaws may have very overcrowded teeth because this combination of teeth and jaws is not compatible.

In some cases, environmental factors influence how the teeth develop. For example, persistent thumb-sucking can move the incisors (the four central teeth in the upper and lower jaws) out of alignment. Teeth may also drift out of position if there is a gap after a tooth is lost because of gum disease or trauma. Nutritional deficiencies and diseases of the jaw also affect the development of the jaws and teeth, although these conditions are rare.

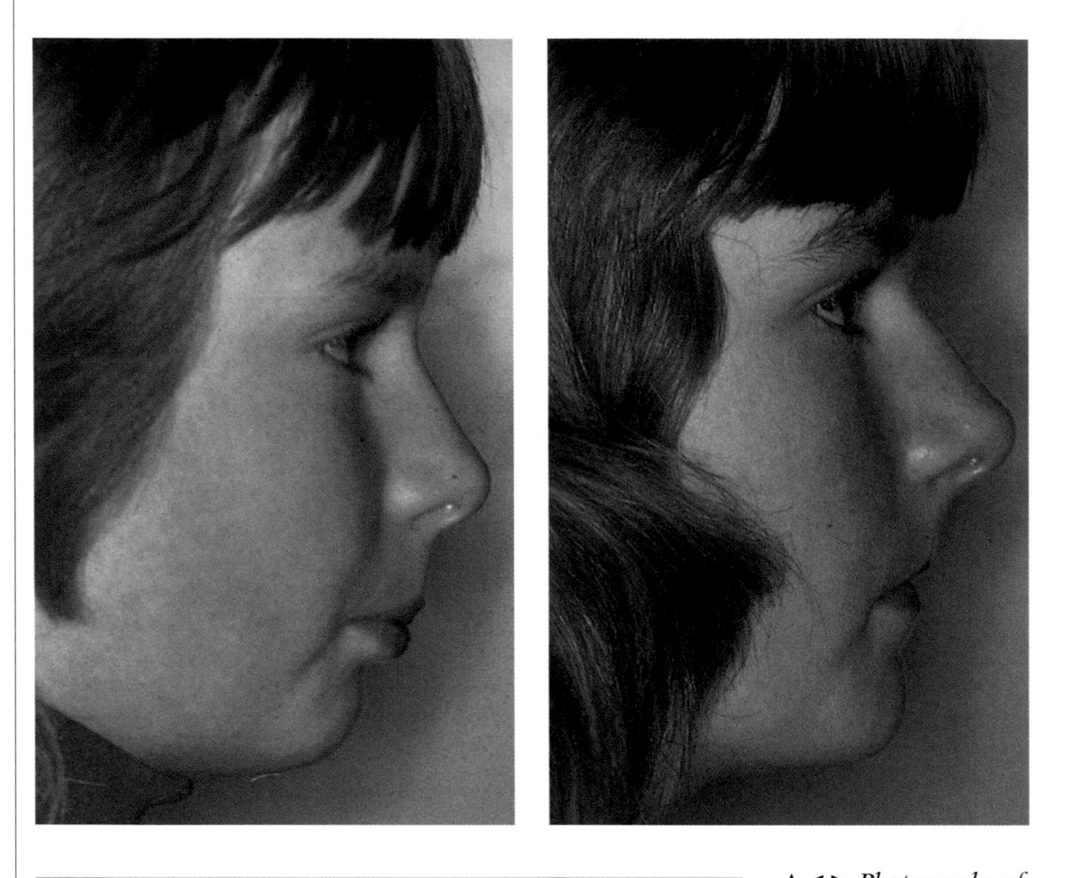

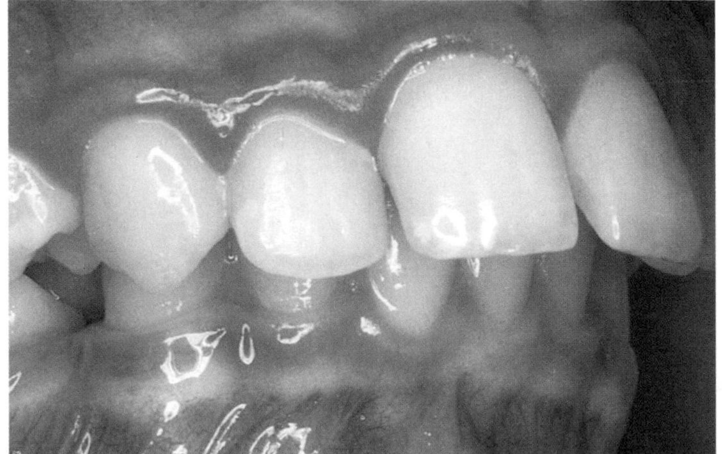

▲◄► Photographs of a girl before and after orthodontic treatment (above) show striking changes in her profile. Images of her teeth before, during, and after treatment (right and left) show how the fixed appliances she wore for three years repositioned her protruding teeth and helped bring her jaws into alignment.

NORMAL BITE OR OCCLUSION

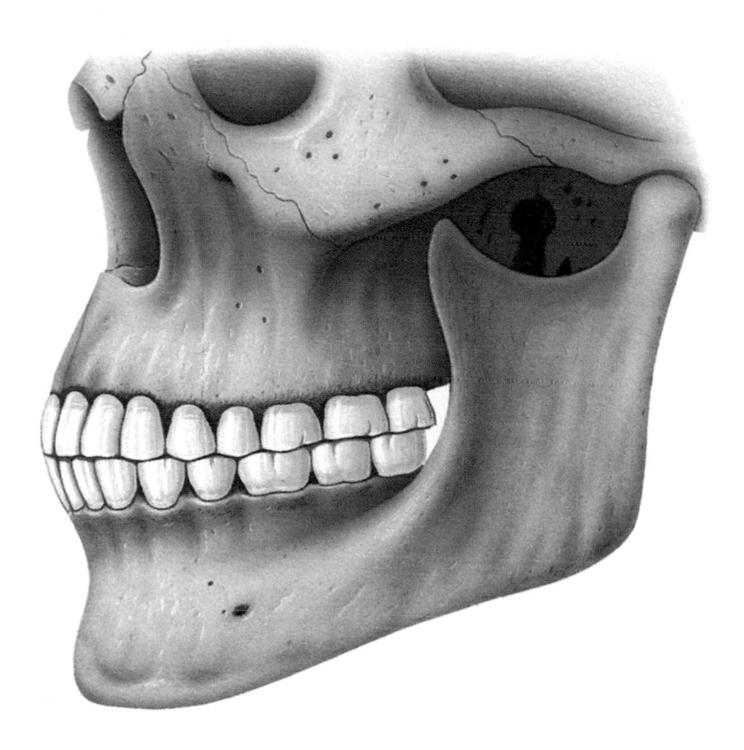

▲ *When a person has a normal occlusion, the upper and lower teeth are symmetrical and evenly spaced, with no overlapping or gaps. The upper arch is slightly larger than the lower arch so that upper teeth fit just around the lower teeth.*

INCORRECT BITE: MALOCCLUSION

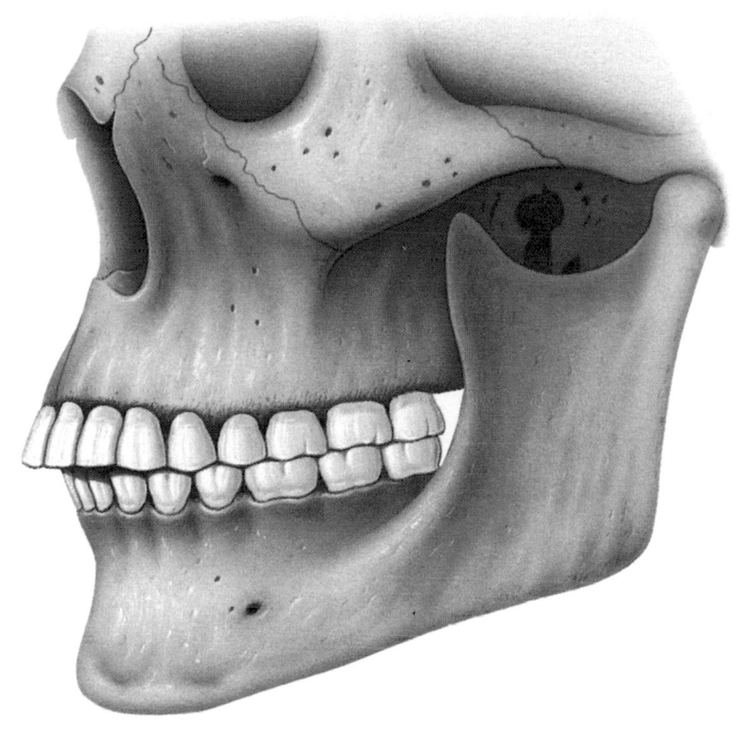

▲ *In malocclusion, the teeth bite incorrectly. There may be spacing, overcrowding, or protrusion of the teeth (as above); the upper or lower jaw may protrude so that the teeth are out of alignment; or the jaws may be unable to close properly.*

Treatment

The age at which orthodontic treatment is given depends on the nature of the problem. Treatment is most commonly started after the premolars (the teeth in front of the molars) and permanent canine teeth (those next to the incisors) come through, usually between the ages of 11 and 12. At this age, the jaws are still growing, so it is easier to move the teeth. In some cases—for example, when there is a severe discrepancy in jaw size that requires the mouth to be gradually reshaped, or when it is necessary to make room in a child's mouth for all the permanent teeth to erupt correctly—treatment may be started before all the baby teeth have fallen out. This type of treatment is known as interceptive orthodontics. Treatment can still be carried out on adults, but it may take longer to achieve the desired result, and any major problems relating to jaw size may require surgery.

First, the orthodontist must discuss the required treatment with the patient (and in the case of a child, with the parents) and obtain consent. He or she will then take impressions of the teeth from which plaster models are made. X rays are used to confirm the presence of, and locate, any teeth that have not yet erupted, and to assess the shape of the jaw (see X Rays). The orthodontist may also photograph the patient's face and teeth; this helps with the assessment and serves as a record to show what has been achieved when the treatment is complete.

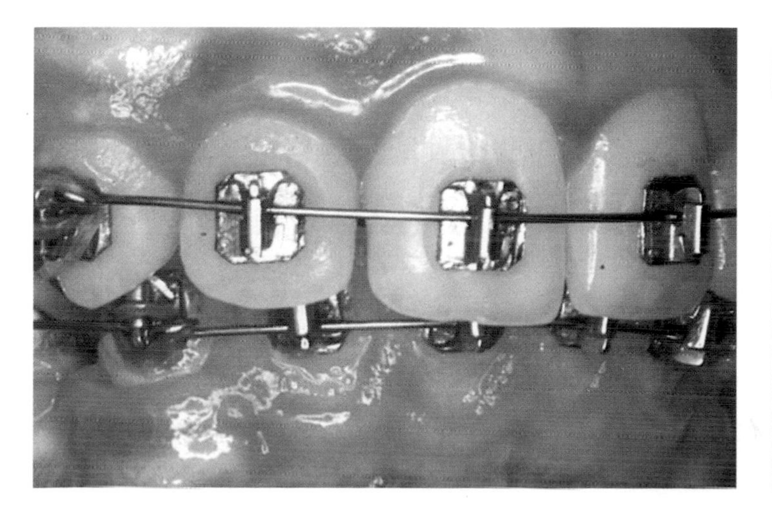

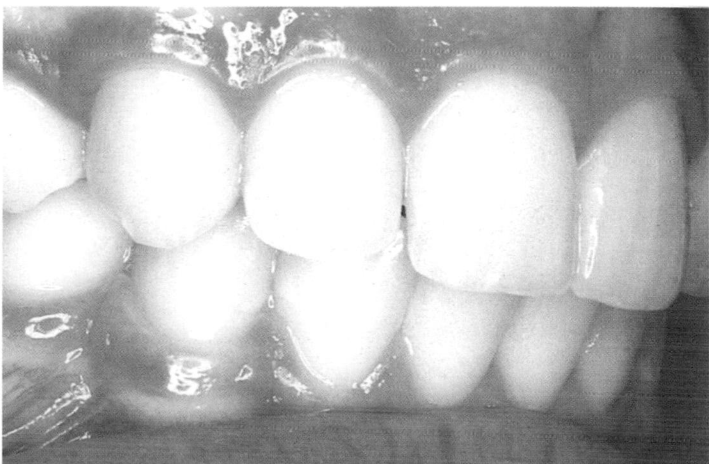

Invisible braces

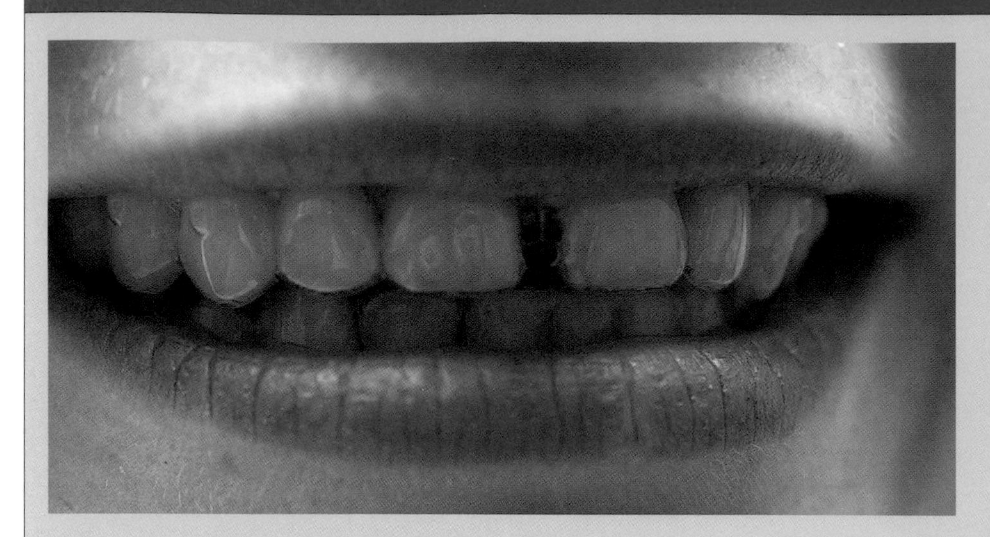

◄ *The new system of invisible braces had its debut in 2000. It provided suitable candidates with an unobtrusive alternative to metal braces.*

"Invisible braces" are one of the latest technologies to be used in orthodontics. Patients are fitted with a series of 12 to 48 clear mouthguards, or aligners, that progressively straighten the teeth over several months. The aligners are worn over the patient's teeth, and a new set is fitted approximately every six weeks.

In addition to being more sightly than metal braces, invisible braces have the advantage that they can be easily removed during eating and for brushing and flossing; thus they may reduce the risk of gum disease and tooth decay when compared with fixed appliances.

However, they are more expensive than traditional appliances, and the treatment time will be increased if they are removed too frequently.

Invisible braces are not suitable for every patient, especially if complicated treatment is required. They are most suitable for adults with slight spacing or crowding; they may also be used as retainers, or used in the later stages of complex treatment.

Orthodontic appliances

There are two main types of orthodontic appliances: functional and mechanical. Functional appliances influence the way in which the jaws develop, often relying on the movements of the muscles and jaws to supply the necessary force. Mechanical appliances move individual teeth. Both types may be either fixed (bonded to the teeth) or removable (the patient can take them out).

Functional appliances: There are numerous types of functional appliance, and they are used to improve the way the upper and lower teeth meet, or bite. Consequently, they are effective only when a child is growing rapidly (see Growth). Some functional appliances move the entire dental arch as one unit: for example, if all the upper teeth are too far forward, a functional appliance can mold the upper arch back as it grows, ensuring a better contact with the lower arch in biting. Others prevent the lips or cheek muscles from pressing on the teeth and influencing their development.

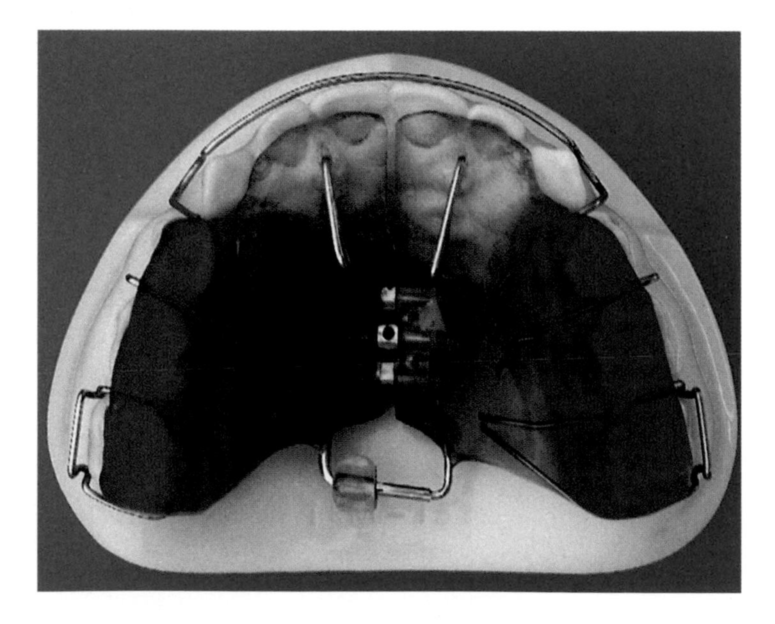

▲ *A colorful removable appliance, fitted around a model of the patient's teeth. The bright acrylic is intended to encourage the child to wear the appliance as instructed.*

In some cases when the upper arch is too narrow, an expander may be used. This type of treatment is usable only while the seam running down the center of the upper jaw has not become fused. The expander is fixed around the back teeth, and special screws are used to gradually push the two halves of the upper jaw apart.

Headgear may be fitted to functional appliances to speed up the treatment by providing extraoral traction (force applied to the teeth from a source outside the mouth). For instance, a metal face bow connected to the appliance may have straps that attach to a neck strap (pulling the upper arch backward) or to a head cap (pulling the upper arch backward and upward). Headgear may be unsightly, but it is highly effective. If the upper jaw needs to be brought forward in relation to the lower jaw, a face mask may be used.

Mechanical appliances: Appliances that move individual teeth do not necessarily need growth to be effective, but they do the job more rapidly during a phase of growing.

Removable appliances are more suitable for cases in which the teeth can simply be moved sideways or tilted back to their correct position. Fixed appliances exert a greater degree of control because they are bonded to each individual tooth and can produce movement in any direction. They tend to be used in more complex cases, particularly when teeth need to be rotated or moved a considerable distance.

Rubber bands or elastic chains may be attached in varying directions to some of the brackets, helping to pull the teeth into place by means of intraoral traction.

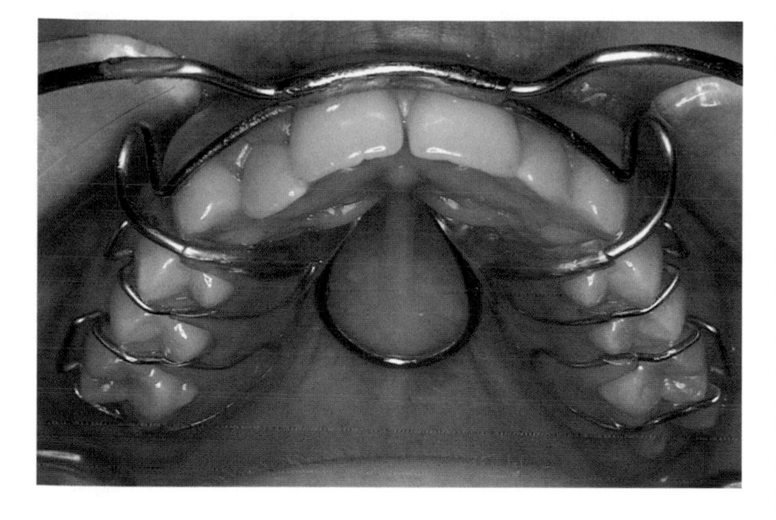

▲ *This shows the front view of a removable appliance with a face bow attached. Straps connected to the face bow and the appropriate headgear provide extraoral traction, molding jaw growth. The whole appliance is worn for 14 hours a day.*

Wearing appliances: Orthodontic appliances and any auxiliary components must be worn for the required number of hours each day if they are to move the teeth effectively. The orthodontist will usually adjust the appliance monthly, and patients may be asked to change components such as elastic bands.

After these adjustments, patients may experience some initial discomfort, but this usually disappears after a few days. Overall, the treatment will normally last between 18 months and two years, depending on the problem.

Retainers: Once the teeth have been moved into the correct position, it is often necessary for the patient to wear retainers for a while afterward. This is because it takes some time for the jawbone to completely remodel around the teeth; without the retainer, the teeth may simply drift back into their original position. Retainers are usually removable, but if there is a continuing problem with stability, the orthodontist may bond a piece of wire to the back of the teeth.

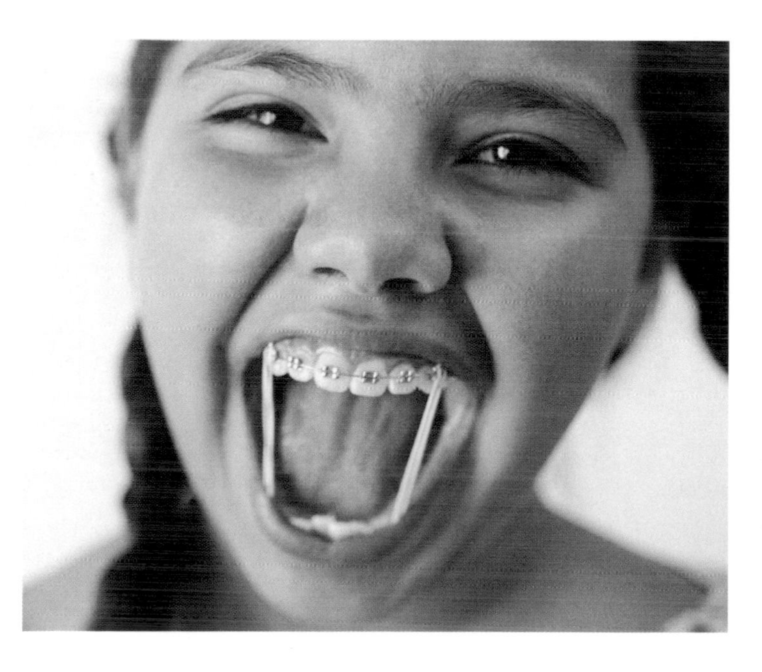

▲ *Elastic bands are used to move the teeth so that the upper and lower teeth fit together correctly. They come in varying colors.*

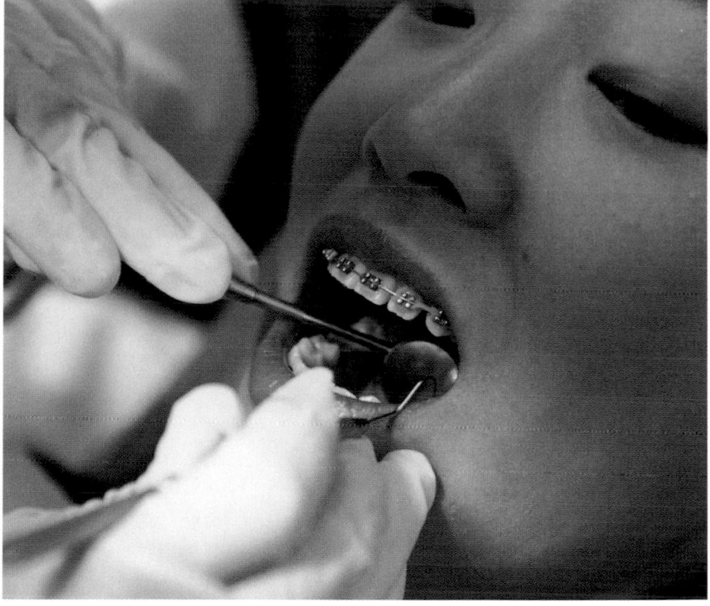

▲ *Fixed appliances need careful monitoring and adjustment by the orthodontist to achieve the desired result.*

Why extractions are necessary

Crowding usually occurs when the teeth are so large that there is not enough space in the jaw for them all to grow normally. If the degree of overcrowding is only slight, patients may be advised to accept the situation. When crowding is more severe, treatment is usually required before all the permanent teeth come through to prevent other problems from developing.

Sometimes crowded teeth can be aligned by enlarging the dental arches. Although this treatment may help in the short term, it has been shown that crowding eventually recurs in many cases. Often, the only successful long-term treatment is to extract some of the existing teeth to make space for the others to develop normally.

When all the teeth are in good condition, it is usually the first premolars that are removed. However, if certain teeth are heavily filled or badly positioned, the orthodontist may decide to extract these instead of the first premolars.

After the teeth have been extracted there is often a spontaneous improvement in the positions of the adjacent teeth, which tend to move into the spaces that have been created. However, the improvement is rarely enough to fully correct the irregularity, so it is usually necessary to fit an appliance.

Outlook

Irregular teeth and malocclusion can usually be treated successfully because the supporting bone responds to light pressure, enabling the teeth to be pushed into place and abnormal jaw growth to be corrected to a large extent. The proportions of the face may also be improved. However, the stability of the teeth may occasionally be affected, and patients with severe discrepancies in the position of their jaws may need surgical treatment.

See also: **Arthritis; Bones; Joints**

Orthopedics

Questions and Answers

My son is in a body cast after an accident. Will his skin suffer?

The skin grows even when it is covered by a plaster cast. When the plaster is finally removed, the skin will look dirty and have the appearance of sandpaper, because it has continued to grow and has shed scales. This is not a long-term problem and should improve within a few weeks.

Is it best to have a bone graft, or have a pin inserted?

It is always better to let things heal naturally whenever possible. A pin, a plate, or another piece of metal is used in the join only if the orthopedic surgeon believes the fracture will not unite firmly without it. A pin holds two bones together, while a graft adds bone pieces that are missing. A cast keeps the injury immobile during the healing process.

I am having a replacement knee joint. Will it have strength and movement like a real knee?

A mechanical replacement can't offer the range of movement of a normal knee joint. There will be some limitation of movement in the twisting and sliding action which an ordinary knee performs, but which the replacement joint cannot do. Although it is limited, the range of motion with a replacement knee will be better than that of your own knee.

After my broken leg mended, I found that it was shorter than the other. Can anything be done?

Your leg is shorter because you suffered a severe fracture and lost bone fragments. If you have any difficulty in walking, it would be a good idea to visit an occupational therapist, who might be able to fit a lift into your shoe.

Orthopedics is the surgical specialty treating diseases and injuries to bones and soft tissues. Orthopedic surgeons deal with a wide range of problems, from fixing sprains and fractures to replacing entire joints.

A broken bone that is left untreated will usually heal, or, in medical terminology "unite." The orthopedic surgeon tries to make sure that the fracture unites in a good position so that the limb will still be able to function well afterward. He or she also ensures that no complications develop (see Fractures).

Treatment of fractures

A limb fracture is usually diagnosed in the hospital emergency room. Any simple fracture can be set there, and a cast may be applied, often under anesthetic. The patient will usually see the orthopedic consultant when he or she visits the outpatient unit so that staff can inspect the cast and take X rays. An X ray will show that the bone ends fit and the splint is strong enough for everyday wear. The orthopedist will decide when the cast should be removed, and whether a new cast is required. Most simple fractures of the arm stay in a cast for four to six weeks. Leg fractures will need a cast for twice as long because the limb is weight-bearing.

A plaster cast is the most common way to treat fractures, but it has its limitations. Some areas of the body, such as the shoulder and hip, are difficult to hold in place. The use of plaster as a cover may cause problems, since the skin itself may have suffered injury and need constant attention. A cast also stops joints from moving, and they may become stiff.

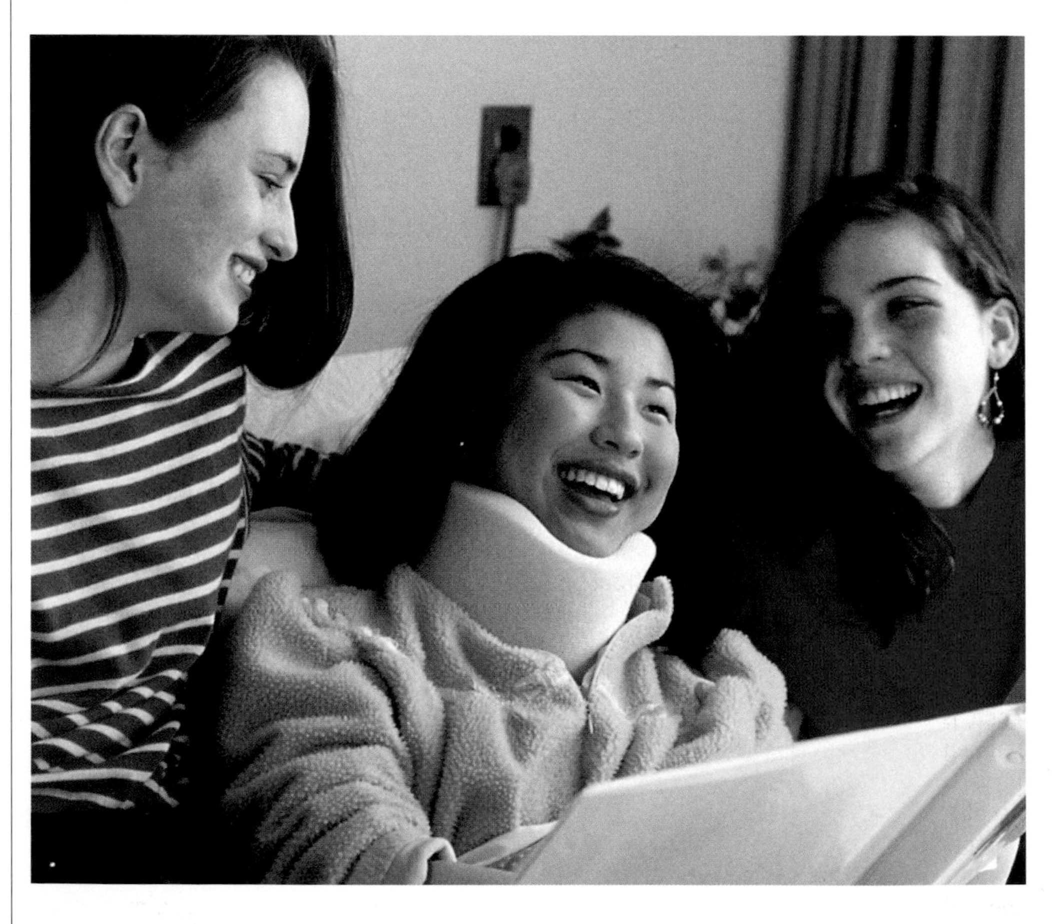

▲ *A cervical collar provides support for the back of the neck and the lower part of the head. Such support is necessary in cases of whiplash or similar types of injury.*

PIN AND PLATE

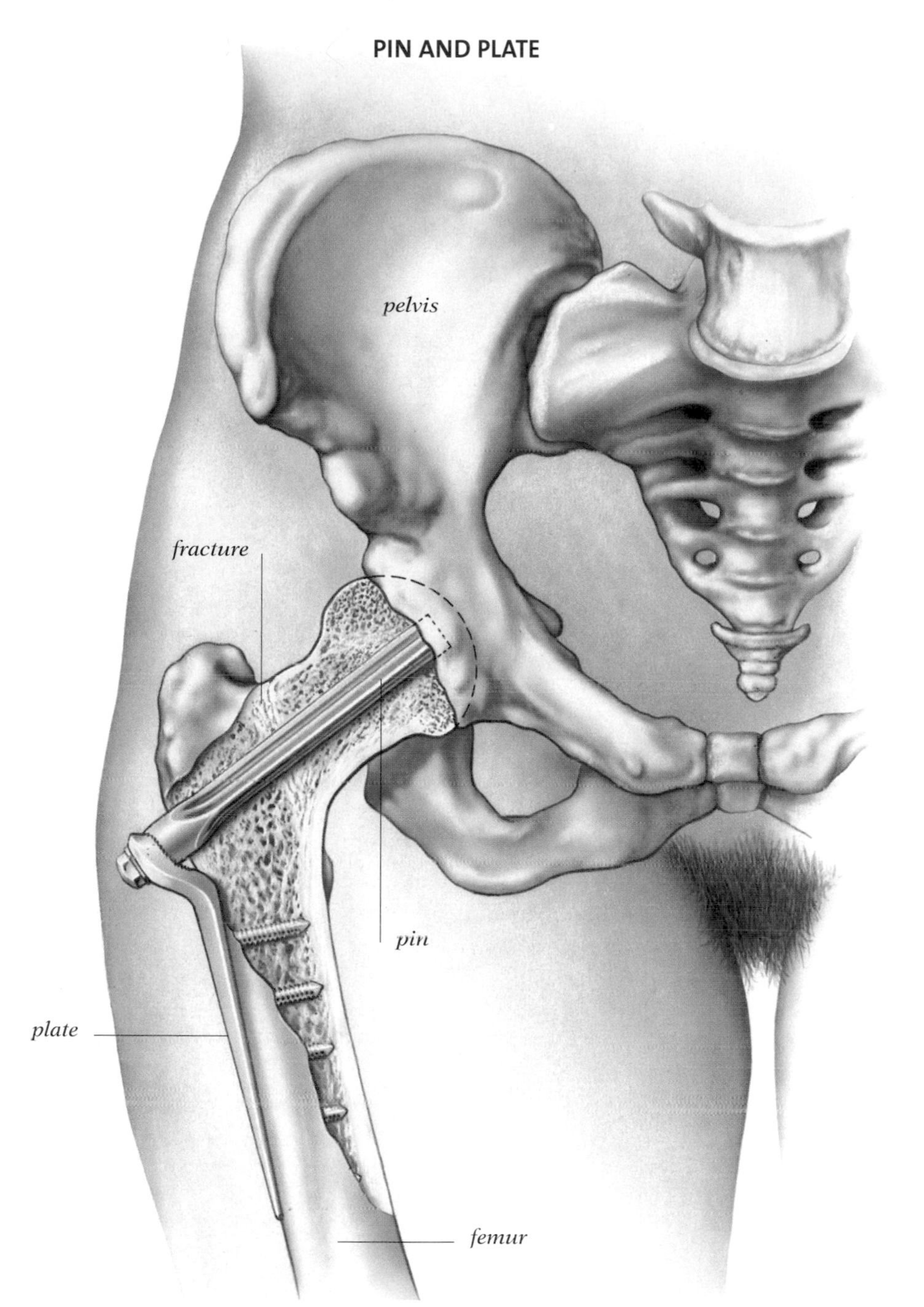

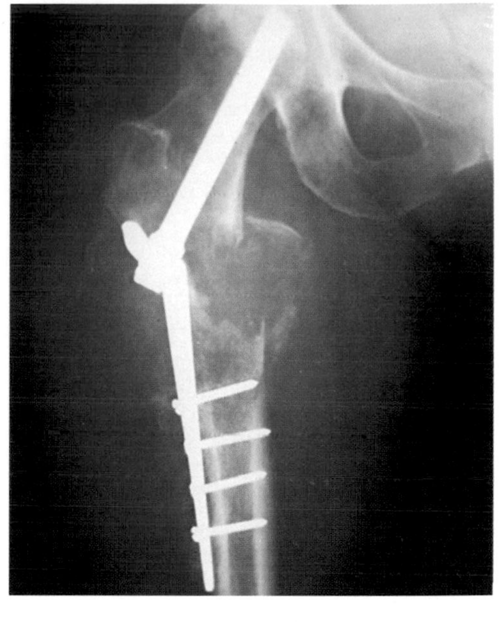

▲ *This X ray shows a femur fracture repaired by pin and plate. The use of metal causes no discomfort to the patient.*

◄ *The pin and plate operation holds a bone rigid as it heals, as in this fracture of the neck of the femur. The operation is especially suitable for older patients.*

Reduction and internal fixation

The orthopedic surgeon may decide that a fracture needs an operation. This may be necessary when the bones cannot be brought into a satisfactory position by other means, or when the fracture would confine the patient to bed for a long time. An incision is made in the skin along the length of the bone, and the surrounding muscles are then pulled back. The periosteum, a layer of tissue that coats the bone, is peeled back from the fracture. The ends of the bones are cleaned and fitted together, or reduced, then joined with a piece of metal using a technique called an internal fixation. A strip of metal is usually screwed along the length of the bone; the strip crosses the fracture site in a procedure called plating. In some cases a long nail is used to hold the bone ends in position, and this is driven up through the hollow shaft of the bone through its entire length.

For difficult or complex fractures of long bones, it is now often found best to maintain alignment and allow mobility by the use of a technique called external fixation. Two or three pins are screwed into the bone above the fracture, and two or three below the fracture. The pins are securely fixed to brackets that can be locked onto a long steel bar. The method is useful for infected fractures, those that are not united, or those in which there is also severe soft tissue injury. Careful daily cleansing of the pins where they pass through the skin is necessary to avoid pin track infection.

Pin and plate operation

When the head of the thighbone is to be fixed, a pin is driven in from the side of the femur and up the center of the broken neck. This ensures that the pin stops just short of the joint. It is held in place with a metal plate screwed to the side of the femur. Such a procedure is called a pin and plate operation.

The advantage of fixation by using pins and plates is that the patient can walk around within days of the operation and a plaster cast is usually unnecessary. Pin and plate surgery is particularly suitable for elderly people who fall and fracture their hips. The metal pin is inert and can remain in the body without causing trouble or discomfort to patients.

Traction for fractures

Traction is used almost exclusively for fractures of the leg. After such an injury the muscles tighten up and pull the bone ends past each other, so that the lower fragment rides up to lie alongside the upper fragment. Unless the bone ends are pulled apart and correctly

Questions and Answers

My young daughter has spina bifida and uses braces on her legs to help her walk. Will she ever be able to do without such prominent supports?

Spina bifida sometimes affects the nerves going to the muscles of the legs, resulting in partial paralysis. There is nothing wrong with the bone. Your daughter may wear braces because she has partially paralyzed legs. As she grows older, however, she should be able to wear less noticeable supports.

I've heard of football players who have had knee cartilage removed. Why is this?

The knee is unique among the joints of the body in that it has two triangular wedges of cartilage that lie within the joint cavity. These act as shock absorbers and take the wear and tear of twisting and running. They are attached firmly to the capsule of the joint (around the edges) and to the bone of the knee joint (at the center).

Unnatural twisting movements, such as those that occur in sports, separate these two points and can tear the cartilage. Because there is no blood supply to the cartilage, once it tears, it can never heal. It then impedes normal joint movement and thus has to be removed. This does not affect the use of the knee joint afterward, but it may lead to osteoarthritis over time.

Is it possible to transplant whole pieces of bone from one patient to another?

Yes. Transplantation of a length of bone, complete with its supplying blood vessels, is possible. The procedure is called a vascularized graft and requires microsurgery to connect a blood supply. These grafts are seldom used, however, because immunosuppression is needed to prevent rejection and there is usually an alternative solution to the problem. They are sometimes used to treat major fractures that will not heal.

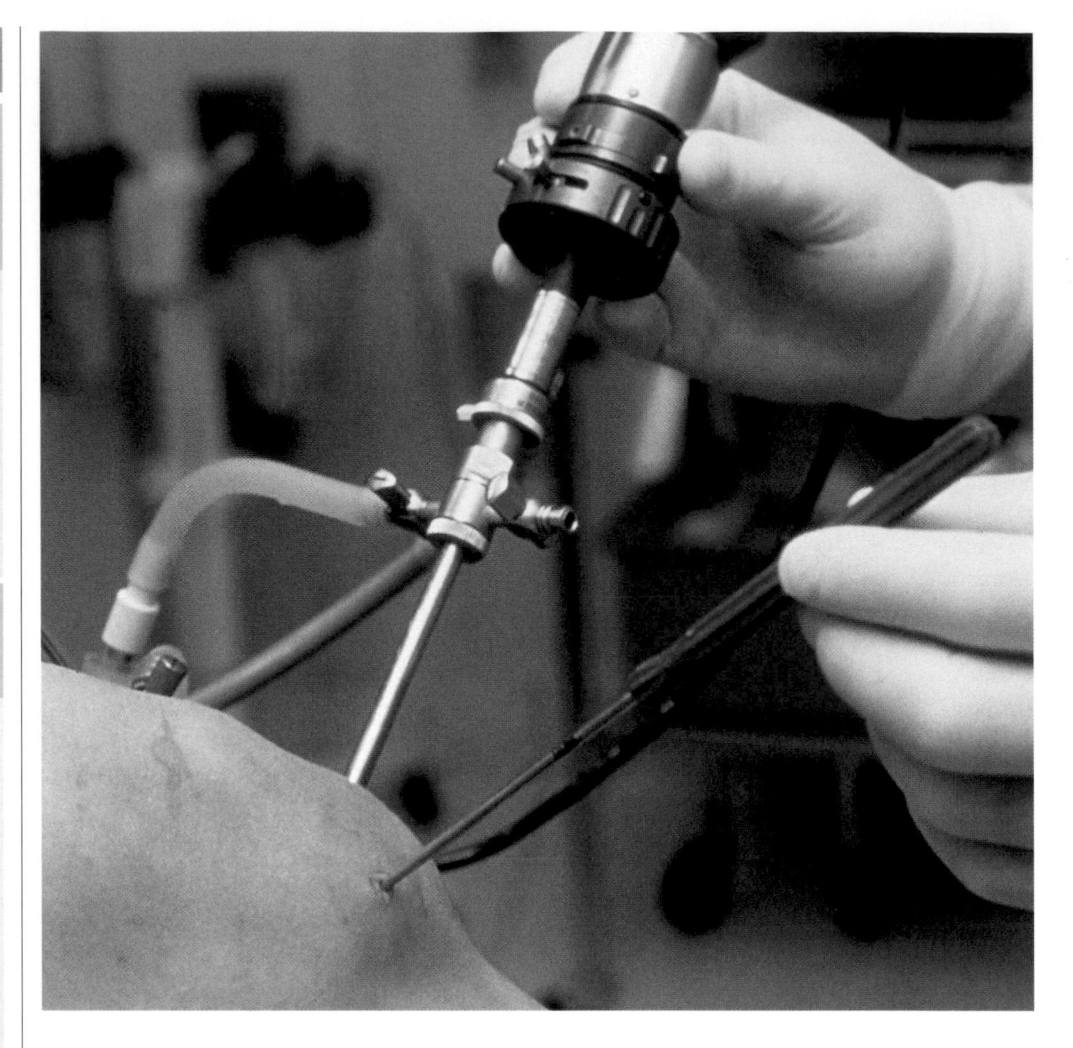

▲ *An arthroscope allows a surgeon access to remove or reshape any damaged cartilage on a patient's knee joint by remote manipulation. This type of surgery is known as minimally invasive keyhole surgery.*

aligned, this will result in union of the fracture with some shortening of the limb. Traction is applied to the lower bone fragment by means of a weight hung from a steel pin that is driven through the shinbone or heel. The weights are usually hung from an arrangement of pulleys placed at the end of the bed. A 200-pound (91-kg) man will need heavier weights than a six-year-old child. To prevent the weights from pulling the patient out of bed, the foot end is sometimes placed on blocks. The advantage of traction is that it leaves the joints free to move, and skin wounds can be monitored (see Traction).

Bone grafting

Some fractures, particularly those located in the tibia, may fail to unite. In such cases, pieces of bone can be taken from another part of the patient's own skeleton and grafted.

A favored site for the donor bone is the pelvis, which is high up on the hip. A strip of bone up to 4 inches (10 cm) long can be cut from this bone without damaging the rest of the skeleton. The fracture is first cleaned thoroughly and small pieces of bone graft are placed inside, causing the body to form strong new bone around the bone graft. After this operation is performed, a sound union of the fracture gradually takes place over the next few weeks.

Compound fractures

A compound fracture, with broken bone ends that penetrate the overlying skin, has a high risk of infection and must be treated carefully. This involves cleaning the wound thoroughly. Dead muscle and skin are cut away, removing the possibility of infection with bacteria and the development of gangrene. After the wound is cleaned, the bone ends can be brought together and the skin sewn into place. Internal fixation is usually avoided, because this makes the possibility of a serious infection more likely. If the skin wound cannot be closed with stitches, skin grafting may become necessary.

Ruptured tendon

A rupture of the Achilles tendon at the back of the heel is a common injury. The patient experiences sudden pain at the time of the injury and suffers considerable disability afterward. This may be treated by stitching the tendon together, or by putting the ankle in a cast.

Tendons can take six weeks to join together, and during this time they may come apart again or become stuck to the surrounding tissue. When tendons are involved that lead to the fingers, this condition is serious; very delicate, complicated surgery may be necessary to restore movement (see Tendons).

Repeated dislocation

Reduction of dislocation is usually simple when a patient is fully relaxed under anesthetic. However, problems can arise when a repeated dislocation occurs.

An example would be after a shoulder injury when the first dislocation has weakened the surrounding tissue. In such a case, surgical reconstruction of the joint capsule is required. Since joint injuries often result in some stiffening, it may become necessary to employ physical therapy. This can greatly improve movement and also strengthen muscles (see Sports Medicine).

Orthopedic surgeons also treat a variety of different conditions that are not actually the result of any injury. These include such serious problems as birth defects and deformities in young children, arthritic conditions, bone cancers, and disorders of the spine.

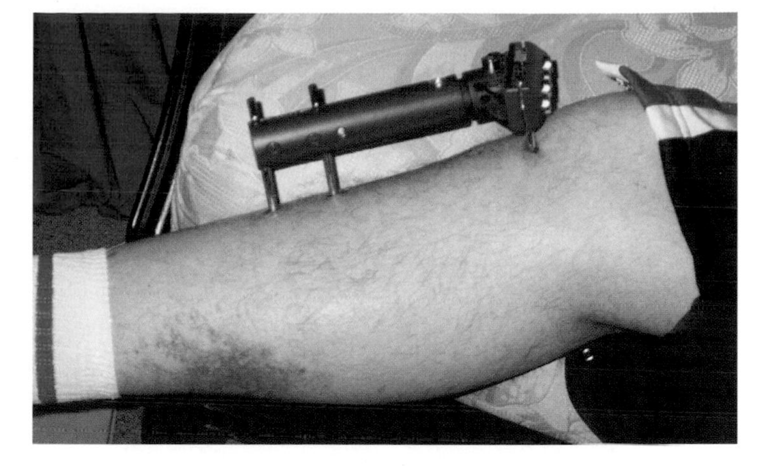

▲ *Pin and plate surgery on this broken leg allows the patient to walk without the weight of a heavy cast.*

PUTTING A LEG IN TRACTION

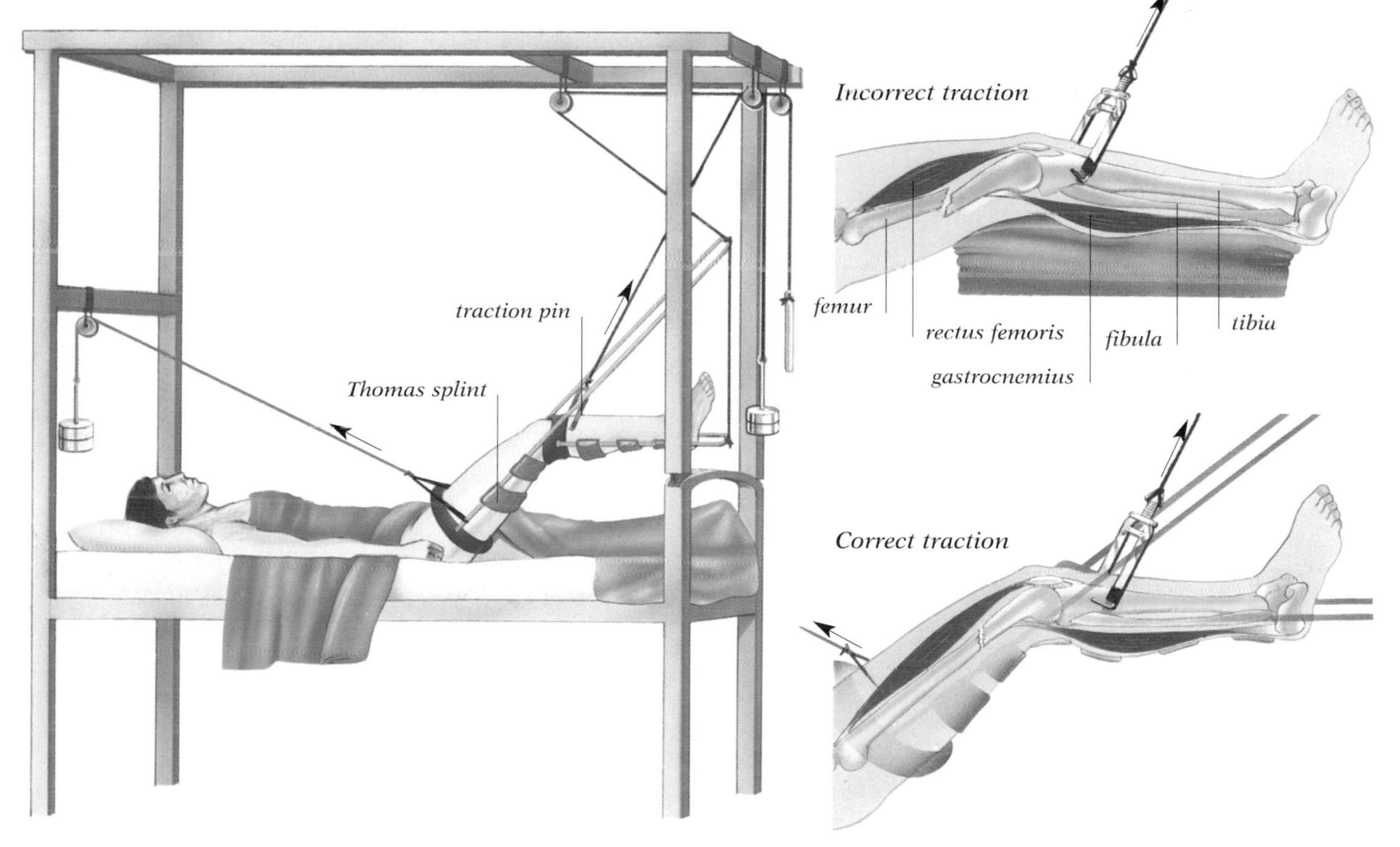

▲ *If the shaft of the femur is fractured, traction must be applied parallel to the fracture to exactly align the fractured bone ends. The calculations are complicated, because various different forces must be counterbalanced to achieve the correct alignment. One factor is the pressure exerted by the leg muscles; the leg must be held in exactly the right position so it can counteract and compensate for the pull of the muscles. The wrong position is shown in the diagram above; it has been corrected below.*

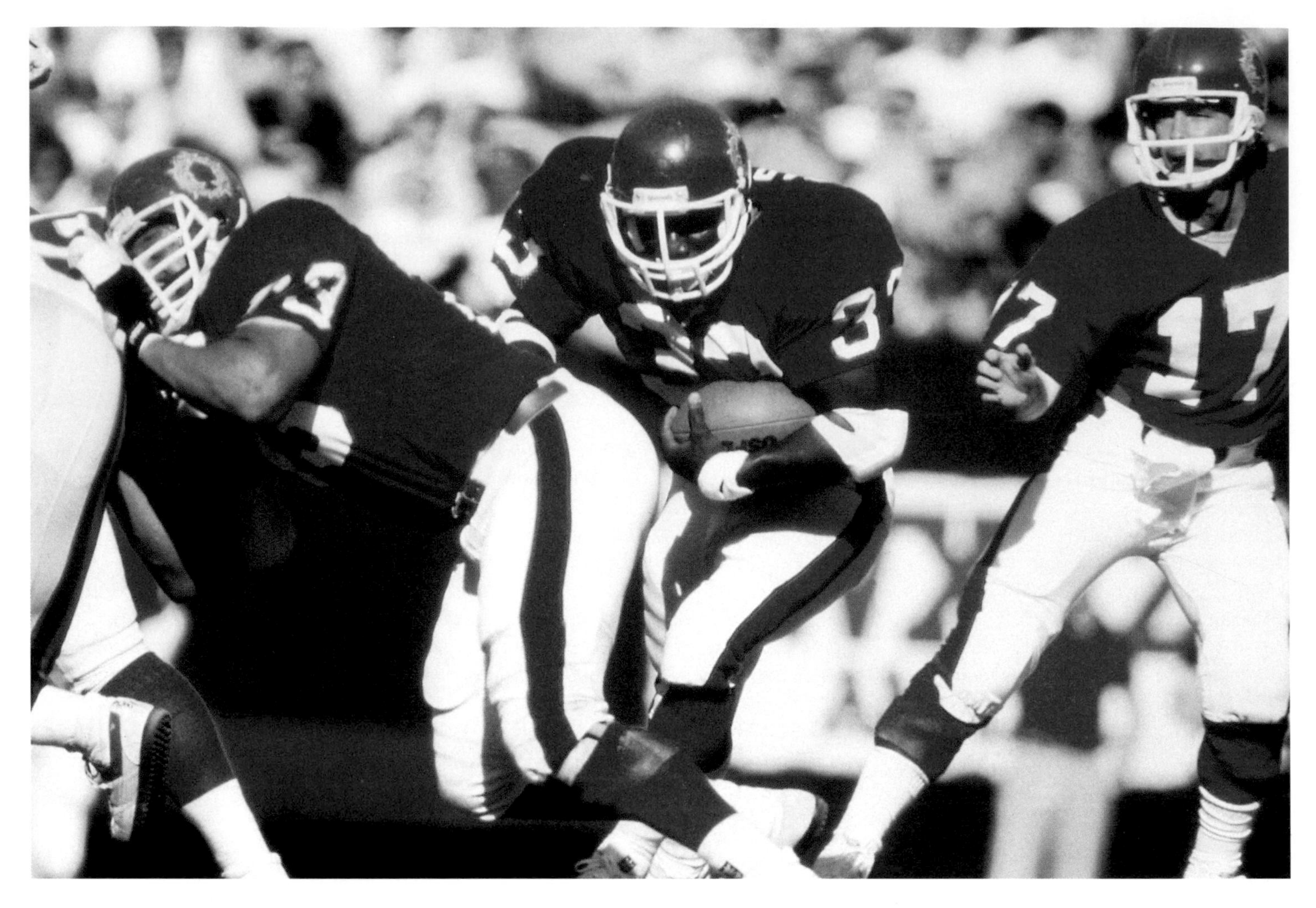

▲ *In sports like football, sudden movements make strenuous demands on the body. Players are likely to suffer common injuries such as torn cartilage.*

Orthopedic surgeons and specialists also treat defects such as a congenital dislocation of the hip, which may run in families (see Genetics). With this condition, the ball of the baby's hip joint either fits poorly in its socket or does not lie in the socket at all. This is usually detected in the first few weeks of life. When it is, the baby is put in a splint or cast to hold the legs apart so that the hip fits firmly in its socket. The hip usually develops normally if treatment is started early enough. If the baby is more than a few months old, surgery may be necessary.

Joint replacement surgery

In the 21st century, durable materials such as plastic, ceramic, and metal have made it possible to replace entire joints (see Joint Replacement). The most common surgery is hip joint replacement, in which a new ball and socket are cemented into the thighbone and hip socket with acrylic cement. Joint replacement surgery is successful in relieving the pain and stiffness due to the wear and tear of arthritis, or the pain of an injury, and artificial hip joints that are made from a new plastic, which has an ultra-high molecular weight, will continue to work efficiently for at least 30 years. As a result, people of 50 or even 60 can have an artificial hip joint and expect it to last for as long as they live (see Arthritis).

The knee, elbow, shoulder, and knuckle joints can also be replaced by joint replacement surgery, using similar techniques.

Recent advances

Many orthopedic surgeons now use an instrument called an arthroscope for looking inside a knee joint. This instrument is like a small telescope that the surgeon can insert into the joint through a small puncture wound (see Endoscopy). He or she can then assess the condition of the joint and cartilages and even perform some surgery without actually having to open the joint. Advances in this field are improving the surgical treatment of many knee injuries.

Some orthopedic surgeons now perform microsurgery using extremely fine stitches to join together severed nerves and blood vessels that are no bigger than a matchstick. This type of surgery is performed using a binocular microscope and very fine surgical instruments. A number of highly publicized operations have shown that even whole severed limbs can be reattached successfully (see Microsurgery).

In addition, there have also been many developments in the design of artificial joints, known as prosthetic articulations, to replace diseased joints other than the hip and knee. Technical developments that improve artificial limbs have given amputees a chance of a better quality of life.

See also: **Bones; Donors; Gangrene; Grafting; Hip; Joints; Surgery; X rays**

Osteoarthritis

Aching and painful joints are a common part of aging, and the cause is often a condition called osteoarthritis. Drugs can relieve the pain of this disease, and in severe cases surgery can offer dramatic improvement.

Osteoarthritis is one of the most common forms of arthritis. Half of the population over the age of 50 has some signs of the disease, which can also affect people in their thirties and forties. Although it is possible to get osteoarthritis in almost any joint in the body, the condition is more likely to occur in certain joints, including the hips, the knees, the hands, the back, and the neck.

Osteoarthritis is extremely painful and can be crippling, since the condition reduces the amount of movement in severely affected joints. Treatment is usually with NSAIDs or other painkillers, and in serious cases surgery may be performed. It is also possible to replace some of the joints that are badly affected.

Structure of the joints

Joints between bones that allow a range of movement are called synovial joints. They are lined with a membrane called the synovial membrane, and this forms a bag that is filled with synovial fluid (see Joints). Bone ends that come into contact with each other within the joint are coated with a tough elastic material called cartilage. It is the action of the two cartilage surfaces coming into direct contact with each other that bears the weight of the joint.

Cartilage itself consists of a hard network of fibers that contains cartilage-producing cells and fluid, providing a well lubricated surface for the moving parts of the joint (see Cartilage). Osteoarthritis is a disease that results when the structure of the cartilage changes.

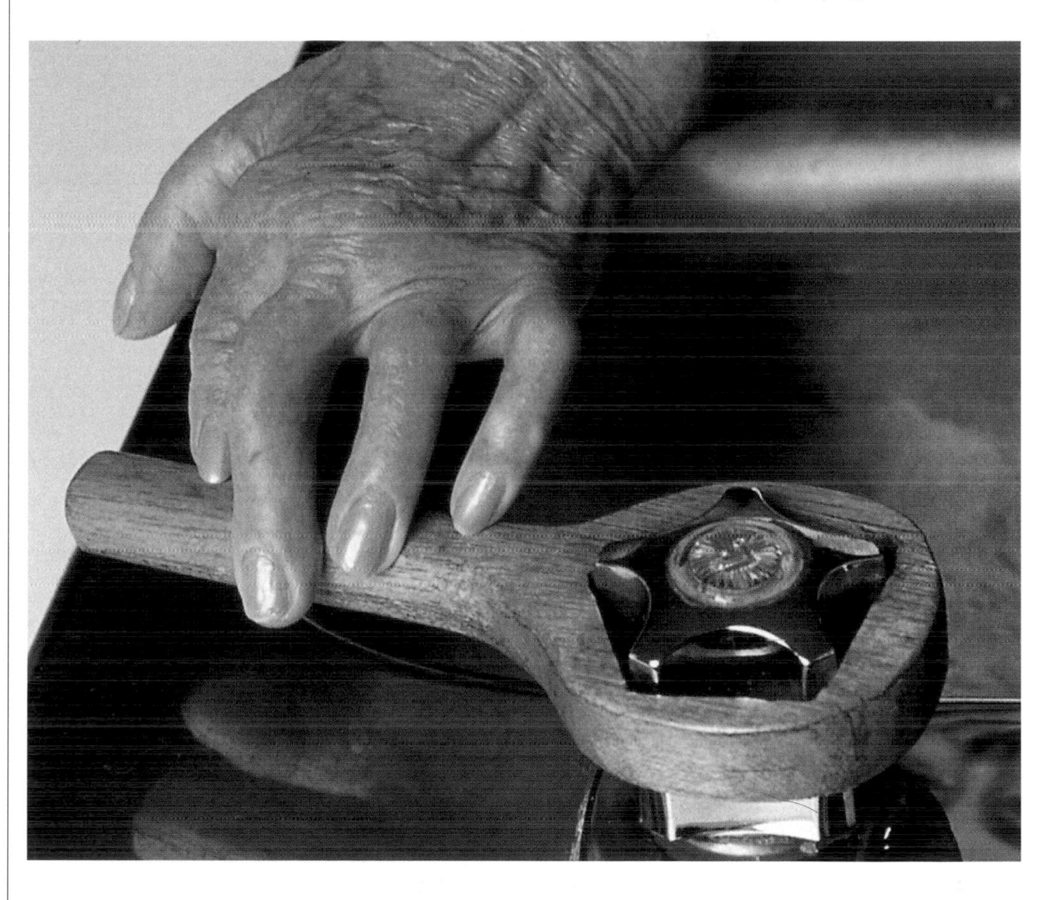

▲ *People who have stiff and deformed osteoarthritic fingers can find everyday activities difficult, but simple mechanical devices can help them maintain their independence.*

Questions and Answers

I have suffered from osteoarthritis for many years. Will my daughter inherit the condition?

Osteoarthritis cannot be inherited, although there is a tendency for people in the same family to develop osteoarthritis of the hands. This might reflect the fact that members of the same family often have similar interests, and thus may subject their hands to the same types of stresses.

I thought that exercise was good for you, but I've read that professional football players often suffer from osteoarthritis. Are some sports considered unhealthy?

Aerobic movement that works your large muscle groups (such as your legs) is very good for you; repeated stresses and shocks to your joints are not. So although exercise is good for you, repeated injuries are not, and may cause osteoarthritis.

For example, gymnasts and ballet dancers land on their bare feet countless times. They land incorrectly when they are learning, and they land harder as they leap higher and swing faster. This repeated shock wears away the cartilage between the joints.

Other sports lead to other complaints. Football players often have a form of arthritis in the middle bones of the foot, and bicyclists often get knee problems —probably because these areas suffer repeated small injuries.

Does cold, damp weather tend to make osteoarthritis worse?

This is such a common complaint that it seems likely to be true. However, there is no logical medical reason to suggest why a cold, damp climate should make the disease more severe. It may be that people are simply more aware of the pain when the weather becomes damp and cold.

Questions and Answers

I have had the cartilage removed from my left knee. Am I likely to get osteoarthritis as a result?

There is no certainty that you will get the disease, but people who have had their cartilage removed have a higher risk of developing osteoarthritis of the knee than those who haven't. The chances also increase if you have injured a knee and torn a cartilage. In both cases, abnormalities in knee function may result, possibly leading to osteoarthritis. To avoid repeated injury to your knee, you should give up contact sports.

After surgery, physical therapy can help mobilize the knee joint. Osteoarthritis is rare under the age of 45, but very common over the age of 60.

I have osteoarthritis and I find that my joints tend to stiffen if I sit down for an hour. Is this a common experience?

Yes. People with arthritis often tend to feel stiff if they have not moved their joints for a while. This is true for people with rheumatoid arthritis and those with osteoarthritis, and both conditions can cause stiffness in the mornings. Osteoarthritis causes stiffness that lasts for about 15 minutes, whereas people with rheumatoid arthritis tend to feel stiff for much longer.

Are men or women more likely to get osteoarthritis, and does it affect the sexes differently?

Osteoarthritis is a disease that particularly affects the elderly. Since women tend to live to a greater age than men, more women appear to suffer from the condition. However, with younger age groups, men and women are almost equally affected—and the condition may even be slightly more common in younger men.

Also, the two sexes tend to get osteoarthritis in different joints. In men it is more common in the hips; in women, the hands, knees, and base of the thumb tend to be affected.

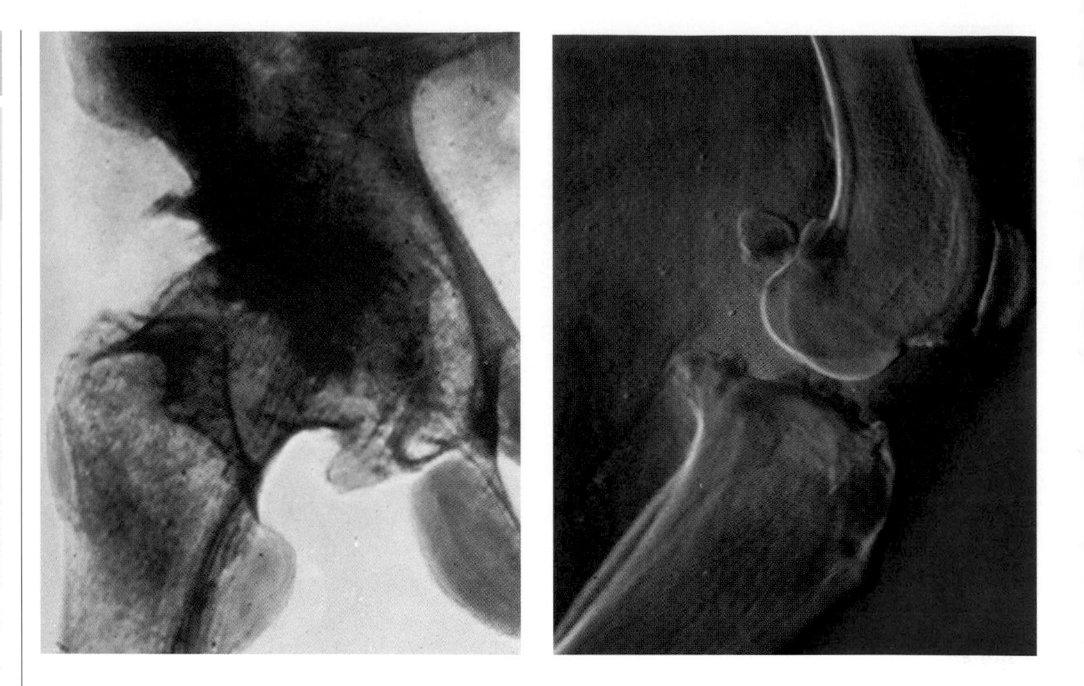

▲ *These X rays of an osteoarthritic hip (left) and knee (right) show how the disease has affected the joints. Normally, bones are capped with cartilage that protects the joints. Here the cartilage caps have worn down and the bone ends bear directly onto each other, so that they, too, are worn down by movement. The result is pain and stiffness.*

Progression of the disease

A great deal is now known about how osteoarthritis develops once it occurs. In the first stage of the disease, small clefts appear on the surface of the cartilage. The number of cells producing cartilage also increases. At this stage patients may not notice any symptoms, or they may experience slight pain and stiffness.

In the next stage, the cartilage caps on the bone ends wear thin, until finally there is no cartilage left and the bone ends bear directly onto one another. Movements of the joint then wear away the bone, causing considerable destruction and thickening of the capsule of synovial membrane that surrounds the joint.

Unlike cartilage, bone is able to repair itself as it is worn away. However, the way in which it manages this around an osteoarthritic joint is disorganized, possibly leading to the formation of rough deposits that do more harm than good to the joint.

Predisposing factors

The causes of osteoarthritis remain obscure. The main factor seems to be the continual stress on the joint, which accounts for the name "wear-and-tear arthritis." However, this theory does not explain why joints that bear the same amount of weight are not always equally affected. For example, although the hip and knee are commonly involved, the ankle is not.

It is possible that certain factors may predispose a person to develop osteoarthritis. For example, a history of repeated small injuries may be a causative factor. For this reason, people who engage regularly in sports such as professional football may be more likely to get osteoarthritis, particularly in their feet. Deformity of a limb or joint may be another contributory factor, since this can lead to severe stresses on the joint, which may cause repeated injury. Another factor making osteoarthritis more likely is that the nerve supply to a particular joint may be interrupted owing to some problem in the nervous system. Since the sensation of pain is interrupted, the patient may injure a joint repeatedly and not be aware of it (see Numbness). However, in most patients showing signs of osteoarthritic disease, there is no obvious cause.

Symptoms

The main symptom of osteoarthritis is pain. This can vary from a dull ache in an affected joint to excruciating pain on movement that can make a patient practically immobile. Usually the pain from an affected joint is more severe during movement, but there may also be a dull pain when

Treating osteoarthritis

SITE	SYMPTOMS	TREATMENT
Hands	Usually affects the joints between the bones of the fingers, producing characteristic lumps on either side of the farthest joint (Heberden's nodes). The thumb is often involved. Joints are painful on movement.	NSAIDs and other pain-relieving drugs. Immobilizing the thumb in a cast may be helpful.
Feet	Pain on walking, most commonly occurring in the joint at the base of the big toe.	NSAIDs and other pain-relieving drugs. Surgical shoes or surgery may help.
Ankles	Very rare, unless there is some bone deformity.	—
Knees	Affects more women than men. Sometimes very little pain. Knock-knees can result.	Basic treatment is with pain-relieving drugs, but very painful or deformed joints can be treated surgically.
Hips	Pain, particularly on walking. Can lead to a limp or a waddle if both hips are involved.	Initial treatment is with NSAIDs or other pain-relieving drugs. A walking stick may be helpful. Surgery such as joint replacement may be used in more severe cases.
Spine	Most common in the neck. Causes pain and limitation of movement. Neck involvement can lead to blackouts or weakness in arms and legs.	NSAIDs and other pain-relieving drugs. A neck collar worn at night may be helpful.
Shoulder	Rare, unless there has been some injury. Immobility and stiffness are usually more of a problem than pain.	Exercises combined with pain-relieving drugs may help to ease shoulder movement.
Elbow	Rare. Pain is the main problem and may occur at rest; there may also be numbness in the arm and hand and loss of muscle power.	NSAIDs and related drugs are used for the pain. Pinched nerves may have to be freed by surgery.

the joint is at rest. This is thought to result from the disorganization of the way the veins drain blood from the joint. Thus pain during rest may be due to the joint's being congested with blood.

As the disease progresses the pain tends to become steadily worse, although not always in the affected joint. For example, it is common for osteoarthritis of the hip to cause pain in the knee on the same side, or in the back.

Osteoarthritis also causes stiffness. This is usually worse in the morning, but it tends to improve within a few minutes. The affected joints may also swell in some cases.

The affected joints may also become considerably deformed as the disease progresses. When badly affected hips and knees creak on movement, doctors call this effect "crepitus." The range of movement in an affected joint may decrease until the joint is almost totally fixed.

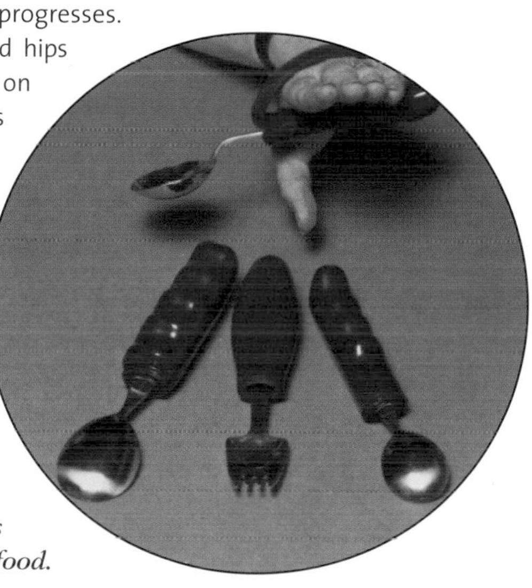

► *The thick molded handles on these utensils can help people suffering from osteoarthritis to perform daily tasks such as preparing food.*

Osteoarthritis may affect one joint in the body or several joints. If only one joint is involved, it is likely to be a large joint such as the knee or the hip. Occasionally, the only joint involved is the one where the palm and wrist meet near the thumb. Common sites for multiple affliction are the hands and the spine.

Dangers

Although unpleasant, osteoarthritis is not a dangerous condition. Serious problems are most likely to arise when the disease affects the spine in the area of the neck, causing pain and stiffness. This condition is called cervical spondylosis.

Three problems can arise from this. The first is pain and stiffness of the neck. The second and third, which are serious but rare, arise from attempts of the bone to repair itself, leading to bone overgrowth. If this overgrowth puts pressure on the blood vessels to the lower part of the brain, it can cut off the blood supply, leading to blackouts and dizziness when a person looks upward or around to the side. Pressure on the spinal cord or the nerves leads to weakness in the arms and legs.

Treatment

Nonsteroidal anti-inflammatory drugs (NSAIDs) are the preferred treatment because they not only stop the pain but also reduce inflammation (see Nonsteroidal Anti-Inflammatory Drugs); acetominophen (Tylenol) reduces pain only (see Painkillers). In some cases, injecting corticosteroids into the affected joint can markedly

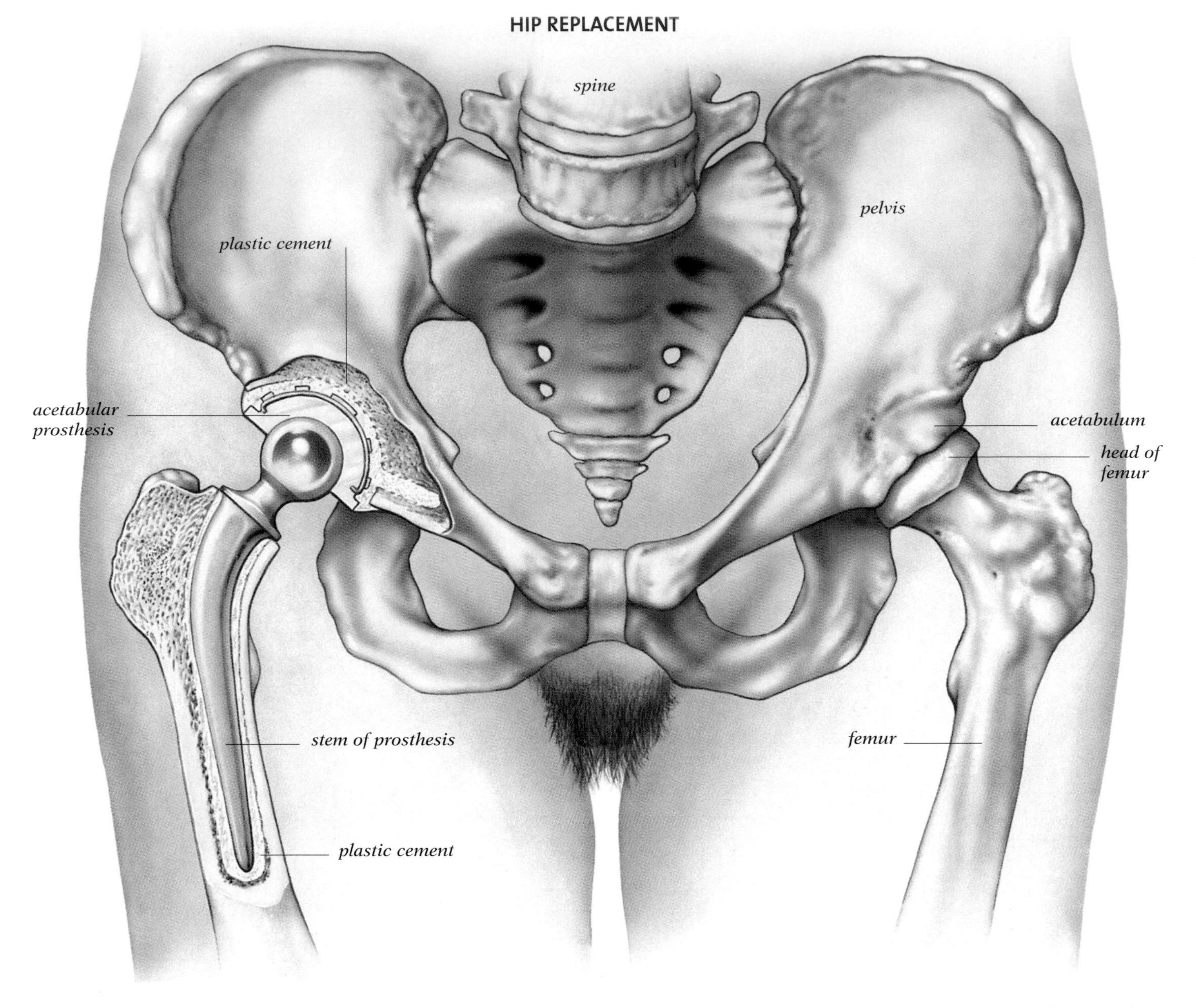

▲ *To replace a hip, the head of the femur is removed, holes are drilled in the femur and the pelvis, and a prosthetic ball and socket are fixed into place. These may be cemented in position or simply pushed tightly into place. Traction may be used to maintain the position of the leg during healing.*

reduce both the pain and the debilitating effects. Using a walking stick can also help if a patient is suffering from osteoarthritis of the knee or hip (see Pain Management).

In severe cases, joint replacement surgery can be performed to lessen pain and improve joint movement. The most successful operation is that on the hip joint, although progress has been made in knee joint replacements (see Joint Replacement).

Since it is uncertain how long replaced joints last, an operation called an osteotomy is likely to be performed on younger patients. This involves remodeling the bones on either side of an affected joint, and it can be of great value in improving the way the joint carries the patient's weight. There is still the option of replacing the joint at some later stage.

Finally, an osteoarthritic joint can be completely fused so that it cannot move and thus cannot cause pain. Although this fusion sounds drastic, it can be extremely successful in some patients, offering tremendous pain relief without too much loss of function in the affected limb, which was probably fairly stiff in the first place.

Outlook

Once osteoarthritis occurs, it does not disappear, and about 80 percent of the population over age 65 has X-ray evidence of the disease. However, only a quarter of those affected show symptoms, and in most cases, these symptoms can be greatly relieved by drugs.

Surgical treatment has advanced greatly in recent decades, bringing great relief to many sufferers, especially those whose hips are affected; they can benefit from replacement surgery. In other joints, surgical treatment is usually regarded as a last resort.

See also: **Arthritis; Back and backache; Bones; Hip; Knee; Neck; Nervous system; Pain; Sports injury**

INDEX

Headings and page numbers in **bold** refer to complete articles. Page numbers in *italics* refer to illustrations or their captions.